Second Edition
The Art, Science, and Technology of Pharmaceutical Compounding

Notices

The inclusion in this book of any drug in respect to which patent or trademark rights may exist shall not be deemed, and is not intended as, a grant of or authority to exercise any right or privilege protected by such patent or trademark. All such rights or trademarks are vested in the patent or trademark owner, and no other person may exercise the same without express permission, authority, or license secured from such patent or trademark owner.

The inclusion of a brand name does not mean the author or the publisher has any particular knowledge that the brand listed has properties different from other brands of the same drug, nor should its inclusion be interpreted as an endorsement by the author or publisher. Similarly, the fact that a particular brand has not been included does not indicate the product has been judged to be in any way unsatisfactory or unacceptable. Further, no official support or endorsement of this book by any federal or state agency or pharmaceutical company is intended or inferred.

The nature of drug information is that it is constantly evolving because of ongoing research and clinical experience and is often subject to interpretation. Readers are advised that decisions regarding drug therapy must be based on the independent judgment of the clinician, changing information about a drug (e.g., as reflected in the literature and manufacturers' most current product information), and changing medical practices.

The author and the publisher have made every effort to ensure the accuracy and completeness of the information presented in this book. However, the author and the publisher cannot be held responsible for the continued currency of the information, any inadvertent errors or omissions, or the application of this information. Therefore, the author and the publisher shall have no liability to any person or entity with regard to claims, loss, or damage caused, or alleged to be caused, directly or indirectly, by the use of information contained herein.

Second Edition

The Art, Science, and Technology of Pharmaceutical Compounding

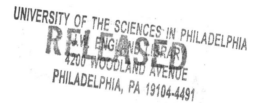
Loyd V. Allen Jr., PhD
Editor in Chief
International Journal of Pharmaceutical Compounding
Edmond, Oklahoma
and
Professor Emeritus
College of Pharmacy
University of Oklahoma Health Sciences Center
Oklahoma City, Oklahoma

American Pharmaceutical Association
Washington, D.C.

American Pharmaceutical Association
Washington, D.C.

Editor: Linda Young
Cover Design: Mary A. Burns
Composition: The Clarinda Company
Editorial Services: Publications Professionals LLC

Library of Congress Cataloging-in-Print Data

Allen, Loyd V.
    The art, science, and technology of pharmaceutical compounding/Loyd V. Allen Jr.
    2nd ed.
        p.; cm.
    Includes bibliographical references and index.
    ISBN 1-58212-035-8
    1. Drugs—Dosage forms.   I. Title.
    [DLNM: 1. Drug Compounding. QV 778 A427a 2002]
    RS200 .A45 2002
    615'.4—dc21

2002018455

How to Order This Book
By phone: 800-878-0729 (domestic) and 802-862-0095 (international) VISA®,
MasterCard®, and American Express® cards accepted.

Contents

Sample Formulations

The following list contains the titles of all the sample formulations included in this edition of *The Art, Science, and Technology of Pharmaceutical Compounding.* The formulations are grouped primarily by dosage form and listed in the order in which they appear in the book.

Powders

Capsules

Tablets

Lozenges/Troches

Suppositories

Sticks

Solutions

Suspensions

Emulsions

Ointments, Creams, and Pastes

Gels

Parenteral Preparations

Biotechnology Preparations

Preparations for Dental Patients

Preparations for Patients with Diabetes

Preparations for Hospice Patients and Patients with Pain

Preparations for Pediatric Patients

Natural, Herbal, and Dietary Supplement Products

Iontophoresis Solutions

Veterinary Preparations

Preface to the Second Edition

The phenomenal growth of pharmaceutical compounding in recent years has been spurred by several simultaneous events. First, the number of discontinued drug products continues to increase. A number of reasons contribute to this increase, including low profits on certain products that are ultimately discontinued, difficulty in manufacturing and formulation processes that lead to a decision to discontinue the product, and the difficulty in obtaining—including importing—certain raw materials used in some commercial products. Despite the reason for discontinuing a product, patients still need the medication; fortunately, in most cases, pharmacists can compound these preparations.

Second, physicians are becoming more aware of use in other parts of the world of various drugs and dosage forms that are not produced and marketed here in the United States. To obtain these preparations, U.S. physicians turn to pharmacists in many cases.

Third, many physicians have patients who can benefit from new drugs or new drug applications. The physicians work with compounding pharmacists to formulate the preparations.

Fourth, the incidence of drug shortages has been increasing in recent years. This increase may be caused by several factors, including just-in-time manufacturing, miscalculations of actual drug usage rates, and difficulty in obtaining some imported raw materials.

We are now in an era of increased emphasis on quality and documentation of compounded formulations. Therefore, it is incumbent on all pharmacists who compound to be intimately familiar with General Chapter ⟨795⟩, "Pharmacy Compounding," of the *United States Pharmacopeia 25/National Formulary 20*. Pharmacists—as well as all personnel involved in compounding—should be trained in the principles outlined in this chapter and should practice within its guidelines.

Colleges and schools of pharmacy are beginning to reinstate laboratory classes in the curriculum; these classes are important as pharmacy compounding requires a strong scientific base in inorganic and organic chemistry, physical pharmacy, pharmaceutics, natural products chemistry, biochemistry, and other physical and life sciences. Approximately 75% of the colleges and schools of pharmacy now have some students who receive specialized training from the compounding support industry.

Compounding of sterile products also continues to grow and should be done only by pharmacists who have been properly trained and validated in aseptic processing. Some states already require specific annual training by pharmacists involved in compounding sterile preparations.

Recent activities related to the Food and Drug Modernization Act of 1997 have served to document the importance of pharmacy compounding and the need for it. The Food and Drug Administration (FDA) recognizes the importance of and supports the ability of pharmacists to compound specific preparations for individual patients. FDA is working closely with the United States Pharmacopeia in continuing to enhance the quality of compounded preparations.

In summary, as this second edition is prepared, pharmacy compounding has regained a place of prominence and importance in the overall provision of pharmaceutical products, patient services, and pharmaceutical care. After all, individualization of individual prescriptions through pharmacy compounding is the actualization of providing total pharmaceutical care.

May 2002

Preface to the First Edition

Historically, compounding has been an integral part of pharmacy practice, as shown by the following definitions and references to pharmacy.

- Pharmacy is the art or practice of preparing and preserving drugs, and of compounding and dispensing medicines according to the prescriptions of physicians.[1]
- Pharmacy is (1) the art, practice, or profession of preparing, preserving, compounding, and dispensing medical drugs and (2) a place where medicines are compounded or dispensed.[2]
- Pharmacy is the science, art, and practice of preparing, preserving, compounding, and dispensing medicinal drugs and of giving instructions for their use.[3]

Compounding is a professional prerogative that pharmacists have performed since the beginning of the profession. Even today, definitions of pharmacy include the "preparation of drugs."[4,5]

The heritage of pharmacy, spanning some 5000 years, has centered on providing pharmaceutical products for patients. Pharmacists are the only health professionals who possess the knowledge and skill required to compound and prepare medications to meet the unique needs of patients.

Compounding Yesterday

The apothecary is listed in the Bible as one of the earliest trades or professions. As one reads through the Bible, it is evident that people experienced pain, disease, and suffering and that they used medicines of various types for healing:

"And thou shalt make it an oil of holy ointment, an ointment compound after *the art of the apothecary:* it shall be an holy anointing oil." Exodus 30:25 [emphasis added]

"Dead flies cause *the ointment of the apothecary* to send forth a stinking savour: so doth a little folly him that is in reputation for wisdom and honour." Ecclesiastes 10:1 [emphasis added]

"From the sole of the foot even unto the head there is no soundness in it; *but wounds, and bruises, and putrifying sores:* they have not been closed, neither bound up, neither mollified with ointment." Isaiah 1:6 [emphasis added]

"And by the river upon the bank thereof, on this side and on that side, shall grow all trees for meat, whose leaf shall not fade, neither shall the fruit thereof be consumed: it shall bring forth new fruit according to his months, because their waters they issued out of the sanctuary: and the fruit thereof shall be for meat, and *the leaf thereof for medicine.*" Ezekiel 47:12 [emphasis added]

In many cases, the medicines used were either topical ointments or products such as wines and plant extracts that were taken internally. The apothecary was noted for the mixing of perfumes, ointments, and some medicines, and the physician was noted for taking care of the sick. In some cases, the same individual performed both functions. The heritage of the compounding pharmacist is well documented throughout history as one involved in preparing products used for treatment of disease and for cosmetic purposes.

Compounding Today

Prescription compounding is a rapidly growing component of pharmacy practice. This change can be attributed to a number of factors, including individualized patient therapy, lack of commercially available products, home health care, intravenous admixture programs, total parenteral nutrition programs, and problem solving for the physician and patient to enhance compliance with a specific therapeutic regimen. Pharmacists are creative and should have the ability to formulate patient-specific preparations for providing pharmaceutical care.

An article by Angel d'Angelo, RPh, editor of the *U.S. Pharmacist,* explains that compounding is our heritage. There is no other professional license that allows for the extemporaneous compounding of therapeutic agents. Complete pharmaceutical care must involve the dosage form, which might necessitate compounding a patient-specific form not available commercially; possibly the preparation of a product without a preservative or a specific allergy-producing excipient that must be removed from the formulation. With pharmacokinetic services, the need for individualized dosage units will be required more frequently to meet these patient-specific needs. Pharmacists who compound have a desirable and needed skill.[6]

Pharmacy is united in the sense that pharmacists have a responsibility to serve their patients and to compound an appropriately prescribed product in the course of their professional practice. It is the right and responsibility of pharmacists to compound medications to meet the specific needs of patients. Pharmacists are ultimately responsible for the integrity of the finished product prepared by them or under their immediate supervision.

Pharmacists are the only health professionals formally trained in the art and science of compounding medications. Consequently, they are expected to possess the knowledge and skills necessary to compound extemporaneous preparations. In 1995, the percentage of compounded prescriptions represented approximately 11% of all prescriptions dispensed,[7] which is a five- to tenfold increase in the percentage of such prescriptions dispensed in the 1970s and 1980s. It is evident that the need for individualized drug therapy for patients has been realized and is resulting in patient-specific prescriptions and the compounding of medications that are not commercially available.

The purpose of this book is (1) to provide a basic foundation of knowledge that will enable pharmacists to sharpen their skills in compounding pharmacy, (2) to serve as an educational tool for those pharmacists who did not receive instruction in compounding in colleges or schools of pharmacy, and (3) to become a textbook for current pharmacy students taking courses in pharmaceutical compounding. This first edition of the book serves as a basic text; it will be revised and developed in greater depth with future editions.

The support of Paddock Laboratories in developing some of the materials used in this book is gratefully acknowledged. Some material was originally published or adapted from materials published in the Secundum Artem series by Paddock Laboratories, Inc., of Minneapolis, Minnesota. Other material, including the cover design, has been adapted from the *International Journal of Pharmaceutical Compounding* (*IJPC*), a bimonthly professional and scientific journal devoted to pharmaceutical compounding and published in Edmond, Oklahoma. Photographs of compounding equipment were graciously supplied by the Professional Compounding Centers of America, Inc. The use of these materials is sincerely appreciated.

References

1. *Webster's Revised Unabridged Dictionary of the English Language.* Springfield, Mass: G & C Merriam Co; 1913:1075.
2. *Webster's Tenth New Collegiate Dictionary.* Springfield, Mass: Merriam Webster, Inc; 1993:871.
3. *International Dictionary of Medicine and Biology.* Vol. III. New York: John Wiley and Sons; 1986.
4. *The Compact Oxford English Dictionary.* 2nd ed. New York: Oxford University Press Inc: 1991.
5. *American Heritage Dictionary of the English Language.* 3rd ed. 1992, in electronic form in Microsoft Bookshelf '95. 1995.
6. Angel d'Angelo. Compounding: our heritage. *Int J Pharm Compound.* 1997;1(4):286.
7. Ray Gosselin. Pharmaceutical care: part of TQM? *Drug Topics.* July 10, 1995;139(13):10.

Introduction

Pharmacists are unique professionals, who are well trained in the natural, physical, and medical sciences and aware that a single mistake in the daily practice of their profession may result in potential tragedy. However, because of their demonstrated expertise, their demeanor, and the manner in which they have practiced their profession over the years, pharmacists continue to be ranked among the most respected individuals in our society. In general, pharmacists have the reputation of being available to residents of the local community in times of need, interacting with and providing needed medications for patients, and working with patients to regain or maintain a certain standard of health or quality of life.

Pharmacists possess knowledge and skills that are not duplicated by any other profession. Their roles in ambulatory care can include dispensing and compounding medications, counseling patients, minimizing medication errors, enhancing patient compliance, monitoring drug therapy, and minimizing drug expenditures.

Pharmacy activities that individualize patient therapy include clinical and compounding functions. The functions are related and equally important to the success of such activities. A pharmacist's expertise must be used to adjust dosage quantities, frequencies, and even dosage forms for enhanced compliance. All pharmacists should be aware of the **drug therapy** options provided by compounding. Pharmacy is united in the belief that pharmacists have a responsibility to serve their patients and compound an appropriately prescribed product in the course of professional practice. It is both the right and responsibility of pharmacists to compound medications (sterile and nonsterile) to meet the specific needs of patients.

What Is Compounding?

The definition of compounding has been the subject of much discussion and has been addressed by the National Association of Boards of Pharmacy.

> Compounding means the preparation, mixing, assembling, packaging, or labeling of a drug or device (i) as the result of a practitioner's Prescription

Drug Order or initiative based on the pharmacist/patient/prescriber relationship in the course of professional practice, or (ii) for the purpose of, as an incident to research, teaching, or chemical analysis and not for sale or dispensing. Compounding also includes the preparation of drugs and devices in anticipation of Prescription Drug Orders based on routine, regularly observed patterns.[1]

Still, compounding may hold different meanings for different pharmacists. It may mean the preparation of suspensions, topicals, and suppositories; the conversion of one dose (e.g., oral to rectal, injection to oral) or dosage form into another; the preparation of select dosage forms from bulk chemicals; the preparation of intravenous admixtures, parenteral nutrition solutions, and pediatric dosage forms from adult dosage forms; the preparation of radioactive isotopes; or the preparation of cassettes, syringes, and other devices with drugs for administration in the home setting.

The pharmacist plays an important role on the hospice team and can greatly enhance quality of life for hospice patients. Pediatric patient compliance is a challenge as children either don't want to, or can't, take tablets or capsules and manufacturers don't provide liquid dosage forms for many medications; this is where the pharmacist steps in. Compounding for the geriatric patient can be a much greater challenge than for almost any other group of patients. Oftentimes there are physical, emotional and social difficulties affecting compliance and many geriatric health problems are chronic rather than acute. Pharmacists have also become intimately involved in working with veterinarians in the treatment of animals (companion, recreational, food and exotic).

Compounding has always been a basic part of pharmacy practice, but today it is one of the most rapidly growing areas, and many pharmacists in all types of practice are becoming involved in compounding sterile and nonsterile products. The dramatic growth of pharmaceutical compounding is attributed to the impact of home health care, unavailable drug products, orphan drugs, veterinary compounding, and biotechnology-derived drug products. Newly evolving dosage forms and therapeutic approaches suggest that compounding of pharmaceuticals and related products specifically for individual patients will become more common in pharmacy practice in the years ahead.

Compounding pharmacy is unique because it allows pharmacists to use more of their scientific, mathematical, and technology background than some other types of practices. Compounding pharmacists develop a unique relationship with the patients they serve. They work hand in hand with physicians to solve clinical problems not addressed by commercially available dosage forms.

It almost seems unbelievable that, as we in health care become more aware that patients are "individuals," respond as "individuals," and must be treated as "individuals," some health care providers appear to be grouping patients into "categories" for treatment and "categories" for reimbursement from third-party payers or "categories" for determining levels of care in managed care organizations. Along the same lines, the trend to use "fixed-dose products" provided by pharmaceutical manufacturers that are available just because the marketing demand is sufficiently high to justify their manufacture and production seems not quite appropriate. Since when should the availability, or lack of availability, of a specific commercially available product dictate the therapy of a patient?

Should Every Pharmacist Compound?

Only properly trained pharmacists should be involved in pharmaceutical compounding. If pharmacists wish to compound but do not possess the required techniques and skills, they should participate in continuing education programs that have been designed to provide the proper training, including the scientific basis and practical skills necessary for sound, contemporary compounding.

Today, any pharmacist is legally qualified to compound, but who is a technically qualified, trained, compounding pharmacist? To be capable of meeting the special or advanced needs of today's patients, whether human or animal, a compounding pharmacist must

- have access to the most recent information available.
- maintain an inventory and provide for proper storage of drugs and flavoring agents and be capable of obtaining any chemical within a reasonable time.
- be dedicated to pharmacy and willing to put forth the necessary financial and time investment.
- have the appropriate physical facilities and equipment to do the job right (the extent and type of compounding may be determined or limited by the facility).
- be committed to lifelong learning and continuing education, since a major advantage of compounded prescriptions is that they provide treatments that are new, undeveloped, and often not commercially available.
- have a willingness to tear down walls and build bridges to share experiences with others for the good of all.

Should You Compound?

When considering whether or not to compound, pharmacists should consider the technical aspects and economic impact of the service.

Technical Considerations

There are three types of compounded prescriptions: isolated, routine, and batch prepared. An isolated prescription is one that the pharmacist is not expecting to receive nor will expect to receive again. A routine prescription is one that the pharmacist may expect to receive on a routine basis in the future; there may be some benefit to "standardize" such preparations to ensure product quality, that is, maintain preparation protocols on file. A batch-prepared prescription is one that is prepared in multiple identical units as a single operation "in anticipation" of the receipt of future prescriptions.

Pharmacists must consider not only their technical qualifications to compound a product, but also the technical validity of the prescription. The box "Technical Considerations for Compounding a Prescription" presents a series of questions designed to aid in evaluating the technical considerations for compounding.

The "batch production" of sterile products, especially in the hospital and home health care environments, has increased noticeably. There are a number of reasons for this increase, including the following:

- The changing patterns of drug therapy, such as home parenteral therapy and patient-controlled parenteral administration.

Technical Considerations for Compounding a Prescription

- Is the product commercially available in the exact dosage form, strength, and packaging?
- Is the prescription rational concerning the ingredients, intended use, dose, and method of administration?
- Are the physical, chemical, and therapeutic properties of the individual ingredients consistent with the expected properties of the ordered drug product?
- Will this compounded product satisfy the intent of the prescribing physician and meet the needs of the patient?
- Is there an alternative (e.g., different dosage form, different route of administration) by which the patient will receive a benefit?
- Is there a bona fide prescriber-pharmacist-patient relationship?
- Can ingredient identity, quality, and purity be assured?
- Does the pharmacist have the training and expertise required to prepare the prescription?
- Are the proper equipment, supplies, and chemicals or drugs available?
- Is there a literature reference that might provide information on use, preparation, stability, administration, and storage of the product?
- Can the pharmacist perform the necessary calculations to prepare the product?
- Can the pharmacist project a reasonable and rational "beyond-use" date for the prescription?
- Is the pharmacist willing to complete the necessary documentation to prepare the product?
- Can the pharmacist do some basic quality control to check the product prior to dispensing (e.g., capsule weight variation, pH, visual observations)?
- What procedures are in place for investigating and correcting failures?
- How long will the patient be using the product and is the expected duration of therapy consistent with an appropriate expiration date? Alternatively, should the product be prepared in small quantities and dispensed to the patient in short intervals?
- Does the patient have the necessary storage facility, if required, to ensure the potency of the product until its beyond-use date?

- The use in hospitals of injectable drug products that are not commercially available to meet individual patient needs or the prescriber's clinical investigational protocols.
- Cost containment, whereby a pharmacy batch produces drug products that are intended to be similar to commercially available products.

Batch compounding can reduce the cost of a medication that must be taken over a long period or continuously for a chronic condition. This process allows the patient to store the product at home and reduce the number of pharmacy visits. Pharmacists who choose to perform batch compounding should be capable and willing to do it properly, particularly when sterile drug products are involved. (See the box "Technical Considerations for Batch Compounding.")

Economic Considerations

Several economic considerations must be weighed when making the decision to compound prescriptions, including the pharmacist's compensation for the service

Technical Considerations for Batch Compounding

- Will the processes, procedures, compounding environment, and equipment used to prepare this batch produce the expected qualities in the finished product?
- Will all the critical processes and procedures be carried out exactly as intended for every batch of the prepared product to produce the same high-quality product in every batch?
- Will the finished product have all the qualities as specified upon completion of the preparation and packaging of each batch?
- Will each batch retain all the qualities within the specified limits until the end of the labeled expiration date?
- Will it be possible to monitor and trace the history of each batch, identify potential sources of problems, and institute appropriate corrective measures to minimize the likelihood of their occurrence?

and the impact of the service on health care costs. Both factors are equally important.

Pharmaceutical compounding is a cognitive service; therefore, appropriate reimbursement is justified. The pricing of a compounded prescription should take into consideration pharmacodynamic/pharmacotherapeutic decision making, formulation expertise, the time involved, and reimbursement for materials. Compounding prescriptions can be attractive for the pharmacist both professionally and financially. Historically, it has been said that compounding is an act whereby the professional and scientific knowledge of a pharmacist can find its expression. For those pharmacists dedicated to performing quality compounding, the professional, psychological, and financial rewards can be substantial.

Compounding prescriptions can be one way of lowering the cost of drug therapy. In some cases it may be less expensive for the pharmacist to prepare a specific prescription for the patient, which may mean that the patient may actually obtain the drug rather than have to do without it. If compounding a prescription will enable a patient to afford the drug therapy, it must be considered.

Another way in which compounding may lower drug costs concerns the economic utilization of very expensive drug products that may have short shelf lives. If a patient does not need the entire contents of a vial or dosage unit, the remaining drug product is often discarded and wasted. In numerous instances, however, the pharmacist can divide the commercial product into smaller usage units, store it properly, and dispense the required quantity on individual prescriptions.

A related economic question involves the commercialization of compounded products. Over the years many compounded products have eventually become commercially available. Examples include fentanyl lozenges, minoxidil topical solution, nystatin lozenges, clindamycin topical solution, tetracaine-adrenalin-cocaine (TAC) solution, erythromycin topical solution, and some premixed intravenous solutions. It is inevitable that a pharmaceutical manufacturer will produce a product when it becomes economically profitable to do so.

Summary

Compounding pharmacists are interested in and excited about their practice. In fact, many pharmacists intimately involved in pharmaceutical care have come to realize the importance of providing individualized patient care through the preparation of patient-specific products. As compounding pharmacy continues to grow, it will provide an opportunity for more pharmacists to use their innovative skills to solve patient's **drug** problems.

Pharmaceutical compounding provides pharmacists with a unique opportunity to practice their time-honored profession. It will become an even more important part of pharmacy practice in the future, particularly for those involved in community, hospital, long-term care, home health care, veterinary care, and specialty practices.

Although pharmacists should not hesitate to become involved in pharmacy compounding, they should be aware of the requirements for and uniqueness of formulating a specific drug product for a specific patient. This service is an important component in providing pharmaceutical care. After all, without the pharmaceutical product, there is no pharmaceutical care.

Reference

1. Good compounding practices applicable to state-licensed pharmacies. In: *Model State Pharmacy Act and Model Rules of the National Association of Boards of Pharmacy.* Park Ridge, Ill: National Association of Boards of Pharmacy; 1993: C.1–C.5.

Abbreviations and Approximate Solubility Descriptions

Abbreviations for Container Specifications

Tightly closed	T
Well closed	W
Light resistant	LR

Abbreviations for Solubility Parameters

Very soluble	VS
Freely soluble	FS
Soluble	Sol
Sparingly soluble	SpS
Slightly soluble	SlS
Very slightly soluble	VSS
Partially soluble	PartSol
Practically insoluble	PrIn
Insoluble	IS
Miscible	Misc
Immiscible	Immisc
Partially miscible	PartMisc
Dispersible	Disp
Swells	Swells

Approximate Solubility Descriptors

Descriptive Term	Parts of Solvent Required for 1 Part of Solute
Very soluble	Less than 1
Freely soluble	From 1 to 10
Soluble	From 10 to 30
Sparingly soluble	From 30 to 100
Slightly soluble	From 100 to 1000
Very slightly soluble	From 1000 to 10,000
Practically insoluble, or insoluble	10,000 and greater

Source: United States Pharmacopeia 24/National Formulary 19. Supplement 1.
Rockville, Md: The United States Pharmacopeial Convention; 1999:2720.

Chapter 1

Guidelines for Compounding Practices

Compounding is an integral part of pharmacy practice and is essential to the provision of health care.[1] Compounding can be as simple as the addition of a liquid to a manufactured drug powder or as complex as the preparation of a multicomponent parenteral nutrition solution. In general, compounding differs from manufacturing in that compounding involves a specific practitioner–patient–pharmacist relationship, the preparation of a relatively small quantity of medication, and different conditions of sale (i.e., specific prescription orders).

The pharmacist is responsible for compounding preparations of acceptable strength, quality, and purity with appropriate packaging and labeling in accordance with good pharmacy practices, official standards, and current scientific principles. Pharmacists should continually expand their compounding knowledge by participating in seminars, studying current literature, and consulting with colleagues.

Definitions

Compounding is the act of preparing, mixing, assembling, packaging, and/or labeling of a drug or device as the result of a practitioner's prescription drug order or initiative based on the practitioner–patient–pharmacist relationship in the course of professional practice, or for the purpose of, or as an incident to, research, teaching, or chemical analysis and not for sale or dispensing. *Compounding* also includes the preparation of drugs or devices in anticipation of prescription drug orders based on routine, regularly observed prescribing patterns.[2,3]

Manufacturing is the production, preparation, propagation, conversion, and/or processing of a drug or device, either directly or indirectly, through the extraction from substances of natural origin or independently through means of chemical or biological synthesis, and the term includes any packaging or repackaging of the substance(s) or labeling or relabeling of its container and the promotion and marketing of such drugs or devices. *Manufacturing* also includes the preparation and promotion of commercially available products from bulk compounds for resale by pharmacies, practitioners, or other persons.[2,3]

To further delineate between manufacturing and compounding, a set of general guidelines has been formulated (see the box "Guidelines to Distinguish Between Manufacturing and Compounding").

Guidelines to Distinguish between Manufacturing and Compounding

▸ Pharmacists may compound, in reasonable quantities, drug products that are commercially available in the marketplace based upon the existence of a pharmacist–patient–prescriber relationship and the presentation of a valid prescription.

▸ Pharmacists may compound nonprescription medications in commercially available dosage forms or in alternative dosage forms to accommodate patient needs.

▸ Pharmacists may compound drugs in limited quantities prior to receiving a valid prescription based on a history of receiving valid prescriptions that have been generated solely within an established pharmacist–patient–prescriber relationship, and provided that they maintain the prescriptions on file for all such products dispensed at the pharmacy.

▸ Pharmacists should not offer compounded medications to other pharmacies for resale; however, a practitioner may obtain compounded medication to administer to patients, but it should be labeled with the following: "For Office Use Only," date compounded, "use by" date, and name, strength, and quantity of active ingredients.

▸ Compounding pharmacies/pharmacists may advertise or otherwise promote the fact that they provide prescription compounding services.

Source: References 4 and 5.

Compounding Facility and Equipment

Pharmacies that engage in compounding should have a designated area with adequate space for the orderly placement of the equipment and materials used in compounding activities. The pharmacist is also responsible for the proper maintenance, cleanliness, and use of all equipment involved in the compounding practice. The reader is referred to Chapter 2, "Facilities, Equipment, and Supplies," for a detailed discussion of the physical facility. Chapter 2 also details the specific equipment and supplies needed in the compounding process.

Personnel

Only personnel authorized by the responsible pharmacist should be in the immediate vicinity of the drug-compounding operation. Any person with an apparent illness or open lesion that may adversely affect the safety or quality of a drug product being compounded should be excluded from direct contact with components, drug product containers, closures, in-process materials, and drug products until the condition is corrected or determined by competent medical personnel to not jeopardize the safety or quality of the product being compounded. All personnel who assist in compounding procedures should be instructed to report to the responsible pharmacist any health conditions that may have an adverse effect on drug products.

Duties

The pharmacist has the responsibility and authority to inspect and approve or reject all components, drug product containers, closures, in-process materials, and labeling, as well as the authority to prepare and review all compounding records to ensure that no errors have occurred in the compounding process. In addition to compounding, the pharmacist provides other services, such as the following:

- Publicizes that both prescription and nonprescription compounding services are available. These services may include chemicals, devices, and alternative dosage forms.
- Provides drug searches on specific chemicals in different dosage forms, strengths, bases, and the like to accommodate physicians' specific needs.
- Provides follow-up information in response to a practitioner's request for information regarding a compounded medication.
- Consults with practitioners regarding a particular dosage form when discussing services with a health care provider.

Qualifications

Pharmacists should possess the education, training, and proficiency necessary to properly and safely perform the compounding duties at the level with which they are involved. All pharmacists who engage in the compounding of drugs should be proficient in the art and science of compounding and should maintain that proficiency through current awareness and training.

Instruction for compounding pharmacists should include, but not be limited to, the following:

- Proper use of compounding equipment such as balances and measuring devices, including guidelines for selecting proper measuring devices, limitations of weighing equipment and measuring apparatus, and the importance of accuracy in measurements.
- Pharmaceutical techniques needed to prepare compounded dosage forms (i.e., comminution, trituration, levigation, pulverization by intervention, and geometric dilution).
- Properties of dosage forms to be compounded and related factors, such as stability, storage considerations, and handling procedures.
- Literature regarding stability, solubility, and other physicochemical properties of the ingredients.
- Handling of nonhazardous and hazardous materials in the work area, including protective measures for avoiding exposure, emergency procedures to follow in the event of exposure, and the location of Material Safety Data Sheets (MSDSs) in the facility. (See Chapter 3, "Records and Record Keeping," for a discussion of this record.)
- Use and interpretation of chemical and pharmaceutical symbols and abbreviations in medication orders and in product formulation directions.
- Review of pharmaceutical calculations.

Attire

Personnel engaged in the compounding of drugs should wear clean clothing appropriate to the operation being performed. Protective apparel, such as coats or jackets, aprons, or hand or arm coverings, should be worn as necessary to protect drug products from contamination. A clean laboratory jacket generally is considered appropriate attire for nonsterile compounding procedures. Work with hazardous materials, such as chemotherapeutic agents, may require the use of goggles, gloves, masks or respirators, double gowns, and foot covers; showers and eyewash stations should be provided.

Ingredient Standards

Throughout history, pharmacists have used chemicals and other materials for prescription compounding. In the past, these chemicals and materials were obtained from natural products, raw materials, and household ingredients. Today, compounding pharmacists use chemicals from various sources, depending on their availability. A standard operating procedure (SOP) to cover chemical purchasing is provided at the end of this chapter.

Some chemical companies place a disclaimer on their chemicals for a number of reasons, including the following:

- Companies do not want to be required to label the materials under the *Food, Drug and Cosmetic Act of 1938 (FDC Act)*; consequently, they state that the materials are not to be used as drugs. This exempts the companies from having to comply with the FDC regulations.
- Source of the chemicals may be companies that do not meet current good manufacturing practices as stipulated in parts 210 and 211 of the *Code of Federal Regulations*; thus, when drugs are repackaged, only select information concerning the levels of potency and impurities and other miscellaneous characterization data are provided.
- Disclaimer protects the companies from liability associated with the use of their products that have not undergone the full safety and effectiveness testing required by the Food and Drug Administration (FDA) for the manufacturing of drug products.

Historically, the FDC Act has not applied to chemicals used for compounding, although it does apply to chemicals used for manufacturing. The selection of a chemical source for compounding is a judgment call on the part of pharmacists. When selecting a supplier of compounding chemicals, pharmacists should obtain and review certificates of analysis for purity, impurities, and so forth as one aspect of the decision-making process. The SOP "Purchasing Chemicals for Pharmaceutical Compounding" provides information on acceptable sources of ingredients, as stipulated in Chapter <795>, "Pharmacy Compounding," which is now official in the *United States Pharmacopeia 25/National Formulary 20 (USP 25/NF 20)*.

Appendix I lists drug products that have been withdrawn or removed from the market because of safety or efficacy concerns. Preparing compounded formulations of any of these products will be subject to enforcement action.

The Compounding Process

Before the actual steps are taken to prepare a product, a number of questions must be considered. The questions most relevant to the process are as follows:

- What are the physical and chemical properties and medicinal and pharmaceutical uses of the drug substance?
- Are the quantity and quality of each active ingredient identifiable?
- Based on the prescribed purpose of the prescription, will the preparation and route of administration provide adequate absorption, either locally or systemically?
- Are excipients present from any source (manufactured products) that may be expected to cause an allergic reaction, irritation, toxicity, or an undesirable organoleptic response from the patient?

▸ For products that are to be administered orally, are the active ingredients stable in the normal gastric pH range, or are they subject to extensive hepatic first-pass metabolism?

Steps in the Compounding Process

A number of steps must be followed before, during, and after the actual compounding activity. These steps can be grouped into five major phases: preparatory, compounding, final check, sign off, and clean up. The box "Steps in the Compounding Process" lists each phase and summarizes its corresponding steps. The following section discusses the steps in detail.

Steps in the Compounding Process

Preparatory
1. Judging the suitability of the prescription in terms of its safety and intended use and the dose for the patient.
2. Performing the calculations to determine the quantities of the ingredients needed.
3. Selecting the proper equipment and making sure it is clean.
4. Donning the proper attire and washing hands.
5. Cleaning the compounding area and the equipment, if necessary.
6. Assembling all the necessary materials/ingredients to compound and package the prescription.

Compounding
7. Compounding the prescription according to the formulary record or the prescription using techniques according to the art and science of pharmacy.

Final Check
8. Checking, as indicated, the weight variation, adequacy of mixing, clarity, odor, color, consistency, and pH.
9. Entering the information in the compounding log.
10. Labeling the prescription.

Sign Off
11. Signing and dating the prescription affirming that all of the indicated procedures were carried out to ensure uniformity, identity, strength, quantity, and purity.

Clean Up
12. Cleaning and storing all equipment.
13. Cleaning the compounding area.

Continuous Quality Improvement

Before dispensing the prescription to the patient, the pharmacist should ensure the accuracy and completeness of the compounded product by reviewing each step in the preparatory, compounding, final check, and sign-off phases. In the preparatory review, the pharmacist checks that all preparations for the compounding process were handled appropriately. Aspects to be reviewed include the following:

▸ Appropriate ingredients, adjuvants, and equipment were selected for the specific preparation.
▸ Calculations are correct.
▸ Measurements were performed accurately with properly functioning equipment.

- The formulation is appropriate for the intended use and stability limits of the preparation.

The pharmacist then reviews the compounding steps to ensure that the procedures and techniques used to prepare the product were faithfully followed and appropriately documented. This review also ensures that the product is reasonably aesthetic and uniform in content.

The pharmacist's review of the final check phase should be comprehensive. It is intended to verify the following:

- The calculated yield is consistent with the actual yield.
- The tolerance for individual dose weight variation has been met by a sampling technique when appropriate (i.e., capsule weight).
- The physical characteristics (clarity, color, odor) of the preparation are consistent with those predicted for the preparation.
- Physical tests were performed when appropriate, and the preparation meets the test limits.
- The preparation is suitably labeled, and the contents have been verified with the prescription order. All legal requirements have been imprinted on the label and in the compounding record.
- The preparation is suitably packaged for patient use, and the container that is selected will protect the preparation from undue environmental exposure until at least the "discard-after" or "beyond-use" date.
- Documentation is appropriate, as listed in Chapter 3, "Records and Record Keeping."
- The patient or caregiver has been adequately informed about ways to identify obvious evidence of instability in the compounded preparation.
- The preparation is labeled with explicit storage and administration instructions.

The pharmacist may also decide to submit samples of compounded products to an analytical testing laboratory. Such analytical testing could include dissolution rates and concentrations of compounded medications. Additional tests, assays, or visual observations of samples of the preparation may also be performed to ensure the content, stability, pH, sterility, nonpyrogenicity, and the like. The pharmacist may use an analytical testing laboratory to perform some of the testing; this would involve testing samples of a compounded product, not every prescription that is compounded via that process.

Packaging, Storage, and Labeling

The pharmacist should inspect and approve all components, drug product containers, closures, labeling, and other materials involved in the compounding process. These materials should be handled and stored in a manner that will prevent contamination.

Packaging

Compounded preparations should be packaged according to the specifications described in the current edition of the *USP 25/NF 20*. The selection of a container depends on the physical and chemical properties of the compounded preparation and the intended use of the product.

To help maintain potency of the stored drug, packaging materials should not interact physically or chemically with the product. Materials that are reactive, additive, or absorptive can alter the safety, identity, strength, quality, or purity of the compounded drug beyond the specifications for an acceptable product. Container characteristics of concern include inertness, visibility, strength, rigidity, moisture protection, ease of reclosure, and economy of packaging.

Plastic containers have become increasingly popular because they are less expensive and lighter in weight than glass. Only plastic containers that meet *USP 25/NF 20* standards should be used.

Storage

Chemicals should be stored according to either the manufacturers' directions or the appropriate monographs in the *USP 25/NF 20*. In general, compounding chemicals should be stored in tightly closed, light-resistant containers at room temperature; some chemicals, however, require refrigeration. Chemicals should also be stored off the floor, preferably on shelves in a clean, dry environment. Commercial drugs to be used in the compounding process should be removed from cartons and boxes before they are stored in the compounding area.

Temperature requirements for storage of substances are detailed in the appropriate *USP 25/NF 20* monographs. The temperatures of the storage areas, including refrigerators and freezers, should be monitored and recorded at least weekly.

Flammable or hazardous products should be stored appropriately in safety storage cabinets and containers; these items are available from many laboratory suppliers.

Labeling

Labeling should be done according to state and federal regulations. Usually, labeling information includes the (1) generic or chemical names of the active ingredients, (2) strength or quantity, (3) pharmacy lot number, (4) beyond-use date, and (5) any special storage requirements.

When a commercial drug product has been used as a source of the drug, the generic name of the drug product, not the proprietary name, should be placed on the label. Inactive ingredients and vehicles should also be listed on the label. If no expiration date is provided on the chemicals or materials that are used, a system of monitoring should be established (e.g., placing the date of receipt of the materials on the label of the container). Monitoring expiration dates will ensure that materials, ingredients, and supplies are rotated so that the oldest stock is used first.

The use of specialty "coined" names or short names for convenience should be discouraged. Such names can cause difficulty in emergency departments if an overdose or accidental poisoning has occurred or if health professionals treating the patient need to know what the patient has been taking. If batch quantities of a product are prepared, a lot number should be assigned and placed on the labels. Surplus prepared labels should be destroyed.

If excess product is prepared or additional quantities are prepared in anticipation of future requests for the product, the pharmacist should have written procedures for the proper labeling of the excess product. Labeling should include the (1) complete list of ingredients, (2) preparation date, (3) assigned beyond-use date, (4) appropriate testing/published data, and (5) control numbers. The product should then be entered into the inventory and stored appropriately to help ensure its strength, quality, and purity. When the compounding process is completed, the excess product should be reexamined for correct labeling and contents.

Quality Control

The pharmacist should review all compounding records for accuracy and conduct in-process and final checks to ensure that errors have not occurred in the compounding process. Written procedures for the compounding of drugs should be available and followed to ensure the identity, strength, quality, and purity of the finished product. Such procedures should include a listing of the ingredients, quantities, order of mixing or preparation, and a detailed description of the compounding process. The equipment and utensils used should be listed, as well as the container and closure packaging system. Information concerning stability and compatibility should be included, along with any documentation related to the product.

Ingredients should be accurately weighed, measured, or subdivided as indicated. The compounding pharmacist should check and recheck these operations at each step in the compounding process to ensure that weights or measures are correct.

SOPs should be prepared that describe the tests or examinations to be conducted on the finished product. These tests could include physical examination; and pH, weight, and volume measurements. Such procedures are established to monitor the output of the compounding pharmacy and to validate the performance of compounding processes that may cause variability in the completed drug product.

Stability, Expiration, and Beyond-Use Dating

USP 25/NF 20 defines *stability* as the "extent to which a dosage form retains, within specified limits and throughout its period of storage and use, the same properties and characteristics that it possessed at the time of its preparation."[4] The compounding pharmacist must avoid formulation ingredients and conditions that could result in a subpotent product that leads to poor clinical results. Knowledge of the chemical reactions by which drugs degrade often provides a means of establishing conditions under which the rate of degradation can be minimized. At all steps in the compounding, dispensing, and storage processes, the pharmacist should observe the compounded drug preparation for signs of instability. A discard-after or beyond-use date is the date after which a compounded product should be discarded. This period should be based on available stability information and reasonable patient needs with respect to the intended drug therapy. When a commercial drug product is used as a source of active ingredients, its expiration date can often be used as a factor in determining a discard-after date.

When determining a discard-after date, a pharmacist may consider the following factors/measures:

- The nature of the drug and its degradation kinetics.
- The container in which the drug is packaged.
- The expected storage conditions to which the preparation may be exposed.
- The expected length of therapy.
- The expiration date of similar commercial products for guidance, if the active ingredient is a USP/NF substance.
- Published literature.
- Telephone call to the manufacturer, if no printed information is supplied with the product.

The beyond-use date assigned to a specific product should be based on the following:

- Physical and chemical properties of the ingredients.
- Use of preservatives and/or stabilizers.
- Dosage form of the product.
- Storage conditions.
- Scientific, laboratory, or reference data.

It is difficult to assign a beyond-use date. The pharmacist should consult all available stability information and then make a conservative estimate for the product. Several general guidelines should also be considered. First, when a manufactured commercial product is used as the source of the active ingredient, the beyond-use date should be no more than 25% of the manufacturer's *remaining* expiration date or 6 months, whichever is less. For example, if a product received on April 1, 2000, has an expiration date of December 31, 2000, 8 months of the expiration date remain. Therefore, the beyond-use date for the compounded product should be 2 months (25% of 8 months) from the date of its preparation. Second, when a USP or an NF pure chemical is used, the beyond-use date should be no more than 6 months for dry products. (See Chapter 4, "Stability of Compounded Products," for cases that do not fall within either of these guidelines.)

All compounded products should be observed periodically for signs of physical instability, including evidence of microbiological and fungal contamination of any products whose formulas lack preservatives. If large quantities of a product have been legitimately prepared, it may be advisable to conduct potency and stability assays on the product to ensure the compounding pharmacist of the product's potency up to the assigned beyond-use date. (See Chapter 4, "Stability of Compounded Products," for more detailed information on beyond-use dates.)

Records and Reports

Pharmacists should maintain at least four sets of records for compounding: (1) formulation records, (2) compounding records, (3) SOPs, including equipment-maintenance records, and (4) ingredients records, including certificates of analysis and MSDSs. Records and reports should be retained for the period of time required by state laws and regulations for the retention of prescription files. All records and reports should be readily available in the pharmacy for authorized inspection during the retention period. The proper recording of information is so vital to ensuring consistent preparation of a formulation that an entire chapter is devoted to the subject; the reader is referred to Chapter 3, "Records and Record Keeping," for a detailed discussion of each type of record.

Patient Counseling

Compounded prescriptions provide an excellent opportunity for patient counseling. The pharmacist can explain that this particular prescription has been prepared especially for the patient and can indicate other steps that are required before its administration. This occasion can also be used to discuss other routine subjects with the patient.

Reference Library

Compounding pharmacists must have ready access to reference materials on all aspects of compounding, including reprints of journal articles. These materials may include on-site books, reprints, and journals, as well as telephone access to information from a compounding or drug information center. Computer access to such information is also important.

Pharmacies should also maintain a limited reference library. The section "Standard Operating Procedures" explains how to establish and maintain a compounding pharmacy reference library; it also provides a list of information resources that should be part of any pharmacy library.

Standard Operating Procedures (SOPs)

Purchasing Chemicals for Pharmaceutical Compounding

Purpose of SOP

The purpose of this procedure is to establish appropriate guidelines and documentation for purchasing chemicals for use in pharmaceutical compounding to ensure that all pharmaceuticals are of appropriate quality.

Regulatory Issues

Chapter <795>, "Pharmacy Compounding," states that "The pharmacist is responsible for compounding preparations of acceptable strength, quality, and purity with appropriate packaging and labeling in accordance with good pharmacy practices, official standards, and relevant scientific data and information."[1] The compounding of quality preparations must involve the use of high-quality chemicals.

Official Compounded Preparations

If USP/NF grade ingredients are used to prepare compounded formulations, the preparation must meet the requirements of compendial monographs.

Other Compounded Preparations

Chapter <795>, "Pharmacy Compounding" also states the following:

> A USP or an NF grade substance is the preferred source of ingredients for compounding all other preparations. If that is not available, or when food, cosmetics, or other substances are or must be used, the use of another high quality source, such as analytical reagent (AR), certified American Chemical Society (ACS), or Food Chemicals Codes (FCC) grade, is an option for professional judgment. For any substance used in compounding not purchased from a registered drug manufacturer, the pharmacist should establish purity and safety by reasonable means, which may include lot analysis, manufacturer reputation, or reliability of source.[1]

Manufactured Drug Products as a Source of Active Ingredients

Manufactured drug products such as injectables, tablets, or capsules may be sources of active ingredients. If such a product is the source of the active ingredient used in the compounding of a prescription, only a manufactured drug from a container labeled with a batch control number and a future expiration date is acceptable. If a manufactured drug product is used, it is important that all the ingredients in the drug product be considered relative to the intended use and the potential effect on the overall efficacy (strength, quality, purity, stability, compatibility) of the compounded preparation.

Professional Judgment

Throughout history, pharmacists have been using chemicals and other materials for prescription compounding that have been obtained from natural products, raw materials, and household ingredients. Today, the responsibility rests on the pharmacist to select the most appropriate quality of chemical for compounding, beginning with the USP/NF grade substance as the first choice and, if this grade is not available, then descending the list of purity grades using professional judgment and discretion. Table 1-1 provides a list of commonly available chemical grades.

Table 1-1. Description of Chemical Grades

Grade	Description
USP/NF	Meets the minimum purity standards; conforms to tolerances set by the *United States Pharmacopeia/National Formulary* for contaminants dangerous to health
ACS reagent	High purity; conforms to minimum specifications set by the Reagent Chemicals Committee of the American Chemical Society
CP (chemically pure)	More refined than technical or commercial grade but still of unknown quality
Technical or commercial	Indeterminate quality

Other high-purity chemical grades include analytical reagent, high-performance liquid chromatography, spectroscopic grade, and primary standard. These grades are used primarily in the analytical chemistry and pharmaceutical analysis field.

For consistent quality in compounded preparations, it is important to use high-quality suppliers of chemicals for compounding. Using the same suppliers will also ensure consistent quality. If different suppliers are used, variations in physico-chemical characteristics, such as particle size, may alter the expected response of drug preparations. It is also wise to have a secondary supplier available in the event of unexpected shortfalls in supply. Figure 1-1 illustrates a record form for suppliers of pharmaceutical chemicals.

Certificates of analysis should be obtained and kept on record as documentation of the quality of chemicals used in compounding preparations. These can be easily maintained in a standard three-ring notebook system.

Establishing and Maintaining a Compounding Pharmacy Reference Library

Purpose of SOP

The purpose of this procedure is to establish appropriate guidelines and documentation for establishing and maintaining a compounding pharmacy reference library.

Pharmaceutical Chemical Suppliers

Substance	Grade	Primary Source/Tel. No.	Secondary Source/Tel. No.

Figure 1-1. Sample record of pharmaceutical chemical suppliers.

Regulatory Issues

Chapter <795>, "Pharmacy Compounding," states that "The pharmacist is responsible for compounding preparations of acceptable strength, quality, and purity with appropriate packaging and labeling in accordance with good pharmacy practices, official standards, and relevant scientific data and information."[1] The compounding of quality preparations requires access to up-to-date, reliable drug information as well as pharmacy compounding information.

The contents of a reference library at a particular practice site will depend in part on the type of compounded formulations being prepared. For example, compounding of sterile products requires specific references related to aseptic compounding practices. However, the following references should be a part of every pharmacy reference library:

- Ansel HC, Allen LV, Popovich NG. *Pharmaceutical Dosage Forms and Drug Delivery Systems.* 7th ed. Baltimore: Lippincott Williams & Wilkins; 1999.
- Ansel HC, Stokksa MJ. *Pharmaceutical Calculations.* 11th ed. Baltimore: Lippincott Williams & Wilkins; 2001.
- Gennaro AR. *Remington: The Science and Practice of Pharmacy.* 20th ed. Philadelphia, Pa: Lippincott Williams & Wilkins; 2000.
- Holdford D, Wick JY, Sethi ML, Kibbe AH. *Handbook of Pharmaceutical Excipients.* 4th ed. Washington, DC: American Pharmaceutical Association; 2002.
- McEvoy GK, Litvak K, Welsh OH. *AHFS Drug Information 2001.* Bethesda, Md: American Society of Health-System Pharmacists; 2001.
- Reynolds JEF. *Martindale: The Extra Pharmacopoeia.* 30th ed. London: The Pharmaceutical Press; 1993.
- *Secundum Artem.* Minneapolis, Minn: Paddock Laboratories [quarterly journal].
- *The Merck Index.* 12th ed. Rahway, NJ: Merck & Co; 1996.
- *United States Pharmacopeia 25/National Formulary 20.* Rockville, Md: United States Pharmacopeial Convention; 2001.

Some editions of these references should be retained in a "previous editions" section of the reference library because they contain valuable information that was not carried forward to new editions; examples include *Remington: The Science and Practice of Pharmacy* and *Martindale: The Extra Pharmacopoeia.* Older editions of some references should be discarded, however, if new research has shown that previously published information is incorrect; examples include *United States Pharmacopeia/National Formulary, Handbook on Injectable Drugs* (L. A. Trissel), and *King Guide to Parenteral Admixtures.*

Procedure for Establishing a Reference Library

1. Determine the books required by the state board of pharmacy. (Place an asterisk by these titles on the Compounding Pharmacy Reference Library Maintenance Form [Figure 1-2].)
2. Determine the scope of practice, or "breadth," required for the pharmacy.
3. Determine the "depth" of the scope of practice.
4. Select the "core" books that will be required (both paper and electronic).
5. Select the "supplemental" books that will be required (both paper and electronic).
6. Individualize the Compounding Pharmacy Reference Library Maintenance Form for your facility.

Compounding Pharmacy Reference Library
Maintenance Form

Title/Author	Date Added	Frequency of Publication[a]	Date(s) Replaced						

[a]Annually, biannually, variable.

Figure 1-2. Sample form for compounding pharmacy reference library.

Procedure for Maintaining a Reference Library

1. Annually (e.g., the first week in January), review the reference library and order "updates" (new book editions or supplements) and recently published new references as required (see step 2).
2. As new editions of pharmacy references are announced, check the edition on hand to determine whether to order the latest edition.
3. Mark the books that should be retained in a "previous editions" section of the reference library.
4. Mark the books that should be discarded when replaced by a new edition.

References

1. Expert Advisory Panel on Pharmacy Compounding Practices. Pharmacy compounding. In: *United States Pharmacopeia 25/National Formulary 20*. Rockville, Md: United States Pharmacopeial Convention; 2001.
2. Good compounding practices applicable to state-licensed pharmacies. In: *Model State Pharmacy Act and Model Rules of the National Association of Boards of Pharmacy*. Park Ridge, Ill: National Association of Boards of Pharmacy; 1993:C.1–C.5.
3. The Food and Drug Administration Modernization Act of 1997. Pub Law 105-115, §127.
4. Stability considerations in dispensing practice. In: *United States Pharmacopeia 25/National Formulary 20*. Rockville, Md: United States Pharmacopeial Convention; 2001.
5. Allen LV Jr. General guidelines for the use of chemicals for prescription compounding. *Int J Pharm Compound.* 1997;1:46.

Chapter 2

Facilities, Equipment, and Supplies

The "tools of the trade" for most professions have changed over the years. Physicians now use computers, laser light, high-technology communications systems, and biotechnology-derived drug products; lawyers conduct large database searches in the courtroom; and pharmacists use computers and handheld pocket computers for such applications as medication dispensing, patient monitoring, patient counseling, drug preparation, high-technology communications, and access to databases and drug delivery devices (pumps).

With the changes that have occurred in the delivery of medical and pharmaceutical care have come changes in the equipment and supplies that are used on a daily basis. As a result, many state boards of pharmacy are revising their regulations to reflect current practice activities, particularly as they apply to the preparation of drug products.

As one looks at the changes in pharmacy, it becomes apparent that the pace of change is quickening, especially as new technology is introduced. Although these new methods and techniques must be mastered as they replace older ones, it is advantageous to retain many of the time-honored approaches, because they are still useful and contribute to patient therapy. Nevertheless, any observer of the future must be cognizant of the role that computerization and robotics will play in pharmacy practices in the years ahead. This new technology will affect counseling, drug utilization review, medication management, and dispensing activities. Pharmacists must know what equipment is available, how to use and maintain it, and how responsibilities and opportunities in health care are changing. As long as drug therapy exists, pharmacists must be involved in the preparation and/or provision and appropriate use of the product to meet the specific needs of the patient. This is especially true for the newer and biotechnology-derived medications and for the provision of patient-specific products that must be compounded.

Historical Review

Historical records show that apothecaries began their ministrations by using very simple equipment and tools—mortars and pestles, knives and axes to obtain plants and plant parts, mixing vessels, and drying tables. Common dosage forms included ointments, oils, and powdered extracts from plants. Later, processes such as distillation and extraction were introduced, which resulted in more complex equipment requirements. The earliest recognized implements of pharmacy are the mortar and pestle, which have become the symbol of pharmacy.

Mortar and Pestle

From the earliest days of pharmacy to the present, the mortar and pestle have been characteristic utensils of the profession. It was selected as the symbol of pharmacy during the 17th century and has been used as a sign for an apothecary's shop or pharmacy. Mortars and pestles are available in different sizes (from several ounces to more than 200 lb) and shapes (e.g., bowl, V, hourglass) and are made of different materials (e.g., wood, brass, glass, porcelain). Some are plain and some are decorated; some are functional and some are fashionable; some are for general use and some are for special use. Grinding (comminution and pulverization) and mixing have always been a part of pharmacy. Formerly, roots, rhizomes, dried herbs, and earth were pulverized before administration in the form of powders, poultices, or ointments. Today, mortars and pestles are used for pulverization of powders and granules and for mixing.

Even pharmacists who do not compound claim the mortar and pestle as the symbol of their profession.

Twentieth-Century Equipment

Equipment used by pharmacists for compounding during the 1940s, 1950s, and 1960s was basic, consisting of mortars and pestles, beakers, conical graduates, prescription balances, hot plates, refrigerators, pill tiles, and spatulas. With the advent of the pharmacist's responsibility for intravenous admixtures in the 1970s, pharmacies added such equipment as laminar flow hoods, aseptic transfer devices and pumps, and sterile filtration units.

The resurgence of compounding in the 1980s and 1990s has led to further expansion into the range of equipment used in pharmacies, depending on the scope of practice. The first contemporary compounding-only pharmacy opened in 1987. Today, there are at least 125 of these pharmacies in North America.

From undertaking traditional compounding activities such as the preparation of syrups, suppositories, troches, and ointments to the high-technology aseptic compounding of total parenteral nutrition solutions that contain 20 or more ingredients and even the programming of ambulatory pumps, pharmacists are entering the world of the technology-based pharmacy.

Despite these tremendous changes in equipment requirements, many regulatory agencies have not "kept up with the profession" in updating practice regulations. Because the practice of pharmacy is now so diverse, it is doubtful that one board-defined list of items will suffice for all practice settings; rather, different equipment lists must be developed based on the type of practice (e.g., community, hospital, home health care, nuclear, traditional and aseptic compounding).

Compounding Facility

The compounding facility should be designed, arranged, and maintained to facilitate quality compounding. The area for compounding sterile drug products should be separate from the area for compounding or dispensing nonsterile drug products.

Traffic in the compounding area should be kept to a minimum, with only designated individuals allowed access. The area should be well lighted and have controlled heating, ventilation, and air conditioning to prevent the decomposition of chemicals and to ensure a comfortable workplace without distractions. The materials used for the floor, walls, shelving and cabinets, and ceiling should not retain dust, odors, or residues from the compounding activities. The area should be free of dust-collecting overhangs (e.g., ceiling pipes, hanging light fixtures, ledges) as well as from infestation by insects, rodents, and other vermin. The actual work area should be level, smooth, impervious, free of cracks and crevices, and nonshedding. The shelving and cabinets should be easy to clean as well.

Surfaces should be cleaned at the beginning and the end of each compounding operation. All equipment that is used should be cleaned thoroughly to avoid cross-contamination between ingredients and preparations. Cleaning should be initiated immediately after the use of any sensitizing, caustic, or dangerous substances. The entire compounding area should be cleaned daily or weekly but not during the compounding process. Pharmacies engaged in only occasional compounding should make adequate preparations before each compounding activity.

Washing facilities should be adequate and easily accessible to the compounding area. These facilities should have satisfactory drainage and provide hot and cold water, cleansing agents, and air-driers or disposable towels. There should be sufficient potable water and a source of purified water USP or other water suitable for the compounding activities. Potable water should be supplied under continuous positive pressure in a plumbing system free of defects that could contribute to the contamination of the product. Sewage, trash, and other refuse in and from the pharmacy and immediate drug-compounding area or areas should be disposed of in a safe and sanitary manner. Trash should be collected and removed daily.

Compounding Equipment/Supplies

Equipment used in the compounding of drug products should be appropriately designed, of adequate size, and suitably located to facilitate compounding operations. The equipment should be of a neutral and impervious composition so that ingredients, in-process materials, or drug products do not react with, add to, or are absorbed by it in such a way that the safety, identity, strength, quality, or purity of the drug product is altered beyond the desired composition.

Equipment and utensils used for compounding should be cleaned and sanitized immediately before use to prevent contamination that would alter the drug product. (See the section "Standard Operating Procedures" for instructions on cleaning glassware.) To ensure that equipment and utensils are clean, they should be inspected by the pharmacist immediately before compounding operations begin.

If the compounding process involves drug products that require special measures to prevent cross-contamination, appropriate precautions must be taken. These precautions include dedication of equipment for these operations and meticulous cleaning of the contaminated equipment.

Automatic, mechanical, or electronic equipment, or other related equipment or systems, may be used in the compounding of drug products. This equipment should be routinely inspected, calibrated if necessary, and checked to ensure proper performance. The maintenance of all equipment should be documented.

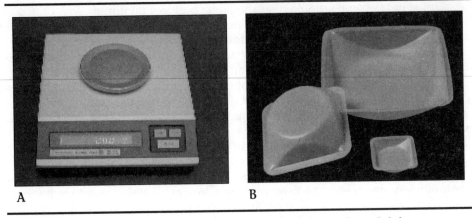

A   B

Figure 2-1. Weighing equipment: A, electronic balance; B, weigh boats.

Equipment for Weighing/Measuring

The accurate weighing and measuring of ingredients is crucial to attain a compounded product that is safe to administer and achieves the desired therapeutic effect. For these reasons, balances and measuring equipment are discussed separately from other compounding equipment.

Balances

Compounding pharmacies use either class A torsion balances or electronic balances to weigh materials used in compounded formulations.

Electronic balances that can weigh quantities as large as 300 g and as small as 1 mg are available (Figure 2-1A). The cost of a balance is generally proportional to the lowest weight that can be accurately measured. Electronic balances weigh small quantities of materials very accurately and at a relatively low investment. These balances are easy to use, clean, and calibrate. They simplify quality control determinations, especially if a printer is attached.

Weight sets for use with prescription balances usually contain both apothecary and metric systems, but the metric system is now the only official measuring system. Brass weight sets should be used with torsion balances only. Materials to be weighed can be placed on weighing papers or in plastic weigh boats (Figure 2-1B).

Balances should be situated in areas of low humidity and placed on flat, nonvibrating surfaces away from vents, fans, and other currents of moving air. The performance of the balances should be checked at least monthly, and the performance should be documented. (See the section "Standard Operating Procedures" for instructions on torsion balance performance tests.)

Measuring Equipment

In addition to the customary measuring equipment consisting of graduated cylinders, pipets, calibrated syringes, and the like, it is becoming more commonplace to use micropipets to accurately measure very small volumes of liquids.

Micropipets eliminate the need to prepare aliquots of drugs when only a very small quantity is required. Because various micropipets are available, the investment can be kept to a minimum. For example, one micropipet can be used for 200 to 1000 μL and another can be used for 5 to 200 μL. Multiple-channel micropipets can be used when it is necessary to deliver up to 12 channels simultaneously (e.g., when 0.5 mL is being placed in a large number of small vials/ampules).

Micropipets should be checked frequently to determine their accuracy in the volume of liquid delivered. This can be easily accomplished by weighing the volume of purified water USP delivered onto a tared receptacle on a balance.

Other Types of Compounding Equipment

The equipment needs of pharmacists vary depending on the type of compounding activities performed. There are four basic areas of involvement: (1) general nonsterile product compounding, (2) advanced nonsterile product compounding, (3) general sterile product compounding, and (4) advanced sterile product compounding. The general equipment requirements for each of these areas are presented in Table 2-1. Many of these items are used for both nonsterile and sterile product compounding; the following discussion is limited to particular items whose applications and use may be unclear or unusual.

General Nonsterile Product Compounding Equipment

A *"hot hand"* is a rubber or plastic molded hand protector that is convenient for picking up very hot or very cold beakers, flasks, and the like.

Capsule-filling devices are available in numerous formats. From inexpensive plastic units for 25 or 50 capsules to the more rugged 100- to 300-capsule machines, these devices are timesavers if a large number of capsules are being prepared. The 100-capsule units can be used to prepare smaller numbers and work well with locking capsules.

Desiccators, containing a desiccant, are important when storing drug products that require a very dry atmosphere. Desiccators are available in glass or plastic and may have a port for a vacuum.

Glass pill tiles are used for the preparation of many different dose forms. Many come with graduated markings on one end to measure lengths of suppositories, pill pipes, and the like. Most glass pill tiles also have a frosted portion that serves as the

Table 2-1. General Compounding Equipment and Supplies

Nonsterile Product Compounding Equipment

General Nonsterile Equipment

Balance—prescription, torsion
Balance—triple beam
Beaker hot hand
Beaker tongs
Beakers—glass/plastic/stainless steel
(50, 100, 150, 250, 400, 600,
1000 mL)
Beakers—with/without handles, glass/
plastic/stainless steel (1000, 2000,
3000 mL)
Capsule-filling equipment
Cylinders—glass/plastic
(graduate 5 to 2000 mL)
Desiccators—glass/plastic
Desiccant (Drier-Rite)

Dishes—with/without handles—
evaporating, porcelain
Funnels—glass/plastic
(2", 3", 4", 5", 6")
Glasses—safety
Graduates—pharmaceutical/conical—
glass/plastic (10, 25, 50, 100, 250,
500, and 1000 mL)
Graters, hand (fine, medium, coarse,
combination)
Gummy gel molds
Hot plates (various sizes and features)
Mortars/pestles—glass/porcelain
(2, 4, 8 oz)
Openers—jar/bottle/tube
Ovens—drying
pH meters

(continued)

Table 2-1. General Compounding Equipment and Supplies (cont.)

General Nonsterile Equipment (cont.)

Pill tiles—glass, frosted
Racks, drying—plastic or epoxy resin
    material
Refrigerator with freezer
Spatulas—plastic/stainless steel,
    assorted (4″, 6″)
Stir plates—magnetic with stir bars
Stirring rods
Strainers—(small, medium, large)
Suppository molds (rectal, vaginal,
    urethral)
Thermometers—glass
Thermometer clips
Troche molds
Weighing dishes—plastic/aluminum
Weighing papers
Weight sets, brass

Advanced Nonsterile Equipment

Balance, electronic (minimum
    sensitivity of 1 mg)
Balance, electronic (minimum
    sensitivity of 10 mg)
Bath, dry—heater/incubator
Beakers, insulated
Beakers, Teflon
Beakers, heat-resistant plastic
Blender (liquify, puree, mix; 12 mL
    to 4000 mL capacities; temperature
    controlled, foam arrestor)
Blender, hand—two-speed lab
    (three blades, with stand)
Blender, hand—variable speed
    (mixing container, stand, various
    blades, at least two speeds)
Boiling chips or beads
Bottles, dispensing fluid—plastic or
    glass
Bottles, drop dispensing—plastic or
    glass
Brushes, cleaning—nylon (various
    sizes/shapes to fit equipment)
Buckets with lids—plastic
Burets (10–50 mL)
Burners, Bunsen or similar (natural
    gas or propane)

Carboys with/without spigots
Carts, plastic/metal
Centrifuge
Chopper/grinder
Coffee grinder
Crimper, hand operated
Desiccator
Desiccator/micromarinader (creates
    vacuum; has desiccator applications)
Dispensing pumps, variable speed
Fat/oil separator (gravy separator)
Food processor (slice, grate, chop,
    puree, mix, knead: various blades)
Heat gun, variable heat outputs
Homogenizers, hand operated or
    electric
Lead sticks, flexible
Light boxes
Magnetic stirrers
Microspatulas, stainless steel,
    Teflon coated
Motorized stirrer
Malt shop mixer (two-speed motor,
    28 oz stainless steel cup)
Mixer—orbital, single/variable speed
Mixer, professional—kitchen
Mortars/pestles (various sizes/shapes)
pH meter
Pipet bulbs
Pipets (1–100 mL)
Pipet fillers, hand operated
Pipets/micropipets (variable sizes:
    5–200 mL, 200–1000 mL)
Pipets—multiple channel
Pipet, motorized
Pitcher, stirring (2000 mL capacity,
    blades attached to handle, plastic)
Powder blender (blends powders in
    dust-free environment and protects
    operator from powder dust)
Repeating dispenser for liquids
Sealers, bag or suppository
Sealers, tube
Sieves, 3″, 5″, 7″ (various mesh sizes)
Solvent dispensing/spray bottles
Spatulas, stainless steel, Teflon coated,
    porcelain, plastic
Sprayer bottles
Tablet press, single punch

Table 2-1. General Compounding Equipment and Supplies (cont.)

Tea/spice ball
Thermometer, digital probe
Thermometer, high-low alarm
Thermometers with alarm
Test-tube rack, four sided
Tongs, beaker/flask/tube
Tool set, cooks' heavy-gauge stainless steel (pasta fork, turner, solid spoon, ladle, server, skimmer, and hanging rack)
Tubing (various sizes/types)
Tubing clamps (various sizes/types)
Ultrasonic cleaner (various capacities)
Vortex mixers
Wash bottles
Water system (high quality)
Workbench protector sheets (plastic, rubber, absorbable paper, matted)

Sterile Product Compounding Equipment

General Sterile Equipment

Ampule openers, disposable
Anemometer, directed reading
Apparel for clean rooms (Class 10,000) (aprons, sleeves, gloves, hoods—open face, hoods—face mask, boot covers, shoe covers, frocks, coveralls, head coverings, lab coats, smocks, shirts/ pants, hats/caps, face masks, beard covers)
Autoclave bags
Autoclave tape
Baggies/pouches/pouch sealers
Biohazard autoclave bags
Biohazard bag holders
Cleaning materials
    Hazardous materials handling equipment
    Pickup roller—cabinet/work space
    Pickup roller—floor
    Pickup roller—wall
Filter unit—repeating syringe with three-way connector and check valve
Filter units, vacuum—disposable

Filters, sterilizing (numerous types/shapes/applications)
Forceps
Impulse or induction sealer for plastic overwraps
Laminar flow hood, horizontal (Class 100)
Laminar flow hood, vertical (Class 100)
Needle destroyer
Pumps, pressure
Pumps, vacuum, electric
Pumps, vacuum, hand operated
Refrigerator
Refrigerator with freezer
Sharps disposal unit
Stainless steel pressure filter holders (various capacities)
Tacky mats
Trash container—gowns/apparel articles
Trash container—plastic/paper articles
Wire racks/shelving

Advanced Sterile Equipment

Autoclave
Cooler/heater for medication transport in automobile (30 L)
Crimper, hand operated
Decappers
Filtration, sterile—equipment
Ice replacement gel (various forms/ types)
Osmometer
Particle counter
Particulate testing equipment
Pump, pressure—vacuum
Pyrogen test materials
Quality control equipment
Sample transporter coolant—pouch (maintains sample at about 5°C [−10°C for 30 minutes])
Smoke sticks
Spatulas and spoons, sterile (plastic for weighing and obtaining drugs)
Sterility test equipment
Ultrafreezer (capable of about −80°C)

primary work area. This area provides a good working surface for comminution with a stainless steel spatula and for mixing ointments.

Ovens (drying) are often required for the drying of various compounded products and for the drying of products that might have adsorbed or absorbed moisture over time. As the potency of the drug increases, the sorption of moisture becomes even more dangerous because of weighing errors; the presence of moisture in the drug gives a greater weight for the same quantity of material than if it had been dried before weighing.

pH meters are commonplace in compounding pharmacies. pH is critical for drug solubility and stability. Many products must be buffered, or the pH must be adjusted to a certain range that requires a greater degree of accuracy than can be provided by pH indicator papers.

Stir plates (magnetic with stir bars) have become standard in pharmacies that compound a large number of fluid preparations. Stir plates enable the pharmacists to perform other duties while ingredients are dissolving and mixing. If the plate has a heating element, it is possible to more easily mix melted ointments and suppository bases to uniformity. The section "Standard Operating Procedures" provides a convenient means of documenting the required calibration information for hot plates.

Suppository , troche, and gummy gel molds that are made of plastic are slowly replacing the older heavy metal molds. Plastic molds may also serve as part of the dispensing package. Because these molds are available in different sizes, unlike many of the metal molds that were reasonably standardized at 2 mL each, they must be used with caution.

Advanced Nonsterile Product Compounding Equipment

Blenders (cabinet top and hand held) are indispensable in the preparation of many products. Kitchen blenders are excellent for preparing solutions, suspensions, emulsions, and even gels (if used properly). They are available in the standard kitchen size of about 28 oz and in laboratory sizes, with vessels ranging from 12 mL to about 4000 mL. Hand-held blenders are suitable for preparing lotions, creams, and other semisolid and liquid preparations. These appliances are available with single, dual, and variable speeds.

Carts (plastic/metal) can be used to move supplies from one area to another. They also provide working surfaces when necessary.

Choppers/grinders and *coffee grinders,* which are available in the kitchen equipment department in large stores and in gourmet shops, can be used for particle size reduction as well as for blending small quantities of powders.

Crimpers (hand operated) are used to attach aluminum tamper-evident safety caps onto containers of prepared products. This system for packaging a product is very convenient when there is a need to ensure that the package has not been opened; it is similar to the seals used for injectables.

Dispensing pumps (variable speed) are invaluable when the same volume of a liquid must be repeatedly measured and dispensed. They are especially useful in packaging finished products into containers.

Dry baths are alternatives to hot plates and are replacing water baths in many facilities. A dry bath is essentially a heated chamber that can be filled with sand, salt, or aluminum blocks designed to hold various sizes of glassware. For example, a beaker can be "wiggled" into the sand after the sand has equilibrated to the temperature required to heat a preparation. Dry baths are easy to use and clean and are virtually maintenance free.

*Fat/oil separator s*can be used to obtain a foam-free liquid from an ingredient that has a foam on top, which makes it difficult to measure. The spout originates at the bottom of the container so the liquid, not the foam, is dispensed. These items are often referred to as "gravy separators."

Food processors capable of slicing, grating, chopping, pureeing, mixing, and kneading, depending on the various blades that are available, have many applications, including the preparation of ointments and pastes.

Heat guns (variable heat) can be used in those situations when heat is required and a hot plate is inconvenient. A heat gun directs the heat to the specific area where it is needed, as in sealing plastic dose containers. It can also be used to apply gentle heat to beakers of liquids and the like.

Homogenizers (hand operated) aid in the preparation of fine emulsions. They can be easily disassembled for cleaning and work with as little as 60 mL of liquid.

Lead sticks (flexible) are convenient for wrapping around beakers, flasks, and other pieces of equipment to prevent them from falling over. The sticks, which are made of soft lead with colorful plastic coatings, are available in many diameters and lengths. They can be easily shaped or formed to fit around almost any item of laboratory glassware or equipment.

Light boxes are excellent aids for determining the completeness of a solution when dissolving solids and for detecting precipitants when working with materials that may be incompatible or are near the limit of solubility. To achieve a similar outcome, one can paint a piece of Masonite half black and half white, using flat paints. When this board is hung on a wall with a fluorescent light placed immediately above it, the dark and light backgrounds help determine the presence of particles in a solution.

Mixers (professional or kitchen) can be used to beat, mix, whip, and knead with flat beaters, dough hooks, and wire whips. They aid in the preparation of products ranging from liquids, including emulsions, to ointments.

Orbital mixers can simultaneously mix a large number of beakers, bottles, flasks, and the like. The containers are fixed in place on a platform that moves in a circular or an orbital motion. These devices are widely used in laboratories and are especially suitable for compounding pharmacies in which a large number of containers must be mixed simultaneously.

Pipet bulbs aid in pipetting and can eliminate many of the dangers associated with pipetting by mouth. There are numerous styles of these bulbs, which may be used not only with measuring pipets but also with transfer pipets when small quantities of liquids must be moved from one vessel to another.

Powder blenders enable pharmacists to blend powders in a dust-free environment and protect the operator from powder dust. These blenders mechanically blend in enclosed plastic bags, which prevents any of the powder from escaping into the environment.

Sealers (bag or suppository) are convenient for sealing plastic bags or certain suppository molds.

Sealers (tube) are widely used for packaging large numbers of ointments, creams, or gels in plastic tubes. They are relatively simple to use and provide reproducible results with products that are attractively packaged.

Tablet presses (single punch) are an easy-to-use method of preparing individual tablets or pellets. A blend of the active drug and excipients can be weighed and placed in the die, the handle lowered, and a tablet produced by compression.

Tea/spice balls hold a flavoring agent while it is being immersed in a liquid until the desired strength is obtained.

Thermometers (with alarm) can audibly indicate when a refrigerator or an oven leaves a preset temperature range. These devices are generally used on freezers and refrigerators, especially ultrafreezers. High–low thermometers, which display the highest and lowest temperatures attained in a given period of time, will become more important as marketing requirements are implemented.

Tool sets (cooks') contain useful implements for compounding, including a pasta fork, turner, solid spoon, ladle, server, and skimmer; often, they are complete with a hanging rack.

Ultrasonic cleaners are useful for cleaning items as well as for accelerating the dissolution of slowly dissolving drugs.

Water system (high quality) may be required if the pharmacy prepares a large quantity of products that require different grades of water.

Workbench protector sheets of plastic, rubber, or absorbable paper are often convenient for defining a work area for a specific project. They can be cleaned or disposed of when finished.

General and Advanced Sterile Product Compounding Equipment

Many of the items listed in the categories of sterile product compounding and advanced sterile product compounding can be placed into one of four general categories. The first group includes items that are used for the preparation of sterile products: ampule openers, impulse sealers, vacuum pumps, sterile filtration equipment, and sterile spatulas and spoons. The second group includes items for quality control, including an anemometer, a particle counter, particulate-testing equipment, pyrogen test materials, and sterility test equipment. The third group encompasses product storage and delivery, including such items as a refrigerator, a cooler/heater for use in an automobile, an ice replacement gel, and an ultrafreezer. The final group includes items used for maintenance of the clean room environment, such as apparel for personnel, cleaning materials, and high-efficiency particulate air cleaner (HEPA) filters.

Standard Operating Procedures (SOPs)

Cleaning Glassware

Purpose of SOP

The purpose of this procedure is to ensure the proper cleaning of all glass compounding equipment used in the pharmacy.

The process of cleaning glass equipment used in compounding is crucial to providing a preparation that is free from contamination by materials used in previous compounding activities.

Equipment/Materials

The facility should have a sufficiently large sink with hot and cold running water, purified water USP, and a suitable draining rack for this activity. Commercial dishwashers generally will work for a portion of the cleaning process.

Cleaning materials include the following:

- Detergent.
- Potable water, hot and cold.
- Purified water USP (distilled water, deionized water, reverse osmosis water).
- Chromic acid cleaning mixture (optional).

Procedure

1. Any residual materials that remain in or on the glassware should be removed, as follows:
   - *Water-soluble materials:* Rinse any residual materials off the item using hot water so the waste flows down the sink. It is important that the materials are not placed into the washing water to avoid potentially contaminating the equipment being cleaned.
   - *Water-insoluble materials:* Using a paper towel or other disposable wipe, remove the materials from the item and discard appropriately. Wet a paper towel or other disposable wipe with alcohol or other suitable solvent for the material, remove any residual material from the item, and discard the waste appropriately.
2. Using an appropriate detergent and hot water, thoroughly wash the item. In the event of stains or difficult-to-remove discoloration, use the chromic acid cleaning mixture (described in the next section) before performing this step.
3. Rinse the item thoroughly with hot water to remove any residual detergent and the like.
4. Rinse the item thoroughly with purified water USP.
5. Place the item on a drain rack to dry.
6. Place the item in its storage unit.

Preparation of Chromic Acid Cleaning Mixture

Ingredients for the cleaning mixture include the following:

- Sodium dichromate 20 g.
- Water 10 mL.
- Sulfuric acid, concentrated 150 mL.

The precautionary measures described in steps 1 and 2 should always be followed when preparing this mixture.

1. Use safety goggles.
2. Prepare this mixture in a hard, borosilicate glass beaker, because the heat produced may cause soft-glass containers to break.
3. Dissolve the sodium dichromate in the water.
4. Very slowly and cautiously, add the sulfuric acid, with stirring.
5. Package in a tightly closed, hard, borosilicate glass container.
6. Because the mixture is extremely corrosive and hygroscopic, store it in a glass-stoppered bottle in a safe place.
7. When mixture removed from the storage bottle acquires a green color, do not return it to the storage bottle; instead, discard the discolored mixture in accordance with hazardous materials procedures.

Glass tends to adsorb the chromic acid, which makes prolonged rinsing imperative. Alkaline cleansing agents such as trisodium phosphate and the synthetic detergents are highly useful but also require prolonged rinsing.

Class A Prescription Torsion Balance Performance Tests

Purpose of SOP

The purpose of this procedure is to ensure that torsion balances are providing accurate weight measurements of compounding ingredients.

Regulatory Issues

Numerous types of balances are available in compounding pharmacies, but all must meet the requirements in Chapter <1176>, "Prescription Balances and Volumetric Apparatus" of the *United States Pharmacopeia 25/National Formulary 20.*

Performance Tests

Torsion balances are commercially available in different models with different features. The four basic tests that must be met are sensitivity requirement, arm ratio test, shift tests, and rider and graduated beam tests. The class A balance should be used in all weighing operations involved in prescription compounding. Most balances have a maximum weight allowable of 120 g; this weight should not be exceeded, because damage to the balance may result.

The balance should be tested in the location in which it is used, which should be away from drafts, traffic, temperature fluctuations, and vibrations. The tests should be performed using a set of test weights at least monthly, and more often if the balance is used extensively. Record all results on the Balance Performance Form for documentation (Figure 2-2).

Sensitivity Requirement. The purpose of the sensitivity requirement is to determine the maximum change in load that will result in a specified change (i.e., one subdivision on the index plate, in the rest position of the indicating element of the balance) when the following steps are followed.

1. Level the balance.
2. Adjust the rest point to zero with the pans empty.
3. Place a 6-mg weight on one of the empty pans.
4. The rest point should be shifted no less than one division.
5. Place a 10-g weight in the center of each of the empty pans.
6. Place a 6-mg weight on one of the pans.
7. The rest point should be shifted no less than one division.
8. Record the results on the Balance Performance Form.

Arm Ratio Test. The purpose of the arm ratio test is to check the equality of length of both arms of the balance.

1. Level the balance
2. Adjust the rest point to zero with the pans empty.
3. Place a 30-g weight in the center of each pan and observe the rest point.
4. If the rest point has changed, place a 20-mg weight on the lighter side; the rest point should move back to the original rest point in step 2.
5. Record the results on the Balance Performance Form.

Shift Test. The purpose of the shift test is to check the arm and lever components of the balance.

1. Level the balance.
2. Adjust the rest point to zero with the pans empty.
3. Place a 10-g weight in the center of the left pan.
4. Place a second 10-g weight in the right pan successively toward the right, left, front, and back sections of the pan.
5. If the rest point differs at any position from that in step 2, place a 10-mg weight on the lighter side; the rest point should move back to the original rest point in step 2.

Balance Performance Log

Brand Name _____

Model No. _____ Serial No. _____

Date	Operator Initials	Sensitivity Requirement Test No. of Div. Moved from Rest Point	Arm Test Ratio		Shift Test		Rider and Graduated Beam Test	
			Pass	Fail	Pass	Fail	Pass	Fail

Figure 2-2. Sample log for testing balance performance.

6. Remove the weights from the pans, and reestablish the zero point, if necessary.
7. Place a 10-g weight in the center of the right pan.
8. Place a second 10-g weight in the left pan successively toward the right, left, front, and back sections of the pan.
9. If the rest point differs at any position from that in step 6, place a 10-mg weight on the lighter side; the rest point should move back to the original rest point in step 6.
10. Remove the weights from the pans, and reestablish the zero point, if necessary.
11. Place a 10-g weight in each pan. Shift both weights simultaneously to the right, left, front, and back sections of the two pans; shift both weights so that one is toward the front and the other is toward the back, one is toward the inside and the other is toward the outside of the pans, and so on until all combinations are checked.
12. If the rest point differs at any position from that in step 10, a 10-mg weight to the lighter side should move the pointer back to the original rest point.
13. Record the results on the Balance Performance Form.

Rider and Graduated Beam Test. The purpose of this test is to determine the agreement of the weights on the rider, or dial, with weights placed on the pans.

1. Level the balance.
2. Adjust the rest point to zero with the pans empty.
3. Place a 500-mg test weight on the left pan.
4. Move the rider, or dial, to the 500-mg point on the beam, or dial, and determine the rest point.
5. If the rest point differs from that in step 2, add a 6-mg weight to the lighter side.
6. The rest point should be brought back to that in step 2.
7. Record the results on the Balance Performance Form.

Implications of Findings

If the balance fails any test, it should not be used but instead should be immediately repaired or readjusted, and performance should be retested.

If the balance has a 6-mg sensitivity, 120 mg would be the minimum quantity of material that should be weighed to provide an error of $\pm 5\%$. If smaller quantities are needed, an aliquot should be prepared.

Calibration of Hot Plates

Purpose of SOP

The purpose of this procedure is to document the actual temperatures of heated liquids at each dial setting of a particular hot plate. It should be kept in mind that variables are involved, such as the size of the container, whether the hot plate is placed in an area where there may be drafts, the heat conductivity of the liquid, and so on. Different liquids may require different times to reach the desired temperature. A thermometer should always be used to determine the actual temperature in the liquid being heated.

Compounding Principle

To compound more efficiently, a compounding pharmacist/technician should know approximately what temperature is reflected by a number on the adjustable dial. This can minimize long waits, which can occur if a desired temperature is approached too slowly, or unnecessary waits for the material to cool down, which can occur due to overshooting the temperature.

As a hot plate ages, the efficiency of the heating elements may deteriorate and the calibration may not remain the same. Consequently, it is important to perform this function at regularly scheduled intervals, such as quarterly intervals, to monitor the performance of the hot plate.

Precautions for Use

The hot plate must be plugged into an outlet that provides the proper voltage so that a fire hazard is not created or circuit breakers are not tripped. If turning on a hot plate trips circuit breakers, a licensed electrician should be contacted.

It is also important to keep the hot plate clean. If there is a chance of boiling over, breakage, or other incidents, it may be wise to set a flat-bottomed metal pan on the hot plate and to set the container to be heated inside the pan. This will prevent soiling the hot plate in case an accident occurs.

It is also good practice to use a thermometer to check the temperature of the material as required and to not totally depend on the calibration settings.

Equipment/Materials

Only a few materials are needed to calibrate hot plates:

- Certified thermometer.
- Beaker of purified water.
- Beaker of suitable oil.
- Marker, tape, or both.

Procedure

1. Clean the hot plate.
2. Place the beaker of purified water on the hot plate, and turn to the first incremental setting on the dial, usually 1.
3. Allow the water to warm to a constant temperature, periodically checking the temperature with a thermometer.
4. When the reading is obtained, record the setting in the Hot Plate Calibration Log (Figure 2-3).
5. Move the dial to the next incremental setting and repeat steps 3 and 4.
6. Continue process until a temperature of 90°C is reached. (Note: A reading cannot be easily made when water reaches the boiling point, as it remains at 100°C even though the dial setting may reflect a higher temperature.)
7. Replace the beaker of water with a beaker of oil, and repeat the process followed in steps 2 through 5.
8. Continue past the 90°C setting and record the temperature of the oil at all the remaining incremental settings on the dial.
9. If the temperature readings at each dial setting are not the same for the water and the oil (for temperatures 90°C and less), then use the appropriate scale depending on the preparation being heated during the compounding process. (Note: The temperatures of the two liquids may not be exactly the same due to heat conductance and the rates of cooling that occur from the sides and surface of the liquid in the containers.)
10. Using a marker, label tape, or both, print the corresponding temperature readings labeled "water" and "oil" adjacent to the dial numbers. Also, affix a calibration date to the hot plate as a reminder of when to recalibrate.

Hot Plate Calibration Log

Hot Plate Brand Name _____

Model No. _____ Serial No. _____

Date	Dial Setting	Temperature of Liquids	
		Water	Oil

Figure 2-3. Sample log for calibrating hot plates.

Chapter 3

Records and Record Keeping

Compounding pharmacists must keep the records required by the states in which they practice, as well as those that are characteristic of a well-operated compounding pharmacy. Records provide documentation of the ingredients of a product; facilitate a product recall, if necessary; and enable other compounding pharmacists to duplicate the product in their pharmacies. They also ensure that the compound produced will be consistent from one pharmacy to another, so the patient has confidence in the quality of the product being administered.

Records that should be maintained include (1) standard operating procedures (SOPs) with sign-off sheets for the procedures used, (2) the formulation record, or "recipe," (3) the compounding record, and (4) ingredient records and Material Safety Data Sheets (MSDSs).

Overview of Standard Operating Procedures (SOPs)

All significant procedures performed in the compounding area should be covered by SOPs and documentation. Procedures should be developed for the facility, equipment, personnel, preparation, packaging, and storage of compounded preparations to ensure accountability, accuracy, quality, safety, and uniformity in a compounding practice. More important, the implementation of SOPs establishes procedural consistency and provides a reference for the orientation and training of personnel. Documentation enables a pharmacy to systematically trace, evaluate, and replicate the steps throughout the preparation process of a compounded preparation whenever necessary.

SOPs provide assurance that (1) equipment is maintained in good working order, calibrated, and documented; (2) supplies are received, logged in, stored properly, disposed of correctly, and maintained fresh and within compendial requirements; and (3) all manipulations and procedures are performed uniformly and then documented. Because numerous forms must be completed at the end of many procedures, notebooks should be maintained to handle these forms.

An important component of SOPs is keeping records of equipment maintenance. These records, which should be updated regularly, include documentation of the performance of balances, refrigerators, freezers, mixers, and all other equipment. Equipment files should be organized and updated regularly. Calibration checks should be maintained for documentation on the performance of the equipment. Refrigerator and freezer thermometers should be routinely checked and documented, and the temperatures of these pieces of equipment should be recorded on a regular basis to document their performance. Some equipment, such as laminar flow hoods, should be periodically certified by qualified personnel.

Figure 3-1 represents the first page of a typical SOP record. Documentation of equipment maintenance and supplies would be filed with this page. To avoid mixing or confusing records for different procedures, the appropriate SOP number and, if applicable, the record's revision date should be marked on each page of the supporting documentation. Numerous SOPs are placed in different chapters throughout this book.

Formulation Record

The formulation record provides a consistent source document for preparation of the formulation, considered the "recipe." The compounding record documents the actual ingredients in the preparation and the person responsible for the compounding activity (Figure 3-2). Records should be maintained in sufficient detail so the preparations can be duplicated. Computerized records are appropriate. Individual formulation records for compounds are generally obtained from a variety of sources, including journals, books, other pharmacists, organizations, and even individual development. The formulation record should include the following information:

- Name, strength, and dosage form of the preparation.
- All ingredients and their quantities.
- Equipment required to produce the preparation.
- Pertinent calculations (see Chapter 5, "Pharmaceutical Compounding Calculations").
- Mixing instructions.
- Quality control procedures.
- Source of the recipe.
- Beyond-use date.
- Container used.
- Storage requirements.

The name, strength, and dosage form actually serve as the title of the product or recipe. The title should express the essence of the product as clearly and succinctly as possible, avoiding "secret" jargon.

Individual ingredients and their quantities should be listed. If it is possible that more than one quantity of the product will be produced in the future, the pharmacist should create a table listing the ingredients and the amounts required for various quantities. Because liquid products should be weighed, a notation should be made to that effect, specifying all the information regarding the quantity to be weighed or volumetrically measured. (The formulation record should also contain the specific gravity of the product for the conversions.)

The use of different equipment yields different results. Therefore, it is necessary to list the exact equipment used so the compounded prescriptions will be uniform in appearance and activity.

Precise mixing instructions are required to produce acceptable and uniform products. Mixing instructions include the order of mixing and any environmental or other conditions that should be monitored, such as the temperature, duration of mixing, and so forth. If the mixing order is important, this order should be listed

Standard Operating Procedures   SOP # _____

Date Effective:

Revision Number:

Person Preparing:

Person Checking:

Purpose of Procedure:

[The purpose of the procedure should be described.]

Procedure:

[The procedure should be detailed in a step-by-step fashion so that it can be easily followed by different individuals with the same results. It should contain sufficient detail and descriptive information to minimize any required interpretation.]

1.

2.

3.

4.

5.

Documentation Forms:

[The results of the SOP may need to be documented on a form and maintained in a notebook for easy retrieval. In this case, the organization of the forms notebook should parallel that of the SOP notebook. The reference point can be the SOP number, which should be placed on each page. Space should be available for a description of the procedure that was performed, date, operator's signature, and the results.]

Figure 3-1. Sample standardized operating procedures form.

Formulation Record

Formulation Title _____

(name, strength, dosage form)

Formula No. _____ Quantity Prepared _____

Ingredient	Quantity	Unit	Calculation/Comments
_____	_____	_____	_____
_____	_____	_____	_____
_____	_____	_____	_____
_____	_____	_____	_____
_____	_____	_____	_____
_____	_____	_____	_____
_____	_____	_____	_____
_____	_____	_____	_____

Equipment Required:

Compounding Instructions:

1._____

2._____

3._____

4._____

5._____

6._____

7._____

8._____

9._____

10. _____

Written by:_____ Checked by:_____

Quality Control Tests:

Test	Results
_____	_____
_____	_____
_____	_____
_____	_____

Figure 3-2. Sample formulation record form.

and explained in detail. Any levigating agents, solubilizing agents, and the like that are used in the preparation must also be cited and described.

Quality control procedures should be described, and a data sheet should be provided to document such information as capsule weights, as detailed in Chapter 6, "Quality Control."

The source of the recipe should be included. If the formulation was derived from the literature, a copy of the article should be appended to the formulation record. It is always good pharmacy practice to document the source for future reference.

The beyond-use date is assigned based on the best available knowledge. Chapter 4, "Stability of Compounded Products," provides some general guidelines for instances in which the beyond-use date is not known.

The container to be used should be listed on the formulation record to ensure uniformity of packaging and stability. Because much of the stability information is predicated on a certain type or composition of container, any variance from this style of container may make the beyond-use date suspect.

Storage requirements for the finished product should also be listed. This information should be transmitted to the patient.

Once the formulation record has been prepared and checked, it should be altered only after careful consideration is given to any changes proposed. It is also advisable to have a second pharmacist review any alterations to the formulation record.

Compounding Record

The compounding record should contain the name, strength, and dosage form as they appear in the formulation record. The compounding record is the "worksheet" for the preparation of an individual product. The following information should be recorded for both types of compounded formulations (individual prescriptions and products prepared in anticipation of orders):

- ▸ Formulation record used for the product.
- ▸ Individual ingredients, their lot numbers, and the actual quantities measured/weighed.
- ▸ Quantity of product prepared (i.e., weight, volume, or number of units prepared).
- ▸ Signature of pharmacist or technician preparing the product.
- ▸ Signature or initials of the pharmacist responsible for supervising the preparation and conducting in-process and final checks of the compounded products if a technician performed the compounding function.
- ▸ Date of preparation.
- ▸ Assigned internal identification number, if applicable.
- ▸ Prescription number.
- ▸ Assigned beyond-use date.
- ▸ Results of the quality control procedures (e.g., the weight range of filled capsules).

In some pharmacies, the formulation record is prepared so that it can be photocopied, and space is left on it for the information required for the compounding record. This practice speeds up the record-keeping process. The compounding records are maintained for easy retrieval according to individual state requirements. Figure 3-3 represents a typical record for compounded prescriptions.

Compounding Record

Formulation Title _____ Quantity _____
                        (name, strength, dosage form)

Formula/Rx No. _____ Prepared by _____ Checked by ____R.Ph

Quantity Prepared _____ Date Prepared _____ Beyond-Use Date ____

Ingredient	Quantity	Unit	Manufacturer	Lot No.	Exp. Date
_____	_____	_____	_____	_____	_____
_____	_____	_____	_____	_____	_____
_____	_____	_____	_____	_____	_____
_____	_____	_____	_____	_____	_____
_____	_____	_____	_____	_____	_____
_____	_____	_____	_____	_____	_____
_____	_____	_____	_____	_____	_____
_____	_____	_____	_____	_____	_____
_____	_____	_____	_____	_____	_____

Compounding Instructions:

1._____
2._____
3._____
4._____
5._____
6._____
7._____
8._____
9._____
10. _____

Quality Control Procedures:

Test   Results

_____   _____
_____   _____
_____   _____
_____   _____

Figure 3-3. Sample compounding record form.

Ingredient Records and Material Safety Data Sheets

The pharmacy should maintain records of ingredients purchased, including certificates of analysis for purity of chemicals. (An example of an SOP for a certificate of analysis and information to be evaluated is shown at the end of the chapter.) MSDSs should also be maintained for any drug substance or bulk chemical located in the pharmacy. These data sheets are not required for commercially available finished products; the ingredient information on the product label will suffice. The ingredient information consists mainly of physicochemical, toxicity, and handling information. Precautions, information about other potential hazards, and shipping instructions are also included. This information should be reviewed for the protection of the pharmacist as well as for that of the patient.

These records should be retained as original hard copy; true copies, such as photocopies, microfilm, or microfiche; or other accurate reproduction of the original records. Computerized records are also acceptable. Employees should be instructed as to the location of the files and their format.

MSDSs can be obtained without charge from suppliers and can be easily filed in three-ring binders. They are commonly shipped with chemicals, often packaged in the same carton. They can also be obtained from the Internet or through facsimile from the suppliers.

Standard Operating Procedure

Certificates of Analysis of Materials Used for Pharmaceutical Compounding

Purpose of SOP

The purpose of this procedure is to establish appropriate guidelines and documentation for the requirement for certificates of analysis for materials/chemicals used in pharmaceutical compounding.

Regulatory Issues

Chapter <795>, "Pharmacy Compounding," in *United States Pharmacopeia 25/ National Formulary 20 (USP 25/NF 20)* states, "The pharmacist is responsible for compounding preparations of acceptable strength, quality, and purity with appropriate packaging and labeling in accordance with good pharmacy practices, official standards, and relevant scientific data and information."[1] The compounding of quality preparations must involve the use of quality chemicals.

Ingredients used to compound official preparations must meet the requirements of compendial monographs. If not available, or when food, cosmetics, or other substances are or must be used, the use of another high-quality source, such as analytical reagent (AR), certified American Chemical Society (ACS), or Food Chemicals Codes (FCC) grade, is an option based on professional judgment. For any substance used in compounding but not purchased from a registered drug manufacturer, the pharmacist should establish purity and safety by reasonable means, which may include lot analysis, manufacturer reputation, or reliability of source.

Chapter <795>, "Pharmacy Compounding," also states that "The bulk drug substances must be accompanied by a valid certificate of analysis. For ingredients other than bulk drug substances, pharmacists should use ingredients that comply with an applicable *USP-NF* monograph and the USP chapter on *Pharmacy Compounding <795>.*"[1]

Management of Certificates of Analysis

Certificates of analysis should be obtained and kept on record as documentation of the quality of chemicals used in compounding preparations. Most certificates of analysis are provided in a standard $8\frac{1}{2} \times 11$-in. format and are reasonably similar in appearance for different manufacturers of bulk substances. These certificates can be alphabetically arranged and maintained in standard three-ring notebooks.

Contents of Certificates of Analysis.

If the bulk drug substance is a USP/NF item, then the specific tests listed in the compendia should be addressed on the certificate of analysis. For example, hydrocortisone USP includes a purity rubric (". . . not less than 97.0% and not more than 102.0% of $C_{21}H_{30}O_5$, calculated on the dried basis"). Also, it has specific tests for which information should be provided, including the following:

- ▸ Identification.
- ▸ Specific rotation.
- ▸ Loss on drying.
- ▸ Residue on ignition.
- ▸ Chromatographic purity.
- ▸ Organic volatile impurities.
- ▸ Assay.

Therefore, the certificate of analysis should address the tests/requirements listed for the specific substance/article. If a bulk drug substance is listed as "USP" or "NF," the inference is that the substance meets the standards and passes the tests required for the USP or NF designation. It should be noted that some of the results of the various tests on the certificates of analysis may be numerical and some may be simply "Passes," as in the following example:

Test	Requirement	Result
Specific rotation (*USP 25/NF 20* Chapter <781>)	Between +150° and +156°	+152°
Organic volatile impurities	Meets the requirements	Passes

If a substance is not available as a USP or an NF item, appropriate tests that are similar to those required for related substances can be used, but in all cases the tests should include a purity rubric and an assay result.

Record Maintenance

Chapter <795>, "Pharmacy Compounding,"[1] designates no specific length of time for maintaining the certificates of analysis, which are lot specific. Pharmaceutical judgment suggests that the certificates be maintained on file for a designated time period after the last of the specific lot of the substance was used that would include the projected time of patient administration. In referring to the recommended beyond-use dates, the maximum time is generally 6 months.

Lot Specificity of Certificates of Analysis

Certificates of analysis are lot specific and must match the current lot of bulk drug substance being used for compounding.

Manufactured Drug Products in Compounding

When manufactured drug products are used in compounding, they will not be accompanied by a certificate of analysis but instead will be accompanied by a product information package insert. This information along with the products' specific lot numbers should be maintained on file to document that specific manufactured drug products were used in compounding a formulation.

Reference

1. Expert Advisory Panel on Pharmacy Compounding Practices. Pharmacy compounding. In: *United States Pharmacopeia 25/National Formulary 20*. Rockville, Md: United States Pharmacopeial Convention; 2001.

Chapter 4

Stability of Compounded Products

Stability is the extent to which a product retains, within specified limits, and throughout its period of storage and use, the same properties and characteristics that it possessed at the time of its manufacture. The *United States Pharmacopeia 25/National Formulary 20 (USP 25/NF 20)*[1] provides definitions for five general types of stability:

- *Chemical.* Each active ingredient retains its chemical integrity and labeled potency, within the specified limits.
- *Physical.* The original physical properties, including appearance, palatability, uniformity, dissolution, and suspendability, are retained.
- *Microbiological.* Sterility or resistance to microbial growth is retained according to the specified requirements. Antimicrobial agents that are present retain effectiveness within the specified limits.
- *Therapeutic.* The therapeutic effect remains unchanged.
- *Toxicological.* No significant increase in toxicity occurs.

Instability describes chemical reactions that are ". . . incessant, irreversible, and result in distinctly different chemical entities (degradation products) that can be both therapeutically inactive and possibly exhibit greater toxicity."[2] Incompatibility is different from instability but must be considered in the overall stability evaluation of a preparation. *Incompatibility* generally refers to visually evident and ". . . physicochemical phenomena such as concentration-dependent precipitation and acid-base reactions, with the products of reaction manifested as a change in physical state, including protonation-deprotonation equilibria."[2]

Factors That Affect Stability

Numerous factors can affect the stability of a drug and dosage form, including pH, temperature, solvent, light, air (oxygen), carbon dioxide, moisture or humidity, particle size, and others.

pH is one of the most important factors that affects the stability of a product. The pharmacist can use published pH/stability profiles to determine the pH that will ensure the maximum stability of the product. After determining the pH range, the pharmacist can prepare buffers to maintain the pH for the expected shelf-life of the product.

Temperature affects the stability of a drug by increasing the rate of reaction speed about two to three times with each 10°C rise in temperature. This temperature effect was first suggested by Arrhenius as follows:

$$k = Ae^{-Ea/RT}$$

or

$$\log k = \log A - \frac{Ea}{2.303} \times \frac{1}{T}$$

where k is the specific reaction rate, A is the frequency factor, Ea is the energy of activation, R is the gas constant (1.987 cal/deg mole), and T is the absolute temperature. As is evident from these relationships, an increase in temperature will result in an increase in the specific reaction rate, or the degradation rate of the drug. Temperature effects can be minimized by selecting the proper storage temperature-room, refrigerated, or freezing.

A *solvent* affects the stability of a product if the preparation is a liquid. The solvent can affect the pH, solubility, and solubility parameter (δ) of the active ingredient. The stability of a product may be compromised if solvents are changed indiscriminately.

Light may provide the activation energy required for a degradation reaction to occur. Many light-activated reactions are zero-order, or constant, reactions. The effects of light can be minimized by packaging products in light-resistant containers; products that are light sensitive during administration can even be covered with aluminum foil or an amber plastic overwrap.

Air (oxygen) can induce degradation via oxidation. Degradation can be minimized by filling the container as full as possible, thereby decreasing the headspace, or by replacing the headspace with nitrogen. Another option is to add an antioxidant to the formulation (Table 4-1).

Carbon dioxide can cause insoluble carbonates to form in the solid dosage form, which decreases the disintegration and dissolution properties of the product. Packaging in tight containers and filling the containers as full as possible minimize this condition.

Humidity, or *moisture*, can result in hydrolysis reactions and degradation of the drug product. Working in a dry environment and inserting a desiccant packet in the packaging of the product can lessen the effects of humidity.

Particle size can have an important effect on the stability of a product. The smaller the particle size, the greater is the reactivity of the product. When working with drugs that are less stable in solid dosage forms, such as powders and capsules, it may be advisable to use a larger particle size, as appropriate.

Other factors that can affect drug stability are *ionic strength* and *dielectric constant*.

Paths of Instability

Physical instability can adversely affect drug products. Some paths through which physical instability can occur include the formation of polymorphs, crystallization, vaporization, and adsorption.

Polymorphs are substances that can crystallize in different forms of the same chemical compound. Their crystallized forms differ in energy and may exhibit variations in such properties as solubility, compressibility, and melting point.

Table 4-1. Suggested Antioxidants for Use in Pharmacy Compounding

Antioxidant	Mechanism	Solubility			Usual Concentration Range/Comments
		Water	Alcohol	Oil	
Acetone sodium bisulfite	Reducing	Yes	No	No	0.2%–0.4%
Acetylcysteine	True	Yes	Yes	No	0.1%–0.5%
α-Lipoic acid (sodium salt)	—	Yes	—	Yes	—
α-Tocopherol (synthetic)	True	No	Yes	Yes	
α-Tocopherol acetate	True	No	Yes	Yes	≤0.001%
D-α-Tocopherol (natural)	True	No	Yes	Yes	0.05%–0.075%
DL-α-Tocopherol (synthetic)	True	No	Yes	Yes	0.01%–0.5%
Ascorbic acid	Reducing/Synergy	Yes	Yes	No	Soluble in glycerin/propylene glycol
Ascorbyl palmitate	True	Yes	Yes	Yes	
Butylated hydroxyanisole	True	No	Yes	Yes	0.005%–0.02%/Soluble in propylene glycol
Butylated hydroxytoluene	True	No	Yes	Yes	0.005%–0.02%/Soluble in mineral oil
Calcium ascorbate	Reducing	Yes	Yes	—	
Calcium bisulfite	Reducing	Yes	—	—	
Calcium sulfite	Reducing	Yes	Yes	—	
Cysteine	True	Yes	Yes	No	0.1%–0.5%
Cysteine HCl	True/Synergy	Yes	Yes	No	0.1%–0.5%/Bad odor
Dilauryl thiodipropionate	True	No	Yes	Yes	
Dithiothreitol	True	Yes	Yes	No	0.01%–0.1%
Dodecyl gallate	True	No	Yes	Yes	
Ethoxyquin	True	—	—	Yes	
Ethyl gallate	True	SlS	Yes	No	
Gallic acid	—	Yes	Yes	Yes	
Glutathione	True	Yes	—	—	
Gossypol	True	No	Yes	Yes	
Hydroquinone	Reducing	Yes	Yes	Yes	
4-Hydroxymethyl-2,6-di-tert-butylphenol	—	Yes	Yes	Yes	
Hypophosphorus acid	—	Yes	—	—	
Isoascorbic acid	Reducing	Yes	—	—	
Lecithin	True	Yes	Yes	Yes	
Monothioglycerol	Reducing	Yes	Yes	—	0.1%–1.0%/Slight odor
β-Naphthol	True	Yes	Yes	Yes	
Nordihydroguaiaretic acid	True	No	Yes	Yes	0.001%–0.01%
Octyl gallate	True	No	Yes	Yes	
Potassium metabisulfite	Reducing	Yes	No	No	
Propyl gallate	True	SlS	Yes	SlS	0.001%–0.15% (≤2.5 mg/kg body weight)
Sesamol	—	—	—	—	
Sodium ascorbate	Reducing	Yes	Yes	No	
Sodium bisulfite	Reducing	Yes	SlS	No	0.05%–1.0%
Sodium formaldehyde sulfoxylate	Reducing	Yes	SlS	—	0.005%–0.15%
Sodium metabisulfite	Reducing	Yes	SlS	—	0.01%–1.0%/Soluble in glycerin
Sodium sulfite	Reducing	Yes	No	No	0.01%–0.2%
Sodium thiosulfate	Reducing	Yes	No	—	
Sulfur dioxide	Reducing	Yes	Yes	Yes	
Tannic acid	Reducing	Yes	—	—	
Thioglycerol	Reducing	Yes	Yes	—	
tert-Butyl-hydroquinone	True	—	—	—	
Thioglycolic acid	Reducing	Yes	Yes	Yes	
Thiolactic acid	Reducing	Yes	Yes	Yes	
Thiosorbitol	Reducing	Yes	Yes	Yes	
Thiourea	Reducing	Yes	Yes	No	0.005%
Tocopherols	True	—	—	Yes	0.05%–0.5%

Knowledge of the causative factors of polymorphs can enable the pharmacist to take steps to prevent them. For example, polymorphs can form if heat and shock-cooling are used.

Crystallization of particles in suspension can alter the size distribution of the particles. Temperature fluctuations often cause such crystallization to occur because increasing temperatures result in greater solubility (which means that smaller particles may dissolve faster) and decreasing temperatures result in some crystallization of the drug on particles that are already present. Such fluctuation cycles will cause a decrease in the proportion of smaller particles and an increase in the proportion of larger crystals present.

Vaporization increases at higher temperatures and will result in loss of solvent. When solvent or liquid is lost, the product's concentration increases. This may lead to overdosage when the product is administered. A loss of solvent could also cause precipitation of the drug if the solubility of the drug in the remaining vehicle is exceeded.

Adsorption of the drug or excipients is a common occurrence and may lessen the amount of the drug available for treatment. Drugs may adsorb to filters, the container, tubing, syringes, or other materials. This is particularly troublesome in the case of low-dose drugs. Sorption can often be minimized by pretreating equipment and containers with silain or silicone; in some instances, adding albumin or a similar material to the vehicle before adding the drug can have the same result.

Containers

When selecting a container or package for the finished compounded preparation, it is important to realize that although a drug may be stable when stored in one type of container (glass), it may not be stable in a plastic (PVC) container or an infusion device made of an elastomer.

Glass is generally considered to be the most inert and stable type of containers, but plastic has gained wide acceptability and usefulness.

Observations of Instability

Pharmacists can often detect evidence of instability in dosage forms through observation. Table 4-2 lists the physical evidence of instability that may occur for a number of dosage forms.

Oxidation and the Use of Antioxidants

Antioxidants are added to minimize or retard oxidative processes that occur with some drugs or excipients on exposure to oxygen or in the presence of free radicals. These processes can often be catalyzed by light, temperature, hydrogen ion concentration, presence of trace metals, or peroxides. Oxidation may be manifested as products that have an unpleasant odor, taste, appearance, precipitation, discoloration, or even a slight loss of activity.

To prevent or minimize oxidation, a number of approaches are listed in Table 4-3. It is important to remove oxygen from the ingredients before formulation and to minimize the entrapment of air during formulation. To minimize entrapment of air during the formulation process, care should be taken to not foam, whip, mix too vigorously, or form a vortex during mixing. Mixing ingredients at lower-than-

Table 4-2. Physical Changes Indicating Instability

Dosage Form	Changes
Capsules	A change in the physical appearance or consistency of the capsule or its contents, including hardening or softening of the shell; also, any discoloration, expansion, or distortion of the gelatin capsule
Powders	Caking or discoloration instead of free flowing; release of pressure upon opening, indicative of bacterial or other degradation
Solutions/elixirs, syrups	Precipitation, discoloration, haziness, gas formation resulting from microbial growth
Emulsions	Breaking, creaming
Suspensions	Caking, difficulty in resuspending; crystal growth
Ointments	Change in consistency and separation of liquid, if contained, and formation of granules or grittiness; drying
Creams	Emulsion breakage, crystal growth, shrinkage caused by evaporation of water; gross microbial contamination
Suppositories	Excessive softening, drying, hardening, shriveling; evidence of oil stains on packaging
Gels	Shrinkage, separation of liquid from the gel, discoloration, microbial contamination
Troches	Softening or hardening, crystallization, microbial contamination, discoloration
Sterile products	Discoloration, haziness, precipitation

normal speed in sealed containers works well. For emulsions, a hand homogenizer (producing strong shear forces in a closed space) works well if the product is collected carefully and protected from air.

The most common approach to minimizing oxidation is to add an antioxidant to the system. The selection of an appropriate antioxidant is dependent on several factors, including solubility, location of the agent in the formulation (emulsions), chemical and physical stability over a wide pH range, compatibility, odor, discoloration, toxicity, irritation, potency, effectiveness in low concentrations, and freedom from toxicity, carcinogenicity, and sensitizing effects.

The actual selection of an antioxidant depends on the (1) type of product, (2) route, dose, and frequency of administration, (3) physical and chemical properties of the preservative used, (4) presence of other components, and (5) properties of the closure and container. The effectiveness of antioxidants may actually be decreased in complex systems such as suspensions and emulsions. This decrease may be due to sorption of the antioxidant onto suspended particles or to partitioning of the antioxidant between the phases of an emulsion. Also, it should be noted that antioxidants may sorb to containers and closures.

Table 4-3. General Approaches to Minimizing Oxidation in Pharmaceutical Products

1. Use de-aerated water. Boil the purified water for 5 minutes and immediately cover it so it does not come into contact with air, which may redissolve in it.
2. Incorporate the antioxidants in the product as early in the process as possible. If a polyphasic system is used, such as an emulsion, place an antioxidant in each phase as early in the process as possible. If this is not done, oxidation may occur and much of the added antioxidant will be consumed in neutralizing the already present oxidation products.
3. Do not use a mixing method or device that incorporates air into the system.
4. Use a mixing container that has minimal headspace, preferably replacing the air in the headspace with nitrogen.
5. Add a buffer system to maintain a desired pH.
6. Use ingredients with low heavy metal content.
7. Decrease temperature during preparation, if possible.
8. Assay for actives and antioxidants and even excipients if preparing a product routinely to determine the effectiveness of the antioxidants.
9. Increase concentration of antioxidants if necessary.

In general, antioxidants are used in relatively low concentrations, usually from 0.001% to 0.2%. The lowest effective concentration should be used. When formulating a product, it should be remembered to incorporate the antioxidant early in preparation of the product to minimize the extent of oxidation, rather than at the end of the preparation, when much of the antioxidant is needlessly used up in counteracting the oxidation that has already occurred. Also, it is generally advisable to use a chelating agent along with an antioxidant to chelate trace metals that may catalyze an oxidative process. Commonly used chelating agents are shown in Table 4-4.

The formulation of an antioxidant system is still accomplished primarily through trial and error. Although still largely empirical, with some experimentation and patience, a suitable, stable system with the required antioxidant properties can be developed.

Q_{10} Method of Predicting Shelf-Life Stability

The Q_{10} method of shelf-life estimation is a tool that the compounding pharmacist can use to quickly calculate a beyond-use date for a drug product that is going to be stored or used under conditions that differ from the labeling requirements. The expression "Q_{10}" is actually a ratio of two different reaction rate constants, defined as follows:

$$Q_{10} = \frac{K_{(T + 10)}}{K_T}$$

where K_T is the reaction rate constant at a specific temperature T, and $K_{(T + 10)}$ is the reaction rate constant at a temperature 10°C higher. The commonly used Q values of 2, 3, and 4 are related to different Ea values of 12.2, 19.4, and 24.5 kcal/mol, respectively. For practical purposes, if the Ea is not known, a median value of 3 has been used as a reasonable estimate.

Table 4-4. Solubility of Chelating Agents and Synergists

Added Substance	Solubility			Usual Concentration Range/Comments
	Water	Alcohol	Oil	
Alkyl gallates	Yes	Yes	Yes	
Ascorbic acid	Yes	Yes	No	0.02%–0.1%
Boric acid	Yes	Yes	No	
Citric acid	Yes	Yes	—	0.005%–0.01% (incompatible with potassium-tartrate, alkali, acetates, and sulfites)
Citraconic acid	Yes	Yes	No	0.03%–0.45%
Cysteine	Yes	Yes	No	
EDTA and salts	Yes	Yes	No	0.02%–0.1% (incompatible with polyvalent metal ions)
Gluconic acid	Yes	Yes	No	
Glycine	Yes	Yes	—	
Hydroxyquinoline sulfate	Yes	Yes	—	0.005%–0.01%
Maleic acid	Yes	Yes	No	
Phosphoric acid	Yes	Yes	—	0.005%–0.01%
Polysorbates	Yes	Yes	No	
Saccharic acid	Yes	Yes	No	
Tartaric acid	Yes	Yes	—	0.01%–0.02%
Tryptophan	—	Yes	No	

The actual equation used for estimating shelf-life is as follows:

$$t_{90}(T2) = \frac{t_{90}(T1)}{Q_{10}^{(\Delta T/10)}}$$

where $t_{90}(T2)$ is the estimated shelf-life, $t_{90}(T1)$ is the given shelf-life at a given temperature $T1$, and ΔT is the temperature difference between $T1$ and $T2$.

It is evident from the equation that increasing the expression $(\Delta T/10)$ positively will decrease the shelf-life and that decreasing the expression will increase the shelf-life of the drug. For example, if a preparation that is normally stored at room temperature (25°C) with an expiration date of 1 week is stored in the refrigerator (5°C), what will be the approximate increase in the shelf-life of the product?

$$t_{90}(T2) = \frac{t_{90}(T1)}{Q_{10}^{(\Delta T/10)}} = \frac{1}{3^{(-20/10)}} = \frac{1}{3^{-2}} = 9 \text{ weeks}$$

because a temperature decline of 25° down to 5°C is 20° in the negative direction, −20°. Thus, the increase in shelf-life will be about 9 times or, in this case, 9 weeks, when there is a decrease in the storage temperature of −20°. This calculation assumes an Ea of about 19.4 kcal/mol.

Conversely, if a preparation that is normally stored at refrigeration temperature (5°C) with a shelf-life of 9 weeks is stored at room temperature (25°C), what will be the approximate decrease in the shelf-life of the product?

$$t_{90}(T2) = \frac{t_{90}(T1)}{Q_{10}^{(\Delta T/10)}} = \frac{9}{3^{(20/10)}} = 1 \text{ week}$$

because a temperature increase of 5° up to 25°C is in the positive direction, +20°. This also assumes an *Ea* of about 19.4 kcal/mol.

It should be noted that this method is applicable for products for which a specific shelf-life has been determined and only the storage temperature, not the formulation, varies.

Beyond-Use Dating

There is a difference in terminology between an expiration date and a beyond-use date. An *expiration date* is a projection of the length of time the product can be expected to retain its purity and potency based on accelerated stability studies. Expiration dates are used for commercial products. A *beyond-use* date is an estimate of the time interval that the compounded preparation can be expected to retain its purity and potency based on general guidelines, literature references, or actual real-time stability studies using prescribed conditions. In general, a maximum beyond-use date of 6 months is used because it more nearly fits into the guidelines of a compounded prescription, involving a patient, physician, and pharmacist.

Numerous sources of information can be used to determine an appropriate beyond-use date, including chemical company information, manufacturers' literature, Trissel's *Stability of Compounded Formulations,* the monographs in the latest edition of *AHFS Drug Information, International Journal of Pharmaceutical Compounding, American Journal of Health-System Pharmacy, Hospital Pharmacy,* other journals, and related books and journals. In general, most pharmacists prepare or dispense small quantities of compounded products, recommend storage at room or cold temperatures, and use a conservative beyond-use date.

Assigning a Beyond-Use Date

"Word-of-mouth" stability information can be dangerous. Even though ensuring that all preparations compounded in the pharmacy have accurate beyond-use dating can be tedious and time consuming, it is vitally important. The following scenarios illustrate word-of-mouth dating:

- ▸ "We dispensed monkeymycin for one of our patients and just put a date of 10 days on it," said a pharmacist at a recent pharmacy meeting. "We never heard that anything bad happened, so I guess a couple of weeks should be okay."
- ▸ "We use a 2-week beyond-use date for pedicycline in glass, so I guess 10 days should be safe for it in plastic."

What is wrong here? There is absolutely no assurance that either scenario is going to result in the proper date being assigned to the preparation. Word-of-mouth beyond-use dating is unsafe, unprofessional, unscientific, and ill advised. It may come back to haunt the compounding pharmacist if an adverse event occurs from use of that preparation.

Unless published data are available to the contrary, the following are the maximum recommended beyond-use dates for nonsterile compounded drug preparations that are packaged in tight, light-resistant containers when stored at a controlled room temperature or as otherwise indicated.

- ▸ *Nonaqueous liquids and solid formulations.* If the source of the ingredient(s) is a manufactured drug product, the beyond-use date should be no later than

25% of the time *remaining* on the original product's expiration date, or 6 months, whichever is earlier. If the source of the ingredient(s) is a USP/NF substance, the beyond-use date is no later than 6 months.

- *Water-containing formulations.* When prepared from ingredients in solid form, the beyond-use date should be no later than 14 days when stored at cold temperatures.
- *All other formulations.* In all other instances, the earlier of 30 days or the intended duration of therapy should be used. If valid supporting stability information is available to support a variation in regard to the specific preparation, the beyond-use date limits may be exceeded. (See Chapter <795>, "Pharmacy Compounding," in the *USP 25/NF 20.*[3])

A flowchart that can be used in assigning a beyond-use date is shown in Figure 4-1.

When evaluating stability studies in the literature, for the results to be valid, the pharmacist must be certain that the products studied are similar to the preparation under consideration in drug concentration range, pH, excipients, vehicle, water content, and the like.

Sources of drug stability and compatibility information for parenteral products (admixtures) include *Handbook on Injectable Drugs* (L. A. Trissel) and *King Guide to Parenteral Admixtures.*

Stability Considerations

In the home-care setting, admixed medications typically require longer expiration dates; patients' homes are often located a considerable distance form the infusion pharmacy, and many doses are delivered at one time to eliminate the expense of additional deliveries. The stability of these medications requires additional study, and many research studies are needed to generate the necessary information.

Reference

1. Stability considerations in dispensing practice. In: *United States Pharmacopeia 25/National Formulary 20*. Rockville, Md: United States Pharmacopeial Convention; 2001.
2. Trissel LA. *Handbook on Injectable Drugs*. Bethesda, Md: American Society of Health-System Pharmacists. 10th ed. 1998.
3. Expert Advisory Panel on Pharmacy Compounding Practices. Pharmacy compounding. In: *United States Pharmacopeia 25/National Formulary 20*. Rockville, Md: United States Pharmacopeial Convention; 2001.

Formulation Title _____

(name, strength, dosage form)

Assigned Beyond-Use Date (BUD)ᵃ _____

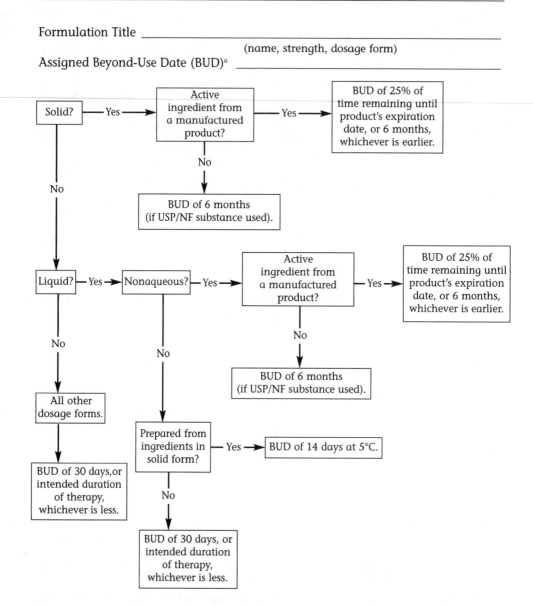

ᵃThe beyond-use-date limits in this flow chart may be exceeded when there is supporting valid scientific stability information that is directly applicable to the specific preparation (i.e., same drug concentration range, pH, excipients, vehicle, water content, etc.), including preparations that have been commercially available.

Documentation/References:

1._____

2._____

3._____

4._____

5._____

Figure 4-1. Flow chart for assigning beyond-use dates.

Chapter 5

Pharmaceutical Compounding Calculations

The preparation, packaging, and dispensing of most compounded prescriptions involve a number of pharmacy calculations. These calculations present one of the greatest potentials for errors in compounding. Even though most of the mathematical processes are relatively simple, misplacing a decimal point or using an estimated value for a medication can have serious consequences, including death. When a unit of measure must be converted to an equivalent value in a different measuring system, exact equivalent values should be used. For example, the correct metric equivalent value for 1 fl oz is 29.57 mL, not 30 mL or even 29.6 mL. Any rounding of values should be saved for the final answer. It is of utmost importance that pharmacists be extremely well grounded in the practice of pharmaceutical calculations because zero tolerance is allowed for errors in these vital operations.

Measurement Systems

The metric system is the official system of measurement used in pharmacy and medicine. Table 5-1 lists the unit of measures commonly used in compounding calculations. Also listed for each unit of measure is its denomination (e.g., liter, meter) abbreviation and its equivalent value to the definitive (i.e., largest denomination for that type of measure). Table 5-2 lists the major denominations and equivalent values for the following measurement systems used in the United States: apothecary, avoirdupois, troy, and household. Table 5-3 lists equivalent values for selected units of measures from the first three measurement systems, whereas Table 5-4 lists equivalent apothecary and metric values for household approximate measures. All four tables are useful references for pharmaceutical calculations.

General Calculations

Weighing, measuring, and diluting ingredients are common preparation steps that require performing calculations. The calculations may include weighing an ingredient on a balance, measuring a liquid ingredient in a graduated cylinder, or using specific gravity values to convert the volume of a liquid to a weight or vice

Table 5-1. Metric Measures

Unit of Measure	Denomination Abbreviation	Equivalent Value to Largest Denomination
Metric Weights		
1 Microgram	μg	0.000001 Gram
1 Milligram	mg	0.001 Gram
1 Centigram	cg	0.01 Gram
1 Decigram	dg	0.1 Gram
1 Gram	g	1 Gram
1 Dekagram	dag	10 Grams
1 Hectogram	hg	100 Grams
1 Kilogram	kg	1000 Grams
Metric Liquid Measures		
1 Microliter	μL	0.000001 Liter
1 Milliliter	mL	0.001 Liter
1 Centiliter	cL	0.01 Liter
1 Deciliter	dL	0.1 Liter
1 Liter	L	1 Liter
1 Dekaliter	daL	10 Liters
1 Hectoliter	hL	100 Liters
1 Kiloliter	kL	1000 Liters
Metric Linear Measures		
1 Nanometer	nm	0.000000001 Meter
1 Micron	μm	0.000001 Meter
1 Millimeter	mm	0.001 Meter
1 Centimeter	cm	0.01 Meter
1 Decimeter	dm	0.1 Meter
1 Meter	M	1 Meter
1 Dekameter	dam	10 Meters
1 Hectometer	hm	100 Meters
1 Kilometer	km	1000 Meters

versa. The reader can use specific gravity values listed in Appendix II in solving this type of calculation. Other common calculations include using the processes of dilution or aliquots to obtain an accurate quantity of material that cannot be directly weighed or measured.

Weighing and Measuring

Weighing or measuring ingredients is one of the first steps in preparing any prescription. One cannot expect to have a properly prepared prescription that complies with USP allowable tolerances unless each ingredient is accurately weighed or measured using properly calibrated equipment. The importance of obtaining accurate weights and measures cannot be overemphasized. In fact, it is a good practice to use a balance that has a printer, so that each weight reading can be printed out and kept as a permanent record.

Table 5-2. Equivalent Values for Other Measurement Systems

Avoirdupois Weights

Pound		Ounces		Grains
1	=	16	=	7000
		1	=	437.5

Troy Weights

Pound		Ounces		Pennyweights		Grains
1	=	12	=	240	=	5760
		1	=	20	=	480
				1	=	24

Apothecary Weights

Pound		Ounces		Drams		Scruples		Grains
1	=	12	=	96	=	288	=	5760
		1	=	8	=	24	=	480
				1	=	3	=	60
						1	=	20

Apothecary Measures

Gallon		Pints		Fluidounces		Fluidrams		Minims
1	=	8	=	128	=	1024	=	61,440
		1	=	16	=	128	=	7680
				1	=	8	=	480
						1	=	60

Table 5-3. Equivalent Values for Selected Units of Measure

Unit of Measure	Equivalent Value
Weight Measures	
1 Kilogram	2.2 Pounds avoir
1 Pound	454 Grams
1 Ounce avoir	28.35 Grams
1 Ounce apothecary	31.1 Grams
1 Pound apothecary	373 Grams
1 Gram	15.432 Grains
1 Grain	64.8 Milligrams
Liquid Measures	
1 Milliliter	16.23 Minims
1 Fluidounce	29.57 Milliliters
1 Pint	473 Milliliters
1 Gallon	3785 Milliliters

Table 5-4. Equivalent Values for Household Approximate Measures

Unit of Measure	Equivalent Value	
	Apothecary	Metric
1 Tumblerful	8 Fluidounces	240 Milliliters
1 Teacupful	4 Fluidounces	120 Milliliters
1 Wineglass	2 Fluidounces	60 Milliliters
2 Tablespoonsful	1 Fluidounce	30 Milliliters
1 Tablespoonful	½ Fluidounce	15 Milliliters
1 Dessert spoonful	2 Fluidrams	8–10 Milliliters
1 Teaspoonful	1 Fluidram	5 Milliliters
½ Teaspoonful	½ Fluidram	2.5 Milliliters

Least Measurable Quantity of Weight

A pharmacy's torsion balance has a sensitivity reading of 5 mg. What is the smallest quantity that can be accurately weighed with a maximum error of 5%?

The formula for calculating this value is expressed as

$$100\% \times \frac{\text{Maximum potential error (sensitivity reading)}}{\text{Permissible error (in percent)}} = \text{Least measurable quantity}$$

$$x = 100\% \times \frac{5 \text{ mg}}{5\%}$$

$$x = 100 \text{ mg}$$

The answer, 100 mg, illustrates the general principle of least measurable quantities with torsion balances: the value of the least measurable quantity is usually 20 times the sensitivity reading of the balance.

The pharmacy's electronic (digital) balance has a sensitivity reading of 0.1 mg. What is the least quantity that can be reasonably weighed on this balance?

A digital balance does not change its readout until a unit of material that equals or exceeds the sensitivity reading is placed on the balance pan. If, in an attempt to weigh 0.1 mg of a drug, 0.14 mg is placed on the pan, the readout will be only 0.1 mg. Therefore, use the same general principle as with torsion balances and do not weigh quantities that are less than 20 times the sensitivity reading of the balance (i.e., 20×0.1 mg = 2 mg).

Quantities of Ingredients

What quantity of each ingredient is required for the following prescription?

℞ Clotrimazole 1% Cream

Clotrimazole powder		1%
Dermabase	qs	30 g

Step 1. Determine the quantity of clotrimazole powder by multiplying its concentration (1% = 0.01) by the total weight of the product:

x = 30 g × 0.01 = 0.3 g of clotrimazole, *answer*

Step 2. Determine the quantity of Dermabase by subtracting the quantity of clotrimazole powder from the total weight of the product:

x = 30 g – 0.3 g = 29.7 g of Dermabase, *answer*

Density Factors in Weighing/Measuring

A pharmacist receives a prescription for 120 mL of a 3% (w/v) hydrochloric acid (HCl) solution. The density of concentrated hydrochloric acid (37% w/w) is 1.18 g/mL. How many milliliters of the concentrated acid would be required for the prescription?

Step 1. Calculate the weight of the required quantity of the 3% HCl solution:

3% (w/v) = 0.03 g/mL

0.03 g/mL × 120 mL = 3.6 g

Step 2. Calculate the volume of the required quantity of the 3% HCl solution:

$$\frac{3.6 \text{ g}}{1.18 \text{ g/mL}} = 3.05 \text{ mL}$$

Step 3. Calculate the volume of the 37% HCl required for the prescription:

37% = 0.37

$$\frac{3.05 \text{ mL}}{0.37} = 8.24 \text{ mL of 37\% HCl, } answer$$

Dilution Aliquots

A pharmacist needs 0.015 mL of a flavoring oil to prepare an oral liquid. Using alcohol as a solvent and a pipet accurate to 0.01 mL, how can this volume of flavoring oil be obtained?

Step 1. Select a multiple of the desired quantity that can be accurately measured with the pipet. For this example, use 10 as the multiple and measure 0.1 mL of flavoring oil (10 × 0.01 mL). Place the oil in a suitable graduated cylinder.

Step 2. Dilute the quantity of flavoring oil calculated in Step 1 with alcohol to a quantity of solution that is divisible by the selected multiple. For this example, add sufficient alcohol to make 50 mL of solution; mix well.

Step 3. Calculate the aliquot of the solution that contains the desired quantity of flavoring oil (0.015 mL) as follows:

$$\frac{0.1 \text{ mL}}{50 \text{ mL}} = \frac{0.015 \text{ mL}}{x}$$

x = 7.5 mL aliquot, *answer*

Step 4. Remove 7.5 mL of the solution that contains the required 0.015 mL of the flavoring oil.

Doses

Calculations concerning doses must also be performed accurately because they have a direct impact on the quantity of a medication that will be administered to a patient. Some of these calculations may involve determining the quantity of medication to be administered (teaspoonful, milliliter, tablet). Others involve converting the dose of a drug to the quantity of the final dosage form that should be administered.

Calibrating Droppers

An anticholinergic liquid has been presented for a toddler at a dose of 0.25 mL. The dropper dispensed with the medication delivers 56 drops of the liquid per 2 mL. How many drops should the parents be instructed to give the toddler?

Step 1. Calculate the number of drops delivered per 1 mL:

$$\frac{56 \text{ drops}}{2 \text{ mL}} = 28 \text{ drops/mL}$$

Step 2. Calculate the number of drops delivered per 0.25 mL:

$$\frac{0.25 \text{ mL}}{1 \text{ mL}} = \frac{x}{28 \text{ drops}}$$

$x = 7$ drops, *answer*

Calculating the Number of Dosage Forms/Volume to Dispense

A pharmacist receives a prescription for Wormaway 1 mg/mL for a family. The medication is to be given the day the prescription is filled and then repeated in 7 days. What total volume of the medication is required if the dose for each person is 0.3 mg/kg of body weight?

Step 1. Convert each person's body weight to kilograms (1 kg = 2.2 lb); multiply those values by 0.3 mg to calculate the number of milligrams per dose for each person; add the values in the last column to calculate the total number of milligrams required for one dose.

Adult 1	$\frac{175 \text{ lb}}{2.2}$	=	79.55 kg × 0.3 mg/kg	=	23.87 mg
Adult 2	$\frac{125 \text{ lb}}{2.2}$	=	56.82 kg × 0.3 mg/kg	=	17.05 mg
Child 1	$\frac{95 \text{ lb}}{2.2}$	=	43.18 kg × 0.3 mg/kg	=	12.95 mg
Child 2	$\frac{75 \text{ lb}}{2.2}$	=	34.09 kg × 0.3 mg/kg	=	10.23 mg
Child 3	$\frac{60 \text{ lb}}{2.2}$	=	27.27 kg × 0.3 mg/kg	=	8.18 mg
Total milligrams required for one dose				=	72.28 mg

Step 2. Calculate the quantity required for two doses:

72.28 mg × 2 = 144.56 mg

Step 3. Divide the quantity for two doses by the concentration of the medication to determine the total volume required:

$$\frac{144.56 \text{ mg}}{1 \text{ mg/mL}} = 144.56 \text{ mL of Wormaway 1 mg/mL, } answer$$

Solutions

Solubility ratios in the literature and in the *United States Pharmacopeia 25/ National Formulary 20* are given as "x:y" and "x in y" (e.g., 1:4 and 1 in 4). These expressions are stated as one part of *solute* plus four parts of *solvent*. The resulting product is described as a 1:5 solution; that is, the product contains one part of *solute* in five parts of *solution*. A *solubility ratio* involves the quantity of solute that will dissolve in a quantity of solvent. This ratio is usually expressed as the number of grams of solute that will dissolve in a certain number of milliliters of solvent. On the other hand, a *solution concentration* involves the quantity of solute in a given quantity of solution. This concentration is usually expressed as the number of grams of solute in a certain number of milliliters of solution. Another example: A substance with a solubility of 1:3 contains 1 g of solute *plus* 3 mL of solvent. The resulting product, a 1:4 solution, contains one part of solute in four parts of solution. In contrast, a 1:3 *solution* contains 1 g of solute in 3 mL of solution (i.e., sufficient solvent is added to make 3 mL of solution).

In pharmaceutical calculations, the concentration of a solution is often expressed as "parts per x." Table 5-5 lists common "parts per x" measurements and their equivalent values in metric measures, percent concentration, and ratio concentration.

Table 5-5. "Parts per x" Measurements and Their Equivalent Values

"Parts per x"	Metric Equivalent	Percent Concentration	Ratio Concentration
1 pp1 (1 part per 1)	1 g/mL	100%	1:1
1 ppt (1 part per thousand)	1 mg/mL	0.1%	1:1000
1 ppm (1 part per million)	1 µg/mL, or 1 g/1,000,000 mL	0.0001%	1:1,000,000
1 ppb (1 part per billion)	1 ng/mL	0.0000001%	1:1,000,000,000

Determining W/W and W/V of Solutions

One gram of boric acid is soluble in 18 mL of water and makes a saturated solution. What is the percentage w/w and w/v of a saturated solution of boric acid?

Step 1. Calculate the total weight of the solution:

1 mL of water weighs 1 g

1 g + 18 g = 19 g

Step 2. Calculate the percentage w/w of the solution by setting up a proportion between the weights and the percentages of saturation:

$$\frac{19\ g}{1\ g} = \frac{100\%}{x\ (\%\ w/w\ of\ solution)}$$

$x = 5.26\%$ w/w, *answer*

Step 3. Because the volume of the solution is between 18 and 19 mL, we know the w/v concentration is greater than 5.26%. Assume the volume is 18.2 mL, and calculate the w/v concentration:

$$\frac{1\ g}{18.2\ mL} = \frac{x\ (\%\ w/v)}{100\%}$$

$x = 5.5\%$ w/v, *answer*

Determining Quantity of Active Drug

What quantity of mannitol is required to prepare 120 mL of a 1:10 solution?

Step 1. Set up a proportion between the ratio concentrations and the quantity of the ingredients:

$$\frac{1 \text{ part}}{10 \text{ parts}} = \frac{x}{120 \text{ mL}}$$

$x = 12$ g of mannitol, *answer*

Step 2. Place 12 g of mannitol in a graduated cylinder and add sufficient solvent to make 120 mL of solution.

A pharmacist receives a prescription for 8 oz of an oral rinse to contain 10 ppm fluoride ion (F⁻) in orange flower water. How much sodium fluoride (NaF) would be required to prepare this compound?

Step 1. Convert ounces to milliliters (1 oz = 29.57 mL) and calculate the total volume of the solution:

8×29.57 mL $= 237$ mL

Step 2. Convert parts per million to a ratio concentration and set up the following proportion to calculate the quantity of fluoride ion required for the prescription:

$$\frac{10 \text{ g}}{1,000,000 \text{ mL}} = \frac{x}{237 \text{ mL}}$$

$x = 0.0024$ g $= 2.4$ mg of F⁻, *answer*

Step 3. Given that 1 mg F⁻ = 2.2 mg NaF, calculate the quantity of NaF required:

$$\frac{1 \text{ mg F}^-}{2.2 \text{ mg NaF}} = \frac{2.4 \text{ mg F}^-}{x \text{ (mg NaF)}}$$

$x = 5.3$ mg NaF

Determining Quantity of Preservatives

How much 95% ethanol would be required to preserve the following prescription?

$\mathbf{R}_x$——————————————————————————————

Active drug #1 (powder)		120 mg
Active drug #2 (aqueous solution)		20 mL
Water		10 mL
Syrup	qs	120 mL

As this prescription is written, the sucrose concentration and preservative properties will decrease because 10 mL of water and 20 mL of aqueous solution are diluting the syrup. To compensate for this decrease, one has a number of options, the simplest of which is the addition of 95% alcohol. The following steps illustrate how to calculate the quantity of alcohol required.

Step 1. Determine the quantity of syrup required for the prescription:

120 mL – (10 mL + 20 mL) = 90 mL

Step 2. Determine the quantity of sucrose present in 90 mL of syrup (w/v of sucrose = 85%):

$$85\% \times 90 \text{ mL} = 76.5 \text{ g}$$

Step 3. Given that 1 g of sucrose preserves 0.53 mL of water, determine the quantity of water that 76.5 g of sucrose will preserve:

$$76.5 \times 0.53 \text{ mL} = 40.5 \text{ mL}$$

Step 4. Given that 1 g of sucrose occupies a volume of 0.647 mL, determine the volume occupied by 76.5 g of sucrose:

$$76.5 \times 0.\,647 \text{ mL} = 49.5 \text{ mL}$$

Step 5. Determine the volume of solution preserved by the sucrose:

$$40.5 \text{ mL} + 49.5 \text{ mL} = 90 \text{ mL}$$

Step 6. Determine the volume of solution that is not preserved:

$$120 \text{ mL} - 90 \text{ mL} = 30 \text{ mL}$$

Step 7. Determine the quantity of absolute (18%) alcohol required to preserve the unpreserved solution:

$$18\% \times 30 \text{ mL} = 5.4 \text{ mL}$$

Step 8. Determine the quantity of 95% alcohol required to preserve the unpreserved solution:

$$\frac{5.4 \text{ mL}}{0.95} = 5.7 \text{ mL of 95\% alcohol, } answer$$

Reducing and Enlarging Formulas

The actual quantity of a formula to be prepared is often not the same quantity that is described in a formulation record. Consequently, in many cases, the quantity must be increased or decreased to achieve the required quantity of product. To ensure that the relative quantities of the ingredients remain consistent, the quantities of all ingredients must be increased or decreased by the same factor.

Solids

A formula for compounding 100 mL of an ibuprofen gel requires 2 g of ibuprofen powder. What quantity of the ibuprofen would be required for 240 mL of the product?

Step 1. Set up a proportion to express the quantities of ingredients per total quantities of product and solve for x:

$$\frac{2 \text{ g}}{100 \text{ mL}} = \frac{x}{240 \text{ mL}}$$

$$x = 4.8 \text{ g of ibuprofen, } answer$$

Partial Dosage Units

How would you determine the quantity of indomethacin required for the following prescription if indomethacin 25 mg capsules are used?

℞ **Indomethacin 5 mg/5 mL Capsules**

Indomethacin		5 mg/5 mL
Ora Plus		60 mL
Ora Sweet	qs	120 mL

Step 1. Determine the total quantity of indomethacin required for the prescription:

5 mg/5 mL = 1 mg/mL

1 mg/mL × 120 mL = 120 mg

Step 2. Calculate the number of capsules required to supply 120 mg of indomethacin:

$$\frac{120 \text{ mg}}{25 \text{ mg/capsule}} = 4.8 \text{ capsules}$$

Step 3. Empty the contents of 5 capsules onto a tared weighing paper and weigh the contents. Given that the weight is 1.6 g, calculate the quantity of mixture to remove to use in the prescription:

$$\frac{x}{1.6 \text{ g}} = \frac{4.8 \text{ capsules}}{5 \text{ capsules}}$$

x = 1.536 g of mixture, *answer*

Hydrated and Anhydrous Crystals

How much MgSO$_4$•7H$_2$O must be weighed to obtain 5 g of MgSO$_4$? (Formula weights: Mg = 24; S = 32; O = 16; H = 1)

Step 1. Using the given formula weights of the elements, calculate the weight of MgSO$_4$:

Weight Mg: 1 × 24 g = 24 g

Weight S: 1 × 32 g = 32 g

Weight O: 4 × 16 g = 64 g

Weight MgSO$_4$ = 24 g + 32 g + 64 g = 120 g

Step 2. Calculate the weight of MgSO$_4$•7H$_2$O:

Weight MgSO$_4$: 1 × 120 g = 120 g

Weight H: 14 × 1 g = 14 g

Weight O: 7 × 16 g = 112 g

Weight MgSO$_4$•7H$_2$O = 120 g + 14 g + 112 g = 246 g

Step 3. Calculate the quantity of MgSO$_4$•7H$_2$O that contains 5 g of MgSO$_4$:

$$\frac{120 \text{ g}}{246 \text{ g}} = \frac{5 \text{ g}}{x}$$

x = 10.25 g of MgSO$_4$•7H$_2$O, *answer*

Stock Solutions

A pharmacist is preparing an ophthalmic decongestant solution in batch form. Each of three bottles will contain 15 mL of the ophthalmic solution. The formula requires 0.01% (w/v) benzalkonium chloride (BAK) as a preservative. The pharmacist has a stock solution containing 17% (w/v) BAK. How much of the BAK stock solution would be required for the three bottles of batch solution?

Step 1. Calculate the total weight of the ophthalmic batch solution:

15 mL × 3 = 45 mL

Step 2. Calculate the weight of the BAK solution required for the batch solution:

0.01% = 0.0001

45 mL × 0.0001 = 0.0045 g

Step 3. Calculate the quantity of the 17% BAK solution required for the batch solution:

$$\frac{0.0045 \text{ g}}{x} = \frac{17 \text{ g}}{100 \text{ mL}}$$

x = 0.026 mL of 17% BAK solution, *answer*

Potency of Salt Forms

Polymyxin B sulfate has a potency of 6000 units/mg. How much polymyxin B sulfate, in milligrams, is required to prepare 10 mL of an ophthalmic solution containing 10,000 units/mL?

Step 1. Calculate the number of units of polymyxin B sulfate required for 10 mL of the solution:

10,000 units/mL × 10 mL = 100,000 units

Step 2. Calculate the milligrams of polymyxin B sulfate required for the prescription:

$$\frac{6000 \text{ units}}{1 \text{ mg}} = \frac{100,000 \text{ units}}{x}$$

x = 16.67 mg of polymyxin B sulfate, *answer*

Mixing Products of Different Strengths

A pharmacist receives an order for 120 g of a 0.1% corticosteroid ointment. Three concentrations of corticosteroid ointment (30 g of 0.1%, 15 g of 0.15%, and 75 g of 0.005%), all in the same ointment base, are on hand. If these three ointments are mixed together, how much additional corticosteroid powder should be added to prepare the prescription. Assume the quantity of corticosteroid powder added will be negligible compared with the total weight of 120 g.

Step 1. Calculate the total milligrams of corticosteroid required for the prescription:

0.1% = 0.001; 0.15% = 0.0015; 0.005% = 0.00005

120 g × 0.001 = 0.12 g = 120 mg

Step 2. Calculate the total milligrams of corticosteroid contained in the three ointments on hand:

x (mg of corticosteroid in 0.1% ointment) = 30 g × 0.001 = 0.03 g = 30 mg

y (mg of corticosteroid in 0.15% ointment) = 15 g × 0.0015 = 0.0225 g = 22.5 mg

z (mg of corticosteroid in 0.005% ointment) = 75 g × 0.00005 = 0.00375 g = 3.8 mg

Total mg of corticosteroid in ointments = x + y + z = 56.3 mg

Step 3. Calculate the amount of additional corticosteroid powder required for the prescription:

120 mg – 56.3 mg = 63.7 mg of corticosteroid power, *answer*

What quantities of a 50% dextrose in water solution ($D_{50}W$) and a 5% dextrose in water solution (D_5W) should be mixed to obtain 900 mL of a 15% dextrose in water solution?

Step 1. Determine the number of parts of $D_{50}W$ and D_5W required for the solution, using the following diagram:

$$50 \searrow \quad \quad \nearrow \frac{10 \text{ (parts of } D_{50}W)}{5} = 2 \text{ parts}$$

$$15$$

$$5 \nearrow \quad \quad \searrow \frac{35 \text{ (parts of } D_5W)}{5} = 7 \text{ parts}$$

Total = 9 parts

This step can also be calculated using the following equations:

Number of parts of $D_{50}W$ = Desired strength (15%) – Strength of weaker component (5%) = 10 parts

Number of parts of D_5W = Strength of stronger component (50%) – Desired strength (15%) = 35 parts

Reduce the number of parts to lowest multiple and calculate the total number of parts:

$$\text{Parts } D_{50}W = \frac{10 \text{ parts}}{5} = 2 \text{ parts}$$

$$\text{Parts } D_5W = \frac{35 \text{ parts}}{5} = 7 \text{ parts}$$

Total = 9 parts

Step 2. Calculate the volumes of $D_{50}W$ and D_5W required for the solution:

$$\frac{2 \text{ parts}}{9 \text{ parts}} = \frac{x \text{ (mL of } D_{50}W)}{900 \text{ mL}}$$

$x = 200$ mL of $D_{50}W$, *answer*

$$\frac{7 \text{ parts}}{9 \text{ parts}} = \frac{y \text{ (mL of } D_5W)}{900 \text{ mL}}$$

$y = 700$ mL of D_5W, *answer*

Reconstituting Powders

The directions to constitute 150 mL of an amoxicillin suspension 250 mg/5 mL call for 111 mL of purified water. The physician has requested the product be constituted at a concentration of 500 mg/5 mL. How much purified water is required for the higher concentration?

Step 1. Calculate the volume of the 250 mg/5 mL solution occupied by the amoxicillin powder:

150 mL – 111 mL = 39 mL

Step 2. Calculate the quantity of amoxicillin present in 1 mL of solution:

$$\frac{250 \text{ mg}}{5 \text{ mL}} = \frac{x}{150 \text{ mL}}$$

$x = 50$ mg/mL $\times$ 150 mL = 7500 mg

Step 3. Calculate the total volume of the requested concentration (500 mg/5 mL) of the solution:

$$\frac{500 \text{ mg}}{5 \text{ mL}} = \frac{7500 \text{ mg}}{x} = 75 \text{ mL}$$

Step 4. Calculate the quantity of purified water to add:

75 mL – 39 mL = 36 mL of purified water, *answer*

Ingredient/Product-Specific Calculations

Some ingredients are prescribed in units of measure other than weight or volume. For example, electrolytes are prescribed in milliequivalents, and certain elements are prescribed in millimoles. Other units of measure are used for products in which activity or potency is of concern. These units of measure can be converted to a metric quantity so that the ingredient can be measured; however, specific calculations and a knowledge of how to use degrees of ionization, potency expressions, and the like are required to convert the units of measure accurately. Further, effervescent mixtures involve the use of stoichiometric ratios to determine the quantities of acids and bases that will react together. Finally, hydrophile-lipophile-balance (HLB) values can be used to determine the proper blending of surfactants for emulsions.

Milliequivalents

A prescription calls for 25 mEq of sodium chloride (NaCl). What quantity of sodium chloride, in milligrams, is required for the prescription? (1 equivalent NaCl = 58.5 g; 1 mEq NaCl = 58.5 mg)

Step 1. Given that 1 mEq of NaCl weighs 58.5 mg, calculate the weight of 25 mEq of NaCl:

25 mEq × 58.5 mg/mEq = 1463 mg of NaCl, *answer*

A pharmacist receives an order for 10 mEq of calcium ion (Ca^{++}). How much of a standard 10% calcium chloride (CaCl$_2$) solution should be used for this order? (Formula weight: Ca^{++} = 40 g; Cl$^-$ = 35.5 g)

Step 1. Calculate the equivalent weight of Ca^{++}. Ca^{++} combines with two Cl$^-$; therefore, the formula weight of Ca^{++} is divided by 2 to obtain the equivalent weight:

$$\frac{40 \text{ g}}{2} = 20 \text{ g}$$

Step 2. Calculate the milliequivalent weight of Ca^{++}:

$$\frac{20 \text{ g}}{1000} = 0.02 \text{ g} = 20 \text{ mg}$$

Step 3. Calculate the quantity of Ca^{++}, in milligrams, required for the prescription:

$$\frac{1 \text{ mEq}}{10 \text{ mEq}} = \frac{20 \text{ mg}}{x}$$
$$x = 200 \text{ mg}$$

Step 4. Calculate the quantity of CaCl$_2$ required to supply 200 mg of Ca^{++}:

$$\frac{40 \text{ g}}{111 \text{ g}} = \frac{200 \text{ mg}}{x}$$

$x = 555$ mg $= 0.555$ g

Step 5. Calculate the quantity of the 10% $CaCl_2$ solution required to supply 555 mg of $CaCl_2$:

10% = 10 g/100 mL

$$\frac{10 \text{ g}}{100 \text{ mL}} = \frac{0.555 \text{ g}}{x}$$

$x = 5.55$ mL of 10% $CaCl_2$ solution, *answer*

A prescription calls for 240 mL of a solution that contains 15 mEq of potassium ion (K^+) as potassium chloride (KCl) and 10 mEq of sodium ion (Na^+) as sodium chloride (NaCl) per tablespoonful of solution. The compound is to be prepared in a suitable vehicle that contains no potassium or sodium ions. How much potassium chloride and sodium chloride would be required for this prescription? (Formula weights: $K^+ = 39$ g; $Cl^- = 35.5$ g; $Na^+ = 23$ g; KCl = 74.5 g; NaCl = 58.5 g)

Step 1. Given that 1 mEq of KCl weighs 74.5 mg, calculate the weight of 15 mEq:

74.5 mg $\times$ 15 mEq = 1118 mg = 1.118 g

Step 2. Calculate the quantity of KCl required for the prescription:

1 tablespoon = 15 mL

$$\frac{15 \text{ mL}}{240 \text{ mL}} = \frac{1.118 \text{ g}}{x}$$

$x = 17.89$ g of KCl, *answer*

Step 3. Given that 1 mEq of NaCl weighs 58.5 mg, calculate the weight of 10 mEq of NaCl:

58.5 mg $\times$ 10 mEq = 585 mg = 0.585 g

Step 4. Calculate the quantity of NaCl required for the prescription:

$$\frac{15 \text{ mL}}{240 \text{ mL}} = \frac{0.585 \text{ g}}{x}$$

$x = 9.36$ g of NaCl, *answer*

Millimoles

How many millimoles of sodium chloride (NaCl) are contained in 1 liter of a 0.9% solution? (Formula weights: $Na^+ = 23$ g; $Cl^- = 35.5$ g; NaCl = 58.5 g)

Step 1. Calculate the quantity of NaCl in the solution:

0.009×1000 mL = 9 g

Step 2. Calculate the millimoles of NaCl contained in the solution:

1 equivalent weight NaCl = 1 mole of NaCl; therefore 1 mole of NaCl weighs 58.5 g

$$\frac{1 \text{ mole}}{58.5 \text{ g}} = \frac{x}{9 \text{ g}}$$

$x = 0.154$ mole = 154 millimoles of NaCl, *answer*

Osmolarity

What is the osmolarity (number of milliosmoles) of 1 L of 0.9% sodium chloride (NaCl) solution? Assume complete dissociation of the ions (NaCl → Na⁺ + Cl⁻). (Formula weights: $Na^+ = 23$ g; $Cl^- = 35.5$ g; $NaCl = 58.5$ g)

Step 1. Calculate the number of millimoles of NaCl in the solution:

Millimoles/L of NaCl = 154 (see previous problem)

Step 2. Calculate the osmolarity of the solution by multiplying the answer in Step 1 by the number of species:

NaCl → Na⁺ + Cl⁻ = 2 species

154 millimoles/L × 2 = 308 mOsmol/L, *answer*

What is the osmolarity of 1 L of a 10% calcium chloride ($CaCl_2$) solution? Assume complete dissociation of the ions ($CaCl_2$ → Ca^{++} + $2Cl^-$). (Formula weights: $Ca^{++} = 40$ g; $Cl^- = 35.5$ g; $CaCl_2 = 111$ g)

Step 1. Calculate the number of millimoles of $CaCl_2$ in the solution:

10% = 100 g/1000 mL

$$\frac{100 \text{ g}}{111 \text{ g}} = \frac{x}{1 \text{ mole}}$$

x = 0.9 moles = 900 millimoles

Step 2. Calculate the osmolarity of the solution:

$CaCl_2$ → Ca^{++} + $2Cl^-$ = 3 species

900 millimoles/L × 3 = 2700 mOsmol/L, *answer*

Units to Weight Conversions

A prescription calls for 150,000 units of nystatin per gram of ointment with 60 g to be dispensed. What quantity of nystatin 4400 units/mg USP should be weighed for the prescription?

Step 1. Calculate the number of units of nystatin required:

150,000 units/g × 60 g = 9,000,000 units

Step 2. Calculate the weight of the required units of nystatin:

$$\frac{9,000,000 \text{ units}}{4400 \text{ units/mg}} = 2045 \text{ mg} = 2.045 \text{ g of nystatin, } \textit{answer}$$

Shelf-Life Estimates

The shelf-life of a compound can be estimated by using the equation

$$t_{90} \text{ New} = \frac{t_{90} \text{ Original}}{Q^{\Delta T/10}}$$

where t_{90} equals the period of time over which a product retains 90% of its potency, ΔT equals change in temperature, and 3 is a reasonable estimate for the "Q" value, based on energies of activation (Ea) from the Arrhenius equation. (See Chapter 4, "Stability of Compounded Products," for a discussion of this equation.)

An antibiotic solution has a shelf-life of 96 hours when refrigerated (5°C). If it were necessary that a patient use the solution in an ambulatory pump at approximate body temperature (30°C) for 6 hours, would the compound still retain at least 90% of its original potency during the entire period of administration?

Step 1. Calculate the change in temperature the solution will undergo:

$\Delta T = 30°C - 5°C = 25°$

Step 2. Calculate the shelf-life of the solution at the new temperature:

$$t_{90} = \frac{96 \text{ hours}}{3^{25/10}} = \frac{96 \text{ hours}}{3^{2.5}} = 6.16 \text{ hours}$$

Step 3. Compare the new shelf-life with the period of administration:

$t_{90} = 6.16$ hours; period of administration = 6 hours; *therefore, the answer is yes*

A prescription is received for an ophthalmic solution with a shelf-life of 4 hours at room temperature (25°C). The preparation is to be administered in a physician's office at 12:00 noon the next day. Can the solution be prepared the evening before at about 8:00 PM and still retain at least 90% of its shelf-life if stored in a refrigerator?

Step 1. Calculate the change in temperature the solution will undergo:

$\Delta T = 5°C - 25°C = -20°$

Step 2. Calculate the shelf-life at the new temperature:

$$t_{90} = \frac{4 \text{ hours}}{3^{-20/10}} = \frac{4 \text{ hours}}{3^{-2}} = 4 \text{ hours} \times 9 = 36 \text{ hours}$$

Step 3. Compare the new shelf-life with the period of refrigeration:

$t_{90} = 36$ hours; period of refrigeration = 16 hours; *therefore, the answer is yes*

A reconstituted antibiotic has a shelf-life at room temperature of 3 days. How long would the preparation be stable if refrigerated (i.e., a reasonable estimate based on t_{90})?

Step 1. Calculate the change in temperature:

$\Delta T = 5°C - 25°C = -20°$

Step 2. Calculate the shelf-life at the new temperature:

$$t_{90} = \frac{3 \text{ days}}{3^{-20/10}} = \frac{3 \text{ days}}{3^{-2}} = 3 \text{ days} \times 9 = 27 \text{ days}, \textit{answer}$$

Effervescent Mixtures

A prescription calls for an effervescent mixture of citric acid/tartaric acid (1:2) molar ratio with sodium bicarbonate to mask the taste of the active drug, potassium chloride (KCl). How much active drug, citric acid ($C_6H_8O_7 \bullet H_2O$), tartaric acid ($C_4H_6O_6$), and sodium bicarbonate (NaHCO_3) would be required for the prescription? (Formula weights: KCl = 74.5 g; NaHCO_3 = 84 g; $C_6H_8O_7 \bullet H_2O$ = 210 g; $C_4H_6O_6$ = 150 g)

℞ **Potassium Chloride 1 mEq/5 g tsp Effervescent Mixture**

Potassium chloride	1 mEq/5 g tsp
Tartaric acid	
Citric acid	
Sodium bicarbonate	
Lime flavor crystals	qs
Dispense 100 g.	

Step 1. Assuming the powder in final form will weigh 5 g per teaspoonful, calculate the number of doses in the prescription:

$$\frac{100 \text{ g}}{5 \text{ g/dose}} = 20 \text{ doses}$$

Step 2. Using the formula weights of each ingredient and assuming the lime flavor crystals contribute negligible weight, calculate the quantity of KCl and the acids required for this prescription:

x (g of KCl required) = 20 doses × 74.5 mg/dose = 1.49 g of KCl, *answer*

y (g of acids required) = 100 g − 1.49 g = 98.51 g

Step 3. Given the ratio of 1 part citric acid to 2 parts tartaric acid, calculate the quantity of sodium bicarbonate that will react with citric acid:

$$3NaHCO_3 + C_6H_8O_7 \bullet H_2O \rightarrow 4H_2O + 3CO_2 + Na_3C_6H_5O_7$$

(3 × 84 g)   (210 g)

$$\frac{1 \text{ part}}{210 \text{ g}} = \frac{x}{3 \times 84 \text{ g}}$$

$x = 1.2$ g (parts)

Step 4. Calculate the quantity of sodium bicarbonate that will react with tartaric acid:

$$2NaHCO_3 + C_4H_6O_6 \rightarrow 2H_2O + 2CO_2 + Na_2C_4H_4O_6$$

(2 × 84 g)   (150 g)

$$\frac{2 \text{ parts}}{150 \text{ g}} = \frac{x}{2 \times 84 \text{ g}}$$

$x = 2.24$ g (parts)

Step 5. Calculate the total quantity of sodium bicarbonate required to react with the acids:

1.2 g + 2.24 g = 3.44 g (parts)

Step 6. Knowing that the prescription requires 98.51 g of the effervescent mixture, calculate the required weight of each ingredient:

Total parts of ingredients = 1 part citric acid + 2 parts tartaric acid + 3.4 parts sodium bicarbonate = 6.4 parts

Quantity of citric acid $= \dfrac{1 \text{ part}}{6.4 \text{ parts}} \times 98.51$ g = 15.39 g, *answer*

Quantity of tartaric acid $= \dfrac{2 \text{ parts}}{6.4 \text{ parts}} \times 98.51$ g = 30.78 g, *answer*

Quantity of sodium bicarbonate $= \dfrac{3.4 \text{ parts}}{6.4 \text{ parts}} \times 98.51$ g = 52.34 g, *answer*

Step 7. Prepare the prescription by accurately weighing the following quantities of the ingredients:

Potassium chloride	1.49 g
Tartaric acid	30.78 g
Sodium bicarbonate	52.34 g
Citric acid	15.39 g
Total weight	100 g

Surfactant Blending

A prescription calls for preparation of 120 g of a cream using 3% Tween 80 and 1% Span 40. What is the hydrophile-lipophile-balance (HLB) value of this mixture? (HLBs: Tween 80 = 15.0; Span 40 = 6.7)

Step 1. Calculate the required weight of each ingredient:

Weight of Tween 80 = 120 g × 0.03 = 3.6 g

Weight of Span 40 = 120 × 0.01 = 1.2 g

Step 2. Calculate the contribution of each ingredient to the total HLB of the mixture:

$$\text{HLB contribution of Tween 80} = \frac{3.6\ g}{4.8\ g} \times 15 = 11.25$$

$$\text{HLB contribution of Span 40} = \frac{1.2\ g}{4.8\ g} \times 6.7 = 1.68$$

Step 3. Calculate the HLB of the mixture:

HLB of mixture = 11.25 + 1.68 = 12.9, *answer*

Dosage Form–Specific Calculations

Solutions

Certain dosage forms (ophthalmic, nasal, and parenteral) must be prepared to be isotonic with body fluids to increase the patient's comfort during administration of the medication and to minimize the damage that can be done when a hypotonic or hypertonic product is administered. The sodium chloride equivalent method can generally be used in calculations dealing with isotonicity. Appendix III, which lists sodium chloride equivalents for many agents, is a useful resource for this type of calculation.

In addition, some preparations must be buffered within a certain pH range to enhance the stability of the active drug(s). Appendix IV, "Buffers and Buffer Solutions," provides tabular data for preparing various types of buffers at specific pH values. Use of this information can speed up calculations dealing with buffer solutions.

Sodium Chloride Equivalents for Nasal and Ophthalmic Solutions

How much sodium chloride is required to render the following prescription isotonic?

℞ Lidocaine Hydrochloride 1% Solution

Lidocaine hydrochloride		1%	(NaCl equiv. = 0.22)
Cocaine hydrochloride		1%	(NaCl equiv. = 0.16)
Epinephrine bitartrate		0.1%	(NaCl equiv. = 0.18)
Sterile water	qs	50 mL	
Sodium chloride		qs	

Step 1. Using the NaCl equivalents provided, calculate the tonicic equivalents of the ingredients required for the prescription:

x (g of lidocaine HCl) = (50 mL × 0.01 g/mL) × 0.22 = 0.5 g × 0.22 = 0.110 g

y (g of cocaine HCl) = (50 mL × 0.01 g/mL) × 0.16 = 0.5 g × 0.16 = 0.080 g

z (g of epinephrine) = (50 mL × 0.001 g/mL) × 0.18 = 0.05 g × 0.18 = 0.009 g

Step 2. Calculate the total NaCl equivalents represented by the ingredients:

Total NaCl equivalents = $x + y + z$ = 0.110 g + 0.080 g + 0.009 g = 0.199 g

Step 3. Calculate the quantity of NaCl required to make 50 mL of water isotonic (NaCl equivalent of isotonic sodium chloride solution = 0.009 g/mL):

50 mL × 0.009 g/mL = 0.45 g

Step 4. Calculate the quantity of NaCl required to make this solution isotonic:

0.45 g – 0.199 g = 0.251 g of NaCl, *answer*

Buffer Solutions and pH

A prescription for optimycin 1% calls for a phosphate buffer with a pH of 6.5. Sorensen modified phosphate buffer will be used to prepare this buffer solution. Sorensen modified phosphate buffer is prepared by mixing the appropriate quantities of a 1/15 M stock acid solution and a 1/15 M stock alkaline solution. What quantities of these two solutions are required to make the phosphate buffer for this prescription?

R_X **Optimycin 1% Solution**

Optimycin   1%
Sodium chloride   qs
Phosphate buffer (pH 6.5)   qs   100 mL

Step 1. Use the table Preparation of Sorensen's Modified Phosphate Buffer Solution with Specific pH in Appendix III to determine the quantity of sodium biphosphate solution and sodium phosphate solution needed to prepare 100 mL of a phosphate buffer with a pH of 6.5:

Required mL of 1/15 M sodium biphosphate solution = 70 mL, *answer*

Required mL of 1/15 M sodium phosphate solution = 30 mL, *answer*

Calibrating a Dropper/Sprayer for Nasal Solutions

The dose for a nasal solution is 250 µg. A 0.5% solution is prepared and placed in a nasal spray bottle. The patient squeezed the bottle 10 times into a plastic bag; the squeezed-out product weighed 500 mg. Assuming the weight of the solution is 1 g/mL (i.e., 500 mg = 0.5 mL), how many squeezes are required to administer the 250 µg dose?

Step 1. Convert percent concentration of the solution to a "parts per x" concentration:

0.5% = 0.5 g/100 mL

Step 2. Calculate the quantity of the solution expelled in 10 squeezes:

$$\frac{0.5 \text{ g}}{100 \text{ mL}} = \frac{x}{0.5 \text{ mL}}$$

x = 0.0025 g/0.5 mL = 2.5 mg/0.5 mL = 2500 µg/0.5 mL

Step 3. Calculate the number of squeezes required to administer the 250 µg dose:

$$\frac{10 \text{ squeezes}}{2500 \text{ µg}} = \frac{x}{250 \text{ µg}}$$

x = 1 squeeze, *answer*

Displacement Factors

When preparing many dosage forms, the volume occupied by the various ingredients must be determined. Some examples are fixed-volume dosage forms such as capsules, molded suppositories, molded troches/lozenges, and molded tablets. Because of the differences in densities of the ingredients, different substances will occupy different volumes in the dosage form. When the actual densities of the ingredients are not known, ratios can be used instead to determine the volumes they occupy. The following problems illustrate both methods of calculating the volume occupied by ingredients.

Powder-Filled Capsules

A pharmacist receives a prescription for forty-eight 15 mg piroxicam capsules. A #1 capsule filled with piroxicam weighs 245 mg; a capsule filled with lactose weighs 180 mg. What quantities of piroxicam and lactose are required for the prescription? Prepare sufficient powder for 50 capsules (2 extra).

Step 1. Calculate the quantity of piroxicam required for 50 capsules:

50 capsules × 15 mg = 750 mg of piroxicam, *answer*

Step 2. Calculate the volume equivalent of lactose that is occupied by the piroxicam in a #1 capsule:

$$\frac{15\ mg}{245\ mg} = \frac{x}{180\ mg}$$

$x = 11$ mg

Step 3. Knowing that 15 mg of piroxicam occupies a similar volume as that of 11 mg of lactose, calculate the quantity of lactose required for the prescription:

Quantity of lactose per capsule = 180 mg – 11 mg = 169 mg

Required quantity of lactose = 169 mg × 50 capsules = 8450 mg = 8.45 g, *answer*

Molded Tablets

A pharmacist receives a prescription for 30 molded tablets. Each tablet is to contain 5 mg of the active drug. The average weight of a tablet containing only base is 65 mg. This value was determined by preparing 30 tablets that contained only the base, weighing the entire batch, and dividing the weight by 30. Because the active drug weighs more than a few milligrams, its density factor should be determined. This factor is equal to the average weight of a tablet containing only active drug, which is 85 mg for this prescription. This value was determined by the same method described for obtaining the average weight of base per tablet.

Determine the quantity of base required for each tablet. Also, determine the total weight per tablet. This value can be used in quality control checks of the finished product.

Step 1. Determine the percentage of the tablet occupied by the active drug by dividing the quantity of drug per tablet by the average weight of the pure drug tablet:

$$\frac{5\ mg}{85\ mg} \times 100 = 5.9\%$$

Step 2. Determine the percent of the tablet occupied by the base:

100% – 5.9% = 94.1%

Step 3. Determine the weight of the base per tablet:

94.1% × 65 mg = 61.2 mg

Step 4. Knowing that each tablet will contain the following quantity of each ingredient, determine the total weight per tablet:

Active drug	5 mg
Base	61.2 mg

Total weight per tablet = 5 mg + 61.2 mg = 66.2 mg, *answer*

Molded Suppositories/Troches/Lozenges

A prescription for 300 mg zinc oxide suppositories calls for cocoa butter to be used as the vehicle. The density factors for cocoa butter and zinc oxide are 0.9 and 4.0, respectively. Given that the suppository mold holds 2.0 g of cocoa butter, what quantities of zinc oxide and cocoa butter would be required to prepare 12 suppositories?

℞ Zinc Oxide 300 mg Suppositories

Zinc oxide	300 mg
Cocoa butter	qs

Step 1. Calculate the total weight of 12 suppositories that contain only cocoa butter:

12 × 2.0 g = 24 g

Step 2. Calculate the density ratio of zinc oxide to cocoa butter:

$$\frac{4}{0.9} = 4.44$$

Step 3. Calculate the weight of zinc oxide required for the prescription:

300 mg × 12 supp. = 3600 mg = 3.6 g of zinc oxide, *answer*

Step 4. Calculate the amount of cocoa butter displaced by the active drug:

$$\frac{3.6\ g}{4.44} = 0.81\ g$$

Step 5: Calculate the weight of cocoa butter required for the prescription:

24 g – 0.81 g = 23.19 g of cocoa butter, *answer*

Determination of Density Factor: Paddock Method

The Paddock Method is a more accurate, but also more time-consuming, method for calculating the replacement value (occupied volume) of the suppository base and ultimately the quantity of active drug required for a prescription. Before these values can be calculated, the density factor, *df*, must be determined, using the following equation:

$$df = \frac{B}{A - C + B}$$

where *A* equals the average weight of a blank, *B* equals the weight of active drug per suppository, and *C* equals the average weight of a medicated suppository.

Each step in this method will be described first, and then a sample calculation for which the values of A, B, and C are given will be taken through each step.

Step 1. Determine the average blank weight (i.e., weight of a suppository containing only the base), A, per mold using the suppository base of interest.

Step 2. Weigh the quantity of suppository base required for 10 suppositories.

Step 3. Weigh 1 g of the active drug.

The weight of active drug per suppository, B, is then equal to

$$\frac{1\ g}{10\ supp.} = 0.1\ g/supp.$$

Step 4. Melt the suppository base and incorporate the active drug. Mix the ingredients, pour into molds, cool, trim, and remove from the molds.

Step 5. Weigh the 10 suppositories and determine the average weight, C.

Step 6. Using the equation provided, determine the density factor, df.

Step 7. To find the replacement value of the suppository base, divide the weight of the medication required for each suppository by the density factor of the medication.

Step 8. Subtract the value in step 7 from the value for the average weight of a blank suppository weight, calculated in step 1.

Step 9. Multiply the value in step 8 by the number of required suppositories to obtain the quantity of suppository base required for the prescription.

Step 10. Multiply the weight of drug per suppository by the required number of suppositories to obtain the quantity of active drug required for the prescription.

A prescription calls for 12 acetaminophen 300 mg (B) suppositories using cocoa butter as the vehicle. The average weight of the cocoa butter blank (A) is 2.0 g, and the average weight of the medicated suppository (C) is 1.8 g. What quantities of cocoa butter and acetaminophen are required for the prescription.

Step 1. Determine the average weight of a blank suppository, A:

A = 2.0 g

Step 2. Determine the quantity of cocoa butter required for 12 blank suppositories:

$12 \times 2.0\ g = 24\ g$

Step 3. Determine the weight of acetaminophen per suppository, B:

B = 0.3 g

Step 4. Melt the cocoa butter and incorporate the acetaminophen. Mix the ingredients, pour into molds, cool, trim, and remove from molds.

Step 5. Weigh the 12 suppositories and determine the average weight of a medicated suppository, C.

C = 1.8 g

Step 6. Determine the density factor:

$$df = \frac{0.3\ g}{2\ g - 1.8\ g + 0.3\ g} = 0.6$$

Step 7. Determine the replacement value of the cocoa butter:

$$\frac{0.3 \ g}{0.6} = 0.5 \ g$$

Step 8. Subtract the replacement value of cocoa butter from the average blank weight:

2.0 g – 0.5 g = 1.5 g

Step 9. Determine the quantity of cocoa butter required for the prescription:

12 × 1.5 g = 18 g of cocoa butter, *answer*

Step 10: Determine the quantity of acetaminophen required for the prescription:

12 × 0.3 g = 3.6 g of acetaminophen, *answer*

Dosage Replacement Factor Method

The Dosage Replacement Factor Method is another method of calculating the quantity of base that will be occupied by the active drug. The dosage replacement factor is determined by the following equation:[1]

$$f = \frac{100 \ (E - G)}{(G)(x)} + 1$$

where *f* equals the dosage replacement factor, *E* equals the weight of a pure base suppository, and *G* equals the weight of a suppository containing *x*% of the active ingredient.

Table 13-5 in Chapter 13, "Suppositories," lists dosage replacement factors for selected active drugs. When this factor is not known, the equation above can be used to calculate it. As illustrated in the following problem, the equation can also be used to calculate the total weight of a prepared suppository or other dosage form.

Prepare a suppository containing 100 mg of phenobarbital (f = 0.81) using cocoa butter as the base. The weight of the pure cocoa butter suppository (E) is 2.0 g. Because 100 mg of phenobarbital is to be contained in an approximately 2.0 g suppository, the phenobarbital will occupy 5% (x) of the total weight. What will be the total weight of each suppository?

Step 1. Use the dosage replacement factor equation to solve for the total weight of each suppository, *G*.

$$0.81 = \frac{100 \ (2 - G)}{(G) \ (5)} + 1$$

G = 2.019 g, *answer*

Primary Emulsions Calculation

If a ratio of 4:2:1 is used for the oil:water:acacia (i.e., the Continental Method) called for in the following prescription, what quantity of acacia is required? (See Chapter 17, "Emulsions," for a discussion of the Continental Method.)

℞ **Acacia Emulsion**

Mineral oil		30%
Acacia		
Flavor		qs
Purified water	qs	120 mL

Step 1. Calculate the volume of mineral oil required for the prescription:

0.3×120 mL $= 36$ mL

Step 2. Using the given ratio, calculate the quantity of acacia required for the prescription:

$$\frac{36 \text{ mL}}{4 \text{ parts}} = \frac{x}{1 \text{ part}}$$

$x = 9$ g of acacia, *answer*

Chapter 6

Quality Control

Quality control is an essential feature of any compounding activity. An effective quality control program must ensure that a product is prepared properly and is stable for the expected duration of its use.

Quality Control Testing in the Pharmacy

Although pharmacies generally do not have fully equipped quality control laboratories, it is still possible to establish an adequate quality control program. Setting up such a program begins with the proper facility, equipment, and supplies. Appropriate standard operating procedures (SOPs) should also be implemented to ensure that equipment is working satisfactorily and that products are prepared properly. At a minimum, SOPs should be in place for electronic balances, pH meters, pipets, air temperature and humidity control, and personnel training.

Equipment Calibration/Maintenance

Electronic Balances

A compounding pharmacy must have access to an accurate, well-maintained prescription balance (preferably an electronic balance) and to a set of calibration weights to assess the performance of the balance. The balance must be placed in an area free of drafts and vibrations and should not be moved around. (See SOP "Electronic Balance Calibration/Maintenance.")

pH Meters

A compounding pharmacy should have access to an accurate pH meter and accompanying pH standard solutions to check the pH of liquid preparations. The pH meter should be calibrated before each use. (See SOP "Use, Standardization, and Care of a pH Meter.")

Pipets

Pharmacies should have manual (and in some cases automatic) pipets for measuring small volumes accurately, as well as a method of ensuring that the pipets are calibrated for delivering the required volumes. (See SOP "Calibration of Pipets.")

Air Quality in Compounding Pharmacy

Procedures must be in place to provide for monitoring of room air temperature and humidity and to ensure air quality in the pharmacy compounding laboratory. (See SOP "Monitoring Air Temperature and Humidity.")

Personnel Training

All personnel involved in compounding, including technicians, must be properly trained. (See SOP "Training Personnel in Compounding SOPs.")

Physical Tests

Pharmacists can perform physical quality control tests to ensure the uniformity and accuracy of many small-scale compounded products. These tests include individual dosage unit weights, average individual dosage unit weights, total product weight, pH, and physical observations such as appearance, taste, and smell. The steps involved in each of these tests are listed below. Table 6-1 indicates which tests are appropriate for the various dosage forms. Chapters on specific dosage forms list appropriate quality control tests.

Table 6-1. Physical Quality Control Tests for Compounded Formulations

Dosage Form	Indiv. Dosage Unit Weights	Avg. Indiv. Dosage Unit	Total Product Weight	pH	Physical Observ. (appearance/odor/taste/texture)
Bulk powder			√		√
Powder papers	√	√	√		√
Capsules	√	√	√		√
Tablets	√	√	√		√
Troches	√	√	√		√
Liquids			√	√	√
Ointments			√		√
Suppositories	√	√	√		√
Gels			√	√	√

Individual Dosage Unit Weights

1. Calibrate and tare the balance to be used.
2. Select 10 dosage units and weigh them individually.
3. Record the individual weights.
4. Determine that none of the individual dosage unit weights are off by more than 5% of the average individual dosage unit weight and that they meet the compendial requirements.

Average Individual Dosage Unit Weights

1. Calibrate and tare the balance to be used.
2. Select 10 dosage units and weigh them all together.
3. Divide the total weight obtained by 10 to get the average dosage unit weight.

Total Product Weight

1. Calibrate and tare the balance to be used.
2. Weigh the prepared product.
3. Enter the value on the product worksheet.

pH

1. Calibrate the pH meter for the pH range to be determined.
2. Determine the pH of the product.
3. Record the value on the product worksheet.

Physical Observations

1. Select an appropriate number of dosage units or the total product.
2. Visually observe the preparation for color, clarity, and uniform distribution if suspended or dispersed materials are present. It may be beneficial to use a "light-dark box." Compare with the expected observations of the product.
3. If appropriate and safe, dip a clean, disposable utensil or glass rod into the product and place a drop on the tongue. After tasting, expectorate the product, rinse the mouth, and discard the tasting utensil or glass rod. Compare with the expected taste of the product.
4. Carefully wave a hand over the product, moving the air immediately above it to detect any odor. Compare with the expected odor of the product.

Tests for Sterile Products

When sterile products are involved, it may also be advisable to conduct pyrogenicity and sterility tests. Table 6-2 indicates the appropriate quality control tests for various types of sterile preparations.

An extract of the horseshoe crab, *Limulus* amebocyte lysate (LAL), is used to test the pyrogenicity of a product. The procedure is involved, and care must be taken to use correct technique to attain the test's end point: a reading of the presence or absence of a gel clot. With practice and careful attention to technique, however, the test can be done easily and routinely. Two types of procedures are used to test the sterility of a product. A physical test of the sterilizing process involves applying autoclave tape to the product containers and checking to see whether the temperature required to kill microorganisms was reached. Also, ampules of viable microorganisms can be included with the products to be autoclaved. After the autoclaving process, a sample from the ampule can be placed on a culture plate. The plate is checked after the appropriate time interval to determine whether any microorganisms survived the sterilization process. No sign of microbial growth indicates the sterilization process was successful. A more appropriate test is to place some of the actual sterilized product on culture plates or in tubes of broth media and, after the appropriate time interval, to check for signs of growth of microorganisms.

Table 6-2. Quality Control Tests for Sterile Products

Dosage Form	Sterility	Pyrogenicity
Ophthalmics	√	
Inhalations	√	
Parenterals	√	√
Nasals	√	

Contract Analytical Laboratories

Pharmacists can also call upon contract analytical laboratories to test products, if needed. Such laboratories are particularly helpful if large quantities of a product are compounded. The pharmacist can periodically send samples of the product for analysis for assay and, if appropriate, content uniformity testing. The results of such testing can serve as documentation of the performance of the compounding pharmacy. Once a good relationship has been established with an analytical laboratory, the pharmacy can initiate a program to ensure product stability. Any product prepared in accordance with a *United States Pharmacopeia* monograph must meet the requirements set forth in that monograph. These requirements are designed to be within the capabilities of the compounding pharmacist.

Standard Operating Procedures (SOPs)

Electronic Balance Calibration/Maintenance

Purpose of SOP

The purpose of this procedure is to document how an electronic balance should be operated and maintained. The procedure additionally describes how calibration weights should be maintained and used to check balance performance. Various brands of electronic balances operate in different ways: this SOP is general in nature and can be modified for specific needs. A balance maintenance routine should be conducted annually; the calibration described here should be done at least weekly and recorded on a "Balance Calibration Log" (Figure 6-1).

Regulatory Issues

A compounding pharmacy must have access to an accurate, well-maintained prescription balance (preferably an electronic balance) and to a set of calibration weights to assess the performance of the balance. The balance must be placed in an area free of drafts and vibrations, and should not be moved around.

Balance Operation/Setup

Basic Setup.

1. Press the ON/OFF key to turn the balance on or off.
2. After the power is turned on, a self-test of all essential electronic functions is automatically run, ending with a display readout of 0.000 g. If a container is being used or if the display does not read 0.000 g, make sure the display is zeroed before weighing.

Balance Calibration Log

Balance Model No.: _____ Manufacturer: _____

Date	Initials	Date	Initials	Date	Initials

Figure 6-1. Sample balance calibration log.

3. The weigh display may show various status messages:
   —STANDBY: The balance has been switched off with the ON/OFF key and is now in the STANDBY mode.
   —POWER OFF: The balance has been disconnected from line power or there has been a power failure.
   —CAL: The calibration function has been called.
   —Other messages vary, depending on the balance model. Users should consult the product manual.

Balance Calibration

Internal Calibration. This feature is not available on all balance models.

1. Unload the balance and zero the display (tare).
2. As soon as the display shows a zero readout, press the MENU key; then press TARE. After a few seconds, the display will read CALIBRATE. The calibration procedure will then start. An acoustic signal indicates the end of the procedure.
3. Enter the date and operator's initials in the "Balance Calibration Log."

External Calibration. This method of calibration requires an accurate calibration weight.

1. Unload the balance and depress the tare control to zero.
2. Place the calibration weight in the center of the pan.
3. Press the CALIBRATION or AUTO CAL key.
4. Enter the date and operator's initials on the "Balance Calibration Log."

Procedure for Weighing Substances

The balance may have two display ranges that can be easily selected at the touch of the soft-key selector. This feature provides a convenient, readily accessible method of selecting an accuracy range without having to access a menu and change codes set in the balance operating program. One range has an accuracy of four decimal places (0.1 mg readability), whereas the second range has an accuracy of five decimal places (0.01 mg readability). The balance will stabilize faster in the display range of four decimal places.

1. After turning on the balance, check the display for the accuracy range. The balance will automatically be in one specific range and may need to be changed before use.
2. To select the alternative range, unload the balance and zero the display (tare).
3. Select the other range by pressing the soft-key selector.

Balance Maintenance/Operating Limits

‣ Always store the balance with the dust cover on and the doors closed (if available).
‣ After concluding all weighings, and before beginning new weighings, clean the balance pan and supporting structures with a camel-hair brush.
‣ Ensure that the balance is serviced by a service representative for preventive maintenance on an annual basis.
‣ Ensure that a set of calibration weights is certified on an annual basis. Certification may be done in conjunction with annual maintenance of the balance.

▸ Maintain weights and keep them in a covered weight box near the balance.

Precautions

▸ When using a balance, especially a top-loading balance, make sure it is away from all drafts and vibrations.
▸ Do not place the balance in the proximity of an air-conditioning vent.
▸ If a sliding door is present on the balance, close it for the final determination in the weighing process.

Use, Standardization, and Care of a pH Meter

Purpose of SOP

The purpose of this procedure is to provide for the use, standardization, and care of a pH meter. The meter should be standardized at each use and the results recorded on the "pH Meter Standardization Log" (Figure 6-2).

Procedure

Use of pH Meter.

1. Use a pH meter with a readability of at least ±0.01 pH units.
2. Standardize the pH meter at each use.
3. Allow sufficient stabilization time for each measurement.
4. Ensure that the sample and buffer solution temperatures are the same.
5. Replace buffer solutions frequently to increase accuracy.
6. If sample pH values vary over a wide pH range, use a pH meter with a slope control to allow adjustment of the span for nonideal electrodes.

Buffer Solutions.

1. Use commercially available pH buffer solutions whenever possible.
2. If commercially available buffer solutions are not available, prepare the following buffer solutions using carbon dioxide (CO_2)-free water:
   —pH 4.01 buffer solution consisting of 0.05 M potassium hydrogen phthalate ($KHC_8H_4O_4$)
   —pH 6.86 buffer consisting of 0.025 M potassium dihydrogen phosphate (KH_2PO_4) and 0.025 M disodium hydrogen phosphate (Na_2HPO_4)
   —pH 9.18 buffer consisting of 0.01 M sodium tetraborate decahydrate ($Na_2B_4O_7 \cdot 10H_2O$)

Standardization of pH Meter. Two standardization methods can be used to standardize pH meters: the one-point method or the two-point method. If all sample pH values are close to the point of standardization (within 1–2 pH units), the one-point method can be used. If, however, the pH values vary somewhat from the point of standardization (greater than 2 pH units) and a high degree of accuracy is required, the two-point method should be used.

To use the **one-point method** of standardization:

1. Measure the temperature of the standard buffer solution.
2. Set the temperature compensator (knob) on the pH meter to that measured temperature.
3. Rinse the electrode with a portion of distilled water or a portion of the standard buffer solution to be used.
4. Place the electrode in a fresh portion of the standard buffer solution and activate the meter.

pH Meter Standardization Log

pH Meter Model No.: _____ Manufacturer: _____

Date	Initials	Date	Initials	Date	Initials

Figure 6-2. Sample pH meter standardization log.

5. Allow the electrode to equilibrate with the standard buffer solution before setting the meter readout to the pH value for that temperature.
6. Set the meter readout to the standard buffer solution value.
7. Place the meter on STANDBY and rinse and blot the electrode.
8. Record the date of the calibration and the operator's initials on the "pH Meter Standardization Log" (Figure 6-2).

The **two-point method** requires a slope control adjustment.

1. When using the two-point method, start the standardization using a pH 7 buffer.
2. Select a second standard buffer with a pH value close to the sample pH value.
3. Measure the temperature of the two standard buffer solutions. They should be similar.
4. Rinse the electrode with a portion of distilled water or a portion of the standard buffer solution to be used.
5. Place the electrode in a fresh portion of the pH 7 standard buffer solution and activate the pH meter.
6. Allow the electrode to equilibrate with the standard buffer solution before setting the meter readout to the pH value of the standard buffer solution.
7. Set the meter readout to the standard buffer solution values.
8. Rinse and blot the electrode.
9. Repeat steps 6–8 with the second standard buffer solution.
10. Place the meter on STANDBY.
11. To make a measurement, place the electrode in the sample and activate the pH meter.
12. Allow the electrode to equilibrate and record the pH value.
13. Place the meter in the STANDBY position.
14. Rinse the electrode with distilled water and blot.
15. Place the electrode in the storage solution.
16. Record the date of the calibration and the operator's initials on the "pH Meter Standardization Log" (Figure 6-2).

Measurement of pH.

1. With the meter in a STANDBY position, remove the electrode from the storage buffer.
2. Rinse the electrode with distilled water or an aliquot of the sample.
3. Measure the sample temperature and set the pH meter temperature compensator (knob) to that measured temperature.
4. Place the rinsed electrode in the sample and activate the meter.
5. Allow the reading to stabilize before recording the pH value.
6. Place the meter in the STANDBY position.
7. Rinse the electrode with distilled water and blot.
8. Repeat for additional samples or place electrode in the storage solution.

Rinsing of the Electrode.

1. To minimize carry-over contamination, rinse the electrode between measurements.
2. Use distilled water and a wiping tissue to blot, not rub, the electrode bulb; or, if a sufficient quantity of sample is available, rinse the electrode with the next sample before actually immersing the electrode in the sample for

a reading. (Note: Rubbing the bulb can impart static electricity to the bulb, resulting in a slow equilibration time for the next reading.)

Care of the Electrode.

1. Keep the electrode wet in a soaking or storage solution, preferably of pH 4 buffer.
2. Use a container for storage that fits around the electrode to provide a tight seal between the electrode and the cap for the container.

Rejuvenation of the Electrode. The response time to obtain a normal pH reading of a buffer solution should stabilize within 10 seconds to 98% of the final reading. If the electrode develops a long lag time (time to stabilize at the value) or slow response time (time meter takes to respond), it may need to be rejuvenated.

1. If the electrode has been used with an organic material, use a suitable organic solvent to remove the material from the electrode bulb.
2. Remove the organic solvent from the electrode by using an intermediate polarity solvent, such as alcohol.
3. Immerse the electrode bulb in 0.1 M HCl for 5 minutes, remove, rinse with distilled water, and blot dry.
4. Immerse the electrode bulb in 0.1 M NaOH for 5 minutes, remove, rinse with distilled water, and blot dry.
5. Immerse the electrode bulb in 0.1 M HCl for 5 minutes, remove, rinse with distilled water, and blot dry.
6. Check the electrode's response. The preceding measures should have made the electrode responsive. If the electrode is still unresponsive, it may need to be replaced.

Calibration of Pipets

Purpose of SOP

The purpose of this procedure is to ensure that all manual and automatic pipets used in the pharmacy are calibrated and are delivering the appropriate volume. At a minimum, pipets should be calibrated every 12 months.

Regulatory Issues

A compounding pharmacy must have access to accurate, well-maintained pipets when measuring small volumes of liquids.

Measure four pipet deliveries gravimetrically at room temperature, average the results, and calculate a percentage error. If the pipet has a single reading out of the individual error range or fails to achieve an average error of less than 4%, adjust it and recheck. For calculations, assume a specific gravity for water of 1.000 g/mL (1.000 mg/μL).

Equipment/Materials

- Electronic balance.
- Weighing boats.
- Beaker of purified water USP.
- Appropriate size pipet tips.
- Pipet.
- "Pipet Calibration Worksheet" (Figure 6-3).

Pipet Calibration Worksheet

Brand/Model: _____

Volume: _____

Person Performing Calibration: _____

Date of Calibration: _____

Weight of Individual
Water Deliveries (mg)

Individual Error Range
for Pipet Volume (Wt)
(see Table 6-3)

#1   _____   _____(mg)

#2   _____

#3   _____

#4   _____

Total   _____

Total divided by 4   _____

Highest recorded weight (H)   _____

Lowest recorded weight (L)   _____

Difference between H and L   _____

Difference divided by highest
recorded weight (H − L/H)   _____

Multiply previous value   _____
by 100 (H − L/H × 100)   (Value should be less than 4%)

Pipet Passes Calibration Test   **YES** _____   **NO**_____

Figure 6-3. Sample pipet calibration worksheet.

Procedure

1. Turn on the electronic balance.
2. Check the calibration on the balance.
3. Put a weighing boat on the balance and tare to zero.
4. Pipet one delivery of water into the boat and record the weight on the form. Retare the balance.
5. Using the same pipet, repeat step 4 three more times and record all readings on the "Pipet Calibration Worksheet" (Figure 6-3). (Note: Each individual reading must fall in the acceptable individual error range for a given pipet. See Table 6-3 for acceptable limits. As shown in the table, the value of the individual error range is equal to a 5% maximum error for all pipets. If the pipet fails to fall into this predefined error range, adjust the pipet and repeat steps 4 and 5.)
6. Average the four weighings and record results.
7. Calculate the average percentage error and record. Calculate by subtracting the low pipet value (L) from the high (H), then dividing the remainder

Table 6-3. Acceptable Individual Error Ranges for Pipets

Expected Pipet Volume	Individual Error Range ($\pm$5% mg)
10 μL	9.5–10.5
25 μL	23.75–26.25
50 μL	47.5–52.5
100 μL	95–105
200 μL	190–210
250 μL	237.5–262.5
300 μL	285–315
500 μL	475–525
1000 μL	950–1050

by the high value and multiplying by 100 to arrive at a final percentage. The calculation is therefore H − L/H × 100. (Note: Average error must be less than or equal to a value of 4% for the pipet to pass.)

8. Record on the "Pipet Calibration Worksheet" whether the pipet passed (all individual *and* average error range limits were satisfied) or failed. Record raw data, even if pipet fails initial tests.

9. If the pipet fails the test, adjust the pipet and repeat steps 4 through 8. Either repair or discard pipets that cannot be calibrated to deliver the appropriate volume.

10. After pipets have been checked, turn off the electronic balance.

Monitoring Air Temperature and Humidity

Purpose of SOP

The purpose of this procedure is to ensure proper monitoring of room air temperature and humidity, and to ensure good air quality in the pharmacy compounding laboratory.

Procedure

Monitoring Air Temperature.

1. Maintain temperatures in the compounding pharmacy between 68°F (20°C) and 77°F (25°C) at all times. This temperature range is important for proper storage and stability of chemicals and products.

2. Determine the temperature of the room daily, using a suitable, nonmobile thermometer located in the immediate vicinity of the compounding area. A digital centigrade thermometer reading to one decimal place is recommended.

3. Record the temperature on the "Air Temperature and Humidity Log" (Figure 6-4).
4. Place form in a notebook.

Monitoring Air Humidity.

1. Determine the humidity in the compounding pharmacy daily using a suitable, nonmobile hygrometer located in the immediate vicinity of the compounding area. A digital hygrometer is recommended. Humidity control is important for proper storage and stability of chemicals and products. It is also important when compounding materials that are hygroscopic, deliquescent, or efflorescent, or that contain water of hydration.
2. Record the humidity on the "Air Temperature and Humidity Log."
3. Place form in a notebook.

Maintaining Air Quality. Routinely cleaning reusable filters or installing new disposable filters in the air-handling system serving the compounding laboratory will ensure appropriately clean, filtered air. Filters should be checked on a scheduled basis, such as every 30 to 60 days, depending on the quality of the air in the laboratory. The following procedures are suggested:

1. Using a nonlinting wiper moistened with 70% isopropanol, clean the outer surface of the air-handling unit.
2. Remove the fastening agents and set the access panel aside.
3. Remove the soiled filter, gently slide it into a plastic bag, and tightly seal the bag.
4. Using a nonlinting wiper moistened with 70% isopropanol, clean the filter housing.
5. Install a new filter, noting the direction for proper airflow.
6. Clean the access panel with 70% isopropanol, replace the panel, and tighten the fastening agents firmly.
7. Attach a label to the exterior of the air-handling unit, noting the date the filter was changed and the next due date for changing the filter.
8. Properly discard the soiled filter, contained in the plastic bag, in the trash.
9. Note in the notebook containing forms for monitoring of air temperature and humidity when the next filter change is due.

Training Personnel in Compounding SOPs

Purpose of SOP

The purpose of this procedure is to establish appropriate guidelines and documentation for all personnel involved in the compounding, evaluation, packaging, and dispensing of compounded preparations.

Applicable Personnel

This procedure applies to all existing employees and to all future employees whose function is related to pharmaceutical compounding.

Air Temperature and Humidity Log

Date	Time	Temper-ature	Humidity		Date	Time	Temper-ature	Humidity

Figure 6-4. Sample log for monitoring air temperatures and humidity of compounding laboratory.

Regulatory Issues

Chapter <795>, "Pharmacy Compounding," of the *United States Pharmacopeia 25/National Formulary 20 (USP 25/NF 20)* states:[1]

> The pharmacist is responsible for compounding preparations of acceptable strength, quality, and purity with appropriate packaging and labeling in accordance with good pharmacy practices, official standards, and relevant scientific data and information. Pharmacists engaging in compounding should continually expand their compounding knowledge by participating in seminars, studying appropriate literature, and consulting colleagues.

It is important that the compounding pharmacist be well trained and that all personnel (pharmacy technicians) involved in compounding also be well trained and participate in training programs. The pharmacist is responsible for ensuring that an ongoing training program has been implemented. Pharmacy practice standards require that every employee be adequately trained in his or her job function and that all of the training be properly documented. Training is advantageous to both the employer and the employee because trained employees are more efficient, safe, and motivated.

Procedure

1. All employees involved in pharmaceutical compounding will read and become familiar with Chapter <795>, "Pharmacy Compounding," of the *USP 25/NF 20*.
2. All employees will read and become familiar with each of the SOPs related to compounding, including those involving the facility, equipment, personnel, actual compounding, and evaluation, packaging, storage, and dispensing of compounded formulations.
3. The pharmacist will meet with employees and review their work and answer any questions the employees may have concerning the SOPs.
4. The pharmacist will first demonstrate the procedures for the employee, and then guide the employee step by step through the procedure. The employee will then repeat the procedure without any help, but under supervision from the pharmacist.
5. When the employee has demonstrated to the pharmacist a verbal and operational knowledge of the procedure, then and only then will the employee be permitted to perform the procedure without supervision.
6. When the pharmacist is satisfied with the employee's knowledge and proficiency, the pharmacist will sign off on the "Compounding SOPs Training Documentation Log" (Figure 6-5) to show that both agree the employee is proficient in compounding SOPs.
7. The pharmacist will continually monitor the work of the employee and answer any questions the employee may have concerning the SOPs.

Reference

1. Expert Advisory Panel on Pharmacy Compounding Practices. Pharmacy compounding. In: *United States Pharmacopeia 25/National Formulary 20*. Rockville, Md: United States Pharmacopeial Convention; 2001.

Compounding SOPs Training Documentation Log

Employee Name: _____   Date Started: _____

Job Title:_____

Date	SOP No.	SOP Title	Employee Signature	Pharmacist Signature

I have read and understand Chapter <795>, "Pharmacy Compounding," of the *United States Pharmacopeia/National Formulary.* I understand that this chapter is the standard of practice for pharmaceutical compounding.

Employee Signature:_____   Date:_____

Pharmacist Signature: _____   Date:_____

Figure 6-5. Sample log for employee training in compounding SOPs.

Chapter 7

Flavors, Sweeteners, and Colors

Flavoring, sweetening, and coloring are vital to patient compliance when medication is administered orally. Many drugs have disagreeable tastes, and the stronger the taste, the more difficult the task of patient compliance. One cannot simply add a flavor to a dosage form containing a bad-tasting drug and expect it to taste good. There is also the challenge of minimizing the taste of a dosage form that remains in the mouth for an extended period of time, such as troches, lollipops, and gummy gels. These dosage forms must also have a smooth surface texture in order for the patient to accept them, but they cannot be disagreeably sticky.

Preparation of an Acceptable Product

A pharmacist willing to spend the time can usually convert a bad-tasting medication into an acceptable product by considering the following techniques:[1]

- Selecting the proper flavor or flavor blends, not necessarily relying on what is traditionally used.
- Replacing or adjusting a vehicle if it is inadequate.
- Selecting a nonoffending preservative.
- Using artificial sweeteners in the proper amount and balance.
- Using desensitizing agents and/or flavor enhancers.
- Obtaining the proper mouth feel, such as smoothness, that results with increased viscosity.
- Complementing any bitterness with an acceptable bitter flavor, such as coffee, chocolate, or maple.
- Masking objectionable tastes by use of the cooling effect of mint and the anesthetizing effect of spices.
- Using acids, such as tartaric, citric, maleic, and the like, to enhance fruit flavors.

Flavor and Taste

The flavor experience is very complex and is a combination of the sensations of taste, smell, touch (texture), sight, and even sound. In general, individuals are more sensitive to odors than to tastes; however, because of a decline in the sense of smell among persons of advanced age, this population may be able to smell only odors at levels that are three to five times greater than that required for young people. Females tend to have a greater sensitivity to odors than do males. Furthermore, disease can alter taste and smell, as evidenced when one has a cold or the flu. Infants and children tend to prefer sweet tastes and do not respond well to things that are bitter. They like flavors such as butterscotch, citrus, berry, and vanilla. Adults accept reasonable levels of bitterness in drug products; thus, wine, spice, chocolate, or anise combinations can be used. For those who fall between the pediatric and advanced-age populations, almost any flavor can be used. Patients who must take a preparation for a long time may require milder flavors, which are less likely to cause flavor fatigue.

Basics of Taste

The four primary tastes are sweet, sour, salty, and bitter. Table 7-1 describes solutions that illustrate these four primary tastes. The chemical structure of a drug can provide an indication of the possible taste the drug might have. Table 7-2 cites some correlations between chemical properties and taste and odor. For example, inorganic salts in solution will result in anions and/or cations in solution, which will elicit a salty taste. Many drugs are organic compounds that have high molecular weights; these compounds have a bitter taste and are among the most difficult to mask. The presence of unsaturated, double bonds results in a sharp, biting taste. Sugars, sorbitol, glycerin, and other polyhydroxyl compounds have a sweet taste, as do alpha-amino acids.

Table 7-1. Solutions That Illustrate the Four Primary Tastes

Solution Strength	Sweet (% sucrose)	Sour (% citric acid)	Salty (% NaCl)	Bitter (% caffeine)
Slight	5	0.05	0.4	0.05
Moderate	10	0.10	0.7	0.10
Strong	15	0.20	1.0	0.20

Source: Reference 1.

Other factors to consider in deriving good-tasting products are as follows: (1) a hot taste is due to a mild counterirritant effect, (2) an astringent taste is due to tannins and acids, (3) coarseness or grittiness is due to texture, and (4) coolness is due to a negative heat of solution. Preservatives also have characteristic flavors, odors, and sensations. Alcohol has a biting taste. Methylparaben has a floral aroma similar to that of gauze pads. Propylparaben and butylparaben produce a sense of numbness in the mouth; thus, it is best to use the lowest concentration possible of these preservatives.

Table 7-2. Correlations between Chemical Properties and Taste and Odor

Taste	Chemical Property
Sour	H⁺
Salty	Simultaneous presence of anions and cations
Bitter	High molecular weight salts
Sweet	Polyhydroxyl compounds, polyhydrogenated compounds, alpha-amino acids
Sharp, biting	Unsaturation

Odor	Chemical Property
Fruity	Esters, lactones
Pleasant	Ketones
Camphoraceous	Tertiary carbon atom

Source: Reference 3.

Flavoring Techniques

Flavoring is both a challenge and an opportunity. It is a challenge because no single correct method exists to solve an ill-defined problem; it is an opportunity because it enables a pharmacist to prepare a product that a patient is willing to take. By following the basic principles presented in this chapter, one should be able to handle successfully many of the flavoring problems that occur in compounding preparations, particularly for pediatric patients.

An acceptable flavor for a patient involves such aspects as (1) immediate flavor identity, (2) rapid full flavor development, (3) acceptable mouth feel, (4) short aftertaste, and (5) no undesirable sensations.[2]

Numerous approaches can be used to prepare an acceptable product that minimizes the bad taste of drugs. These approaches include blending, overshadowing, physical methods, chemical methods, and physiological methods.[3]

Blending is the use of a flavor that blends with the drug taste. In other words, drugs with an acidic taste can be blended with citrus fruit flavors. An example might be the use of orange to blend with ascorbic acid. Salty, sweet, and sour tastes can be used to blend with a bitter taste. The addition of a slightly salty taste may actually decrease sourness and increase sweetness. Bitter tastes can also be partially overcome by adding a sour flavor.

Overshadowing, or overpowering, involves the use of a flavor with a stronger intensity and longer residence time in the mouth than the original product. Examples are wintergreen oil and glycyrrhiza.

Physical methods include (1) the formation of insoluble compounds as a suspension (a drug cannot be tasted if it is not in solution); (2) the emulsification of oils (i.e., placing the bad-tasting drug in the internal phase of an emulsion and flavoring or sweetening the external phase that will be in contact with the oral cavity); (3) the use of effervescent additives, which is a good approach for salty-tasting drugs; and (4) the use of high-viscosity fluids, such as syrups, which tend to keep the flavor in the mouth longer.

Chemical methods of overcoming bad tastes include adsorbing or complexing the drug with an ingredient that eliminates the undesirable taste.

Physiological techniques involve the cooling sensation experienced by mannitol, which is caused by its negative heat of solution, or the anesthetic action of products such as menthol, peppermint, and spearmint. These products serve as desensitizers, which means they reduce the sensitivity of the taste buds to bitterness. Some spices, such as clove and cinnamon, can achieve the same end since they introduce heat and numbness, creating a mild pain reaction.

Flavor intensifiers, such as monosodium glutamate, can serve as flavor enhancers. Citrus enhancers include citric, maleic, or tartaric acids. Flavor enhancement by adding small amounts of vanilla to the basic flavor is a technique long used in the flavor industry. Vanilla seems to intensify and stimulate other flavors to a quicker taste response without altering their basic taste or adding its own taste.

Different flavors and sweeteners can provide different sensations in the mouth. Saccharin may create a rapid bitter sensation followed by a sweet flavor sensation. Sucrose gives a fast sweet sensation that intensifies the full-bodied taste of other flavors. This reaction might also be related to the high viscosity of the product. Many natural flavors do have a "prominent" ingredient. For example, the primary active constituent in cherry is benzaldehyde; in banana, isoamylacetate; in spearmint, L-carvone; and in orange, lemonene. Table 7-3 cites selected flavors that mask some basic tastes.

Table 7-3. Representative Flavors Used to Mask Some Basic Tastes

Taste	Flavor
Sweet	Vanilla, fruit, grape, bubblegum, berry
Acid/sour	Lemon, lime, orange, cherry, grapefruit, raspberry, acacia
Salty	Nut, butter, butterscotch, spice, maple
Bitter	Licorice (anise), coffee, chocolate, mint, grapefruit, cherry, peach, raspberry, orange, lemon, lime
Oily	Peppermint, anise, wintergreen
Metallic	Berry, mint, grape, marshmallow

Source: References 2 and 3.

Lozenges and gummy gels present another problem because of their long residence time in the mouth. To compensate, it is recommended that the quantity of flavoring for these medications be about 5 to 10 times that used in candy products.

If flavoring oils are to be added to aqueous-based products, the oils can be dissolved in a small quantity of glycerin or sorbitol and then incorporated into the product. This technique can also be used to incorporate an oily drug into a lozenge, lollipop, or gummy gel. The solvent technique often uses a ratio of 1 part of solvent, such as glycerin, for 3 to 5 parts of the drug. Example flavors for various classes of drugs are provided in Table 7-4.[4]

Table 7-4. Suggested Flavors for Selected Drug Classes/Populations

Drug Class/ Populations	Flavors
Antibiotics	Cherry, maple, pineapple, orange, raspberry, banana-pineapple, banana-vanilla, coconut-custard, strawberry-vanilla, lemon-custard, cherry-custard, fruit-cinnamon
Antihistamines	Apricot, black currant, cherry, cinnamon, custard, grape, honey, lime, loganberry, peach-orange, peach-rum, raspberry, root beer, wild cherry
Barbiturates	Banana-pineapple, banana-vanilla, black currant, cinnamon-peppermint, grenadine-strawberry, lime, orange, peach-orange, root beer
Decongestants and expectorants	Anise, apricot, black-currant, butterscotch, cherry, coconut-custard, custard-mint-strawberry, grenadine-peach, strawberry, lemon, gooseberry, loganberry, maple, orange, orange-lemon, coriander, orange-peach, pineapple, raspberry, strawberry, tangerine
Electrolytes	Cherry, grape, lemon-lime, raspberry, wild cherry syrup
Patients of Advanced Age	Black currant, grenadine-strawberry, lime, root beer, wild strawberry

Source: Reference 4.

Flavoring Agents

Definitions and Properties

Some terms used to describe flavors and their definitions are as follows.

- *Natural flavor:* Essential oil, oleoresin, essence or extractive, protein hydrolysate, distillate, or any product of roasting, heating, or enzymolysis, which contains the flavoring constituents derived from a spice, fruit or fruit juice, vegetable or vegetable juice, edible yeast, herb, bark, bud, root, leaf or similar plant material, meat, seafood, poultry, eggs, dairy products, or fermentation products thereof whose significant function in food is flavoring rather than nutritional.[5] (The exact composition of "all natural" flavors is unknown.)
- *Artificial flavor:* Any substance used to impart flavor that is not derived from a spice, fruit or fruit juice, vegetable or vegetable juice, edible yeast, herb, bark, bud, root, leaf or similar plant material, meat, fish, poultry, eggs, dairy products, or fermentation products thereof.[6]
- *Spice:* Any aromatic vegetable substance in whole, broken, or ground form, except those substances which have been traditionally regarded as foods, such as onions, garlic, and celery; whose significant function in food is seasoning rather than nutritional; that is true to name; and from which no portion of any volatile oil or other flavoring principle has been removed.[7]

Flavors can be obtained as oil- or water-soluble liquids and as dry powders; most are diluted in carriers. Oil-soluble carriers include soybean and other edible oils; water-soluble carriers include water, ethanol, propylene glycol, glycerin, and emulsifiers. Dry carriers include maltodextrins, corn syrup solids, modified starches, gum arabic, salt, sugars, and whey protein.

Flavors can degrade as a result of exposure to light, temperature, headspace oxygen, water, enzymes, contaminants, and other product components.

Flavors are regulated as follows: the Food and Drug Administration regulates food and pharmaceutical products; the U.S. Department of Agriculture, meat products; and the Bureau of Alcohol, Tobacco, and Firearms, alcoholic products.

Commercial Flavor Designations

Some commonly used commercial designations and their components include the following. (Note: ABCD would be the flavor name, such as cherry.)

Flavor Designation	Components
Natural ABCD	Flavor All components derived from ABCD.
ABCD Flavor—Natural and Artificial No definition of natural to artificial ratio.	At least one component derived from ABCD.
ABCD Flavor—With Other Natural Flavors (WONF) At least one component derived from ABCD.	All components are natural.
Natural Flavor—ABCD Type No components derived from ABCD.	All components are natural.
ABCD Flavor—Artificial Flavor	All components are artificial.
Conceptual Flavors No reference point. May have to declare only in ingredient declaration.	May contain artificial flavors.

Table 7-5 lists some general techniques for selecting flavors.

Effect on Drug Stability

Not all drugs are stable in the presence of flavoring materials. Flavors are complex mixtures that are made up of many chemicals. For example, natural cherry flavor contains more than 70 components and artificial cherry flavor has more than 20; natural banana flavor has more than 150 components and artificial banana has more than 17; natural grape flavor has about 225 components and artificial grape flavor has more than 18. Since each component is a chemical, it may potentially affect the stability of the drug(s) in the formulation. Many natural flavors do have a "prominent" ingredient, for example, benzaldehyde in cherry, isoamylacetate in banana, L-carvone in spearmint, and lemonene in orange.

Another factor to consider is whether the flavors adsorb to containers during preparation of the drug product or during storage. Another problem involves the sorption of flavors to suspended materials or the partitioning of the flavor into the internal phase of emulsions. Any flavor loss should be investigated and corrected.

Table 7.5 Techniques for Selecting Flavors

Type of Flavoring	Test Medium	Preparation
Water-soluble flavors: Generally start at 0.2% for artificial and 1%–2% for natural flavors	Sweetened water containing 8%–10% sugar	Add sugar to water, then add flavoring. Add 0.2%–0.3% citric acid if a fruit flavor
	Sugar syrup, high-fructose corn syrup, or corn syrup	Add flavor to choice of sweetener. Heat mixture in a microwave for 10–20 seconds. Cool before tasting
Oil-soluble flavors: Generally start at 0.1% in finished product for artificial flavors and 0.2% for natural flavors	Powdered sugar and melted shortening in 1:1 ratio	Mix sugar and melted shortening. Add flavor, and taste
	Vegetable oil (especially good for butter and nutty tastes)	Mix oil and flavoring, and taste
Powdered flavors: Generally start at 0.1% in finished product for artificial flavors and 0.75% for natural flavors	Fruit flavors: sugar 98% and citric acid 2%	Mix sugar, citric acid, and flavoring. Add about 75 g/L of water to mixture
	Other flavors: sugar	Mix sugar and flavoring. Add about 75 g/L of water to mixture

Sweeteners

A number of agents are commonly used as sweeteners, including sucrose, dextrose, corn syrup, sorbitol, mannitol, and other sugars. Since many sugars are used in relatively high concentrations, their viscosity effect may retard the rate of dissolution of some drugs. Therefore, it is often advisable to dissolve the active drugs and other excipients in the aqueous vehicle before adding the sugar(s).

Noncaloric sweeteners include saccharin (sodium) and aspartame. Saccharin is about 250 to 500 times as sweet as sucrose, but its bitter aftertaste must be addressed. Aspartame is approximately 200 times sweeter than sucrose and is very widely used. It does not have a prominent aftertaste, but it does have a stability profile that is pH and temperature dependent. For example, aspartame is most stable between pH 3.4 and 5 at refrigerated temperatures. Since it is often used in products that are heated (e.g., syrups, troches), one must be aware of its potential degradation at elevated temperatures. Because the preparation time of most pharmaceutical products is relatively short, the product does not remain at an elevated temperature for long and hence the aspartame should be stable.

A number of agents are commonly used as sweeteners, including sucrose, dextrose, corn syrup, sorbitol, mannitol, and other sugars. Since many sugars are used in relatively high concentrations, their viscosity effect may retard the rate of dissolution of some drugs. Therefore, it is often advisable to dissolve the active drugs and other excipients in the aqueous vehicle prior to adding the sweetener(s).

A wide variety of sweeteners is available for liquid, semisolid, and solid dosage forms. The *United States Pharmacopeia 25/National Formulary 20* does not list all commonly used sweeteners, but it lists 15 monographs in the category of Sweetening Agents, including Aspartame, Dextrates, Dextrose, Dextrose Excipient, Fructose, Mannitol, Saccharin, Saccharin Calcium, Saccharin Sodium, Sorbitol, Sorbitol Solution, Sucrose, Sugar Compressible, Sugar Confectioner's, and Syrup. Table 7-6 contains information on the properties of some of the sweetening agents.

Acesulfame potassium, an intense sweetening agent that is also a flavor enhancer, can be effectively used to mask some unpleasant tastes. It is quite stable in the solid state, in solution, and at elevated temperatures. Synergism with other sweeteners has been effectively used, especially with aspartame or sodium cyclamate.[1]

Aspartame has an intensely sweet taste. It is stable when dry, but can hydrolyze in the presence of moisture. It degrades during prolonged heating; using higher temperatures for short time periods, followed by rapid cooling, can minimize the problem. Aspartame can be used synergistically with saccharin, sucrose, glucose, and cyclamate, and its taste can actually be enhanced with sodium bicarbonate, gluconate salts, and lactose. It does not have the aftertaste associated with saccharin, but it does have a pH- and temperature-dependent stability profile. For example, it is most stable between pH 3.4 and 5 at refrigerated temperatures.

Dextrates is a purified mixture of saccharides from the controlled enzymatic hydrolysis of starch. Dextrates may be heated at 50°C without any appreciable darkening in color.

Dextrose is widely used as a sweetening and tonicity-adjusting agent and as a tablet diluent and binder. It is a stable material and should be stored in a cool, dry place. One gram of anhydrous dextrose is approximately equivalent to 1.1 g of dextrose monohydrate.

Fructose is used as a flavor enhancer, sweetening agent for syrups and solutions, and tablet diluent. Fructose is sweeter than mannitol and sorbitol and is effective at masking unpleasant flavors in tablet formulations; its sweetness profile is experienced more rapidly in the mouth than that of sucrose and dextrose. Also, its greater solubility in alcohol is sometimes an advantage.

Liquid glucose can be used to provide body and sweetness to liquid formulations. It contains dextrose and smaller amounts of dextrins and maltose, being prepared by the partial hydrolysis of starch with acid. Although not a pure, specific chemical entity, it is reasonably uniform from batch to batch.

Glycerin is about two thirds as sweet as sucrose. It is a hygroscopic liquid and should be stored in airtight containers in a cool place. It is not prone to oxidation but will decompose on heating. When glycerin is mixed with water, ethanol, and propylene glycol, the mixtures are chemically stable.

Maltitol solution is an aqueous solution of a hydrogenated, partially hydrolyzed starch that is used as a sweetening and suspending agent. It is noncrystallizing and prevents cap-locking in syrups and elixirs. It is a colorless, odorless, clear viscous liquid that is sweet tasting.

Mannitol is a hexahydric alcohol related to mannose and is isomeric with sorbitol. It imparts a cooling sensation in the mouth (due to its negative heat of solution). It is used as a sweetening agent, tablet and capsule diluent, tonicity agent, and bulking agent and is especially useful for chewable tablet formulations.

Saccharin is odorless or has a faint aromatic odor, and its solutions are acid to litmus. Its relative sweetening power is increased by dilution.

Saccharin calcium is odorless or has a faint aromatic odor. Saccharin sodium is an intense sweetening agent. Saccharin sodium is a white, odorless or faintly

Table 7-6. Usual Concentrations and Solubilities of Sweetening Agents

Sweetener	Usual Con-centration (%)	Sweetness[b]	Solubility (mL solvent/1 g sweetener)[a]		
			Water	Alcohol	Other
Acesulfame potassium	—	180–200	3.7	1000	100 (50% alcohol)
Aspartame	—	180–200	SpS	SlS	
Cyclamate calcium	0.17	30	FS	PrIn	
Cyclamate sodium	0.17	30	5	250	Propylene glycol (25)
Dextrates	—	0.5	1	PrIn	
Dextrose	—	0.65	1	60	Sol (in glycerin)
Fructose	—	1.17	0.3	15	
Liquid glucose	20–60	—	Misc	PartMisc	
Glycerin	≤20	—	Misc	Misc	
Maltitol solution	—	0.75	Misc	Misc (<55% ethanol)	
Mannitol	—	0.5	5.5	83 (18)	Glycerin
Saccharin	0.02–0.5 w/w	500	290	31 (50)	Glycerin
Saccharin calcium	0.075–0.6	300	2.6	4.7	
Saccharin sodium	0.075–0.6	300	1.2	50	Propylene glycol (3.5)
Sorbitol	20–70	0.5–0.6	0.5	25	
Stevia powder	<0.3	30	Sol		
Stevioside	<0.03	300	Sol		
Sucrose	≤85 w/v	1	0.5	170	
Sugar, compressible	10–60	0.98	0.5 (sucrose)	170 (sucrose)	
Sugar, confectioner's	10–50	0.95	0.5 (sucrose)	170 (sucrose)	
Syrup	—	0.85	Misc	Misc	
Xylitol	—	1.0	1.6	80	Propylene glycol (15)

[a]At 20°C unless otherwise specified.
[b]Sweetness relative to sucrose, with sucrose being "1.0."

aromatic, efflorescent, crystalline powder with an intensely sweet taste and a metallic or bitter aftertaste. It decomposes upon heating to a high temperature (125°C) at a low pH (about pH 2).

Sodium cyclamate can be used to enhance flavor systems and to mask some unpleasant taste characteristics; it is often used in combination with saccharin.

Sorbitol occurs as a white, hygroscopic powder, granules, or flakes with a sweet taste. It is also commercially available as a 70% solution.

Stevia (honey leaf, yerba dulce) powder is a relatively new sweetening agent. It is the extract from the leaves of the *Stevia rebaudiana* Bertoni plant. Its sweet taste is attributed to sweet glycosides such as the steviosides, rebaudiosides, and a dulcoside. It is natural, nontoxic, and safe and occurs as a white, crystalline, hygroscopic powder. It can be used in both hot and cold preparations. The source of stevia is important, as some countries (e.g., Paraguay) produce a sweeter and higher-quality product than that obtained from other countries.

Sucrose has a long history of use and is available in highly purified form at a reasonable cost. It is obtained from sugar cane, sugar beet, or other sources. When finely divided, it is hygroscopic and can absorb up to 1% water. Sucrose is stable at room temperature. When heated, it caramelizes at temperatures greater than 160°C. Its dilute solutions support microbial growth and can be sterilized by filtration or autoclaving. When sucrose is used in candy-based products, at temperatures rising from 110°C to 145°C, some inversion of sucrose to dextrose and fructose occurs; one potential problem is that fructose may cause stickiness, but it will inhibit cloudiness/graininess. This inversion process is enhanced in the presence of acids and at temperatures greater than 130°C. The tendency of sucrose to crystallize as seen in cap-locking (i.e., sucrose crystallizes on the threads of the bottle cap and makes cap removal difficult) can be minimized if sucrose is used in conjunction with sorbitol, glycerin, or other polyols.

Syrup NF is a solution of 85% w/v sucrose in purified water. It may be prepared by the use of boiling water or, preferably, using the percolation method, which requires no heat. Unless used when freshly prepared, it should contain a preservative; it has a specific gravity of not less than 1.30.

Xylitol is a noncariogenic sweetening agent used in tablets, syrups, and coatings. It has a sweet taste, and imparts a cooling sensation in the mouth. It is heat stable but can caramelize if heated for several minutes near its boiling point (215°C–217°C).

The cooling sensation of some sugars is due to their negative heats of solution; for example, the following comparisons are given in joules per gram (J/g): mannitol (−120.9), sorbitol (−111.3), sucrose (−18.0), xylitol (−153.1).

Coloring Agents

It is not always necessary to color a product. If a coloring agent is used, however, it should be selected to match the flavor (i.e., green for mint, red for cherry). Better results are generally obtained by using minimal quantities of dyes, which will produce light-to-moderate color densities.

References

1. *The PFC Index—A Guide to Flavor and Fragrance Elegance.* Camden, NJ: The Pharmaceutical Flavor Clinic, Division of Foote & Jenks: 10, 16–17.
2. Reiland TL. Physical methods of taste-masking. Presented at the 1990 Annual

Meeting of the American Association of Pharmaceutical Scientists, Las Vegas, November 4–8, 1990.

3. Reilly WJ Jr. Pharmaceutical necessities. In: Gennaro AR, ed, *Remington: The Science and Practice of Pharmacy.* 20th ed. Baltimore: Lippincott Williams & Wilkins; 2000: 1015–50.

4. Neuroth MI. Liquid medications. In: Martin EW. *Dispensing of Medication.* 7th ed. Easton, Pa: Mack Publishing Co; 1971: 859.

5. *Code of Federal Regulations.* April 1, 2001;21CFR101.22(a)(3). Available at: http://vm.cfsan.fda.gov/~lrd/CF101-22.HTML. Accessed March 19, 2002.

6. *Code of Federal Regulations.* April 1, 2001;21CFR101.22(a)(1). Available at: http://vm.cfsan.fda.gov/~lrd/CF101-22.HTML. Accessed March 19, 2002.

7. *Code of Federal Regulations.* April 1, 2001;21CFR101.22(a)(2). Available at: http://vm.cfsan.fda.gov/~lrd/CF101-22.HTML. Accessed March 19, 2002.

Chapter 8

Preservation, Sterilization, and Depyrogenation

Many pharmaceutical products are injected into the body or applied to compromised areas. If a product containing microorganisms is introduced into or applied to the body, severe infections may result. Such infections could result in the loss of an organ (e.g., an eye) or a limb, or even death. Consequently, certain pharmaceutical preparations must be sterile and contain preservatives to maintain their sterility. Parenteral medications must also be free of pyrogens and have endotoxin levels within allowable limits.

Preservation

Preservation is the prevention or inhibition of microbial growth. In pharmacy, preservatives are typically added to a product either to minimize microbial growth, as is the case with oral liquids, topicals, and the like, or to prevent microbial growth, as is necessary for sterile preparations such as parenterals.

Methods of Preservation

Preservation involves the addition of a substance to a product; however, the type of preservative to be added will vary depending on the characteristics of the product and its acceptability to the patient. Table 8-1 lists the different preservatives that can be used in various preparations.

Selection Factors

When selecting a preservative, a number of factors must be considered, including concentration, pH, taste, odor, and solubility. Some preparations, such as syrups, are inherently preserved by their high concentration of sugar, which acts as an osmotic preservative. This method is discussed in more detail in Chapter 15, "Solutions." For most preparations, however, a suitable preservative is necessary; when choosing a preservative, the pharmacist must ensure that the product prepared is stable. A preservative must be nontoxic, stable, compatible, inexpensive, and have an acceptable taste, odor, and color. It should also be effective against a wide variety of bacteria, fungi, and yeasts.

Table 8-1. Concentrations of Preservatives Used in Pharmaceutical Products

Preservative	Concentration (%)				
	Liquids	Emulsions	Ointments/ Creams	Paren- terals	Ophthalmic/ Nasal/Otic Products
Alcohol/ethanol	15–20	15–20			
Benzalkonium chloride	0.004–0.02	0.002–0.1		0.01	0.013
Benzethonium chloride	0.004–0.02	0.005–0.02		0.01	0.01
Benzoic acid and salts[a]	0.1–0.3	0.1–0.3			
Sodium benzoate	0.1–0.3	0.1–0.3			
Benzyl alcohol	1.0–3.0	1.0–4.0	1.0	2.0	
Boric acid and salts	0.5–1				
Cetylpyridinium chloride	0.01–0.02	0.01–0.02			
Cetyltrimethyl ammonium bromide	—	0.01–0.02			
Chlorobutanol[b]	0.3–0.5	0.5		0.25–0.5	
Chlorocresol	0.05–0.1			0.1–0.3	
Cresol	0.3–0.5	0.3–0.5	0.3–0.5		
Imidazolidinyl urea	—	0.05–0.5			
Metacresol				0.1–0.3	
Myristylgamma picolinium chloride				0.17	
Nitromersol	0.001–0.1				
Parabens[c]	0.001–0.2	0.001–0.2	0.001–0.2		0.1
Benzyl					
Butyl				0.015	
Methyl				0.1–0.2	
Propyl				0.02–0.2	
Phenol[d]	0.2–0.5	0.2–0.5	0.2–0.5		
o-Phenyl phenol	0.005–0.01				
β-phenylethyl alcohol	0.2–1				
Phenylmercuric acetate/nitrate	0.002–0.005	0.002–0.005		0.002	0.004
Sorbic acid and salts	0.05–0.2	0.05–0.2			
Thimerosal	0.001–0.1	0.005–0.02		0.01	0.01

[a]Benzoic acid/sodium benzoate are most effective at a pH of 4 or below.

[b]The anhydrous form of chlorobutanol should be used if a clear solution is desired in liquid petrolatum. Chlorobutanol needs a pH<5; it will also sorb to plastic.

[c]Parabens are usually used in pairs. They have low water solubility and poor taste. May degrade at a pH >8; they are best used at a pH range of 4–8. The parabens may interact with certain macromolecular compounds and bind, resulting in a loss of some effectiveness.

[d]Phenol forms a eutectic mixture with a number of compounds and may soften cocoa butter in suppository mixtures. Phenol may precipitate albumin, gelatin, and collodion. A green color may be produced in the presence of alum or borax.

Dosage Form Considerations

Emulsions. Preservatives may partition into the oil phase and lose their effectiveness. Bacterial growth normally will occur in the aqueous phase. Consequently, the preservative should be concentrated in the aqueous phase. Additionally, since the un-ionized form of the preservative will be more effective against bacteria, the majority of the preservative should be present in the non-ionized state. The preservative must neither be bound nor adsorbed to any agent in the emulsion or the container in order to be effective. In summary, only the preservative in the aqueous phase in the free, unbound, unadsorbed, un-ionized state will be effective in emulsions. The parabens (methylparaben, propylparaben, butylparaben) are among the most satisfactory preservatives for emulsions.

Gels. When added to an aqueous system, 0.1% methylparaben or propylparaben is an acceptable preservative and does not affect the efficiency of the polymer to maintain viscosity.

Oral Inhalations. Any preparation that is not in unit dose containers should contain a preservative, especially with the latest requirement of sterility for this class of dosage forms. The minimum amount of preservative that is still effective should be used. If too high a concentration is used, it may initiate a cough reflex in the patient. Also, too high a concentration of certain preservatives that are also surfactants may result in foaming that may interfere with the delivery of the complete dose.

Lozenges/Troches. A few comments are in order concerning the flavors and effects of preservatives, if included in the product formulation. For example, a 0.08% solution of methylparaben has an odor described as "floral," "gauze pad," or "face powder" sweet. A 0.015% solution of propylparaben has an effect that is tongue numbing, producing a slight sting and a minimal aroma. A 0.125% butylparaben solution has the least aroma of all. Preservatives may have a tendency to partition into flavors since preservatives are not always water soluble and most flavors are oily in nature.

Physicochemical Considerations for Common Preservatives

Preservatives have unique characteristics that must be taken into account during the selection process. For example, the anhydrous form of chlorobutanol should be used if a clear solution is desired in liquid petrolatum. In other examples, ethylenediamine may irritate the skin and mucous membranes and thus should be used with caution, sodium benzoate is most effective at a pH of 4 or below, and a green color may be produced in the presence of alum or borax. Further, the parabens may interact with certain macromolecular compounds and bind, thereby losing some effectiveness (Table 8-2). Finally, phenol forms a eutectic mixture with a number of compounds and may soften cocoa butter in suppository mixtures. Phenol may precipitate albumin, gelatin, and collodion.

Quaternarium Ammonium Compounds

Benzalkonium chloride is an antimicrobial agent commonly used as a preservative. It acts by emulsification of the bacterial cell walls, probably the cell membrane lipids. Ethylenediaminetetraacetic acid (EDTA) is often added in a concentration ranging from 0.01% to 0.1% to enhance the activity of benzalkonium chloride against *Pseudomonas aeruginosa*. Listed incompatibilities include aluminum, anionic materials, citrates, cotton, fluorescein, hydrogen peroxide, hydroxypropyl methylcellulose, iodides, kaolin, lanolin, nitrates, high concentrations of

Table 8-2. Binding Percentages of Parabens with Macromolecular Compounds

Compound	% of Methyl-paraben Bound	% of Propyl-paraben Bound
Gelatin	8	11
Methylcellulose	9	13
Polyethylene glycol 4000	16	19
Polyvinylpyrrolidone	22	36
Polyoxyethylene monostearate	45	84
Polyoxyethylene sorbitan monolaurate	57	86
Polyoxyethylene sorbitan monooleate	57	90

nonionic surfactants, permanganates, protein, salicylates, silver salts, soaps, sulfonamides, tartrates, zinc oxide, and zinc sulfate.

Benzethonium chloride is a detergent antiseptic with the same limitations and behavior characteristics as benzalkonium chloride. It is incompatible with soaps. One advantage to benzethonium chloride is that its germicidal activity increases with an increase in pH. For example, at pH 10 it is several times more active against selected bacteria than at pH 4.

Chlorobutanol

Chlorobutanol is both antibacterial and antifungal. Its antibacterial effectiveness is reduced above pH 5.5. Aqueous solutions of chlorobutanol will degrade in the presence of hydroxide ions. Chlorobutanol aqueous solutions have good stability at pH 3, but stability decreases with an increase in pH. Chlorobutanol may diffuse through polyethylene or other porous containers, resulting in a decreased concentration and effectiveness. Incompatibilities include plastic vials, rubber stoppers, bentonite, magnesium trisilicate, polyethylene, and polyhydroxyethylmethacrylate (in some soft contact lenses). Some antimicrobial activity is lost on contact with carboxymethylcellulose or polysorbate 80 due to sorption or complex formation. Greater antimicrobial effectiveness can be obtained by combining 0.5% chlorobutanol with 0.5% phenylethanol. The anhydrous form of chlorobutanol should be used if a clear solution is desired in a liquid petrolatum vehicle.

Parabens

Methylparaben is most effective in solution between pH 4 and 8, and its efficacy decreases at higher pH levels. In aqueous solution, it can be autoclaved and is stable in aqueous solution in the pH range of 3 to 6 for up to 4 years at room temperature. Methylparaben is incompatible with nonionic surfactants (its antimicrobial activity is reduced), bentonite, magnesium trisilicate, talc, tragacanth, sodium alginate, essential oils, sorbitol, and atropine. It may sorb to some plastics and is discolored in the presence of iron.

Propylparaben is also most effective in solution between pH 4 and 8, and its efficacy decreases at higher pH levels. It can be autoclaved in aqueous solutions of pH 3 to 6 without decomposition; aqueous solutions within this pH range are stable for up to 4 years. Propylparaben is incompatible with nonionic surfactants (reduced effectiveness); in addition, sorption has been reported to magnesium aluminum silicate, magnesium trisilicate, yellow iron oxide, and ultramarine blue.

Discoloration in the presence of iron and hydrolysis by weak alkalis and strong acids can also occur. Some plastics will adsorb propylparaben. Sodium propylparaben is a more water-soluble form of propylparaben that may be used in place of propylparaben, but the pH of the formulation may be increased.

Phenylmercuric Acetate/Nitrate

Phenylmercuric acetate should be protected from light. It is reported to be incompatible with anionic emulsifying agents and suspending agents, tragacanth, starch, talc, sodium metabisulfite, sodium thiosulfate, disodium edetate, the silicates, halides, and some types of filter membranes used for sterilization.

Phenylmercuric nitrate is effective over a broad pH range against both bacteria and fungi and is the preferred form in acidic solutions.

The phenylmercuric salts are used in preference to benzalkonium chloride in solutions of salicylates and nitrates, as well as in solutions of physostigmine and epinephrine that contain sodium sulfite. Its solutions can be autoclaved, but significant amounts of the salt may be lost; therefore, they are best sterilized by filtration. Incompatibilities include anionic emulsifying agents and suspending agents, tragacanth, starch, talc, sodium metabisulfite, sodium thiosulfate, disodium edetate, the silicates, halides, and some types of filter membranes used for sterilizations.

Thimerosal

Thimerosal is an antibacterial agent with weak bacteriostatic and mild fungistatic properties. It is affected by light.

Preservative Effectiveness Testing

Although not required, USP tests for the effectiveness of antimicrobial preservatives should be conducted on any product that is expected to be prepared in quantity and used for an extended period of time. The purpose of the tests, which can be conducted by a testing laboratory, is to demonstrate effectiveness against five different organisms (*Candida albicans, Aspergillus niger, Escherichia coli, Pseudomonas aeruginosa,* and *Staphylococcus aureus*). The results would be applicable only to the specific product prepared and packaged in the original, unopened containers.

Sterilization

Sterilization is the process of destroying or eliminating microorganisms that are present in or on an object or a preparation. Sterility is defined as the absence of all viable life forms. Parenterals and ophthalmics have long had sterility requirements, but now a number of different dosage forms have sterility requirements, including oral inhalations, nasal solutions, implants, irrigations, metered sprays, and certain swabs.

Methods of Sterilization

There are at present five basic methods of sterilization: moist heat, dry heat, chemical, filtration, and radiation. Of these, moist heat, dry heat, some forms of chemical sterilization, and filtration are appropriate for pharmacists to use. Pharmacists can, however, use contract facilities for gaseous and radiation forms of sterilization. The pharmacy should validate all of these methods on a regular basis; the routine use of devices or kits that indicate sterility is also recommended. Heat is the most reliable method of sterilization. The efficiency of heat in destroying microorganisms is dependent on temperature, time, moisture, and pressure. Heat sterilization consists of both moist-heat and dry-heat sterilization processes.

Moist-Heat Sterilization

Moist-heat sterilization (steam under pressure) uses an autoclave that provides a saturated steam environment, typically 121°C at 15 psi. This environment can be varied, depending on the autoclave being used. After the correct temperature and pressure are reached, the sterilization process continues for an additional 20 minutes, at which time the pressure and temperature are allowed to return to ambient at a rate depending on the load or items in the autoclave.

The saturation of water, or steam, at high pressure is the foundation for moist-heat sterilization effectiveness. When steam makes contact with a cooler object, it condenses and loses latent heat to the object. Under autoclaving conditions, the amount of energy released is approximately 524 cal/g, whereas 1 cal/g of energy is released in dry-heat sterilization. The difference explains why moist heat under pressure is more effective than dry heat at the same temperature in destroying microbial life. It also helps explain why objects or products to be sterilized in an autoclave must contain water or permit saturated steam to penetrate and make contact with all surfaces to be sterilized; therefore, air pockets are of great concern. The steam must reach all sites to be effective and is the reason air pockets are of great concern in the steam sterilization process. It also explains why sealed containers must contain water in order to be sterilized. Sealed, dry containers will reach only 121°C inside, and the heat will not be moist; thus, sterilization will likely not occur. Similarly, anhydrous and oily solutions that contain no water will reach only 121°C and the heat will be dry. Moist-heat sterilization is the desired method of sterilization for any item that can withstand high temperatures, including rubber closures, high-density plastic tubing, filter assemblies, sealed-glass ampules containing solutions that can withstand high temperatures, stainless-steel vessels, gowning materials, and various hard-surface equipment items.

Dry-Heat Sterilization

Dry-heat sterilization requires heat in excess of that experienced by autoclaving and involves the use of a high-temperature oven. The following operating conditions have been established: at 160°C, 120 to 180 minutes; at 170°C, 90 to 120 minutes; and at 180°C, 45 to 60 minutes. Sufficient time at the various temperatures must be determined to achieve the desired sterilization. One should not assume that any of the three conditions will automatically suffice for all formulations. Dry-heat sterilization is used to sterilize glass, stainless steel, and other hard-surface materials, as well as dry powders not labile to high temperatures. Injectable oily solutions also can be dry-heat sterilized, if the active ingredient remains potent and stable, using a time/temperature cycle that produces a validated finished sterile product. See the SOP "Operation and Validation of Operation of a Dry-Heat Sterilizing Oven."

Chemical Sterilization

Chemical sterilization involves the use of a gas, such as ethylene oxide, or chemical solutions such as isopropanol and ethanol. The items to be sterilized are placed in an apparatus that is specially designed to expose them to the sterilizing agent. After sterilization, the items are aerated to remove any residual chemical agent. Gaseous sterilization is employed primarily to sterilize items like medical devices and plastic materials that cannot withstand heat or radiation sterilization. Gases commonly used include β-propiolactone, propylene oxide, methyl bromide, formaldehyde, and ethylene oxide. Contract facilities can be located on the Internet that will do small lots of sterilization on a fee basis. Approximately 75% of all single-use, disposable devices are sterilized by ethylene oxide. Two other agents that are gaining in popularity include peracetic acid and vapor-phase hydrogen peroxide. Peracetic acid decomposes to nontoxic products of acetic acid and water without leaving adsorbable residues. Vapor-phase hydrogen peroxide is a powerful antimicrobial and is very effective in killing spore-forming bacteria.

Filtration Sterilization

Filtration, one of the oldest methods of sterilization, is a process whereby particulate matter from a flowing liquid is removed by the use of a filter. Filtration is not actually a terminal sterilization process because the product is then aseptically packaged in the dispensing container. The filter retains the particulate because the particulate is unable to penetrate the smaller pores in the filter matrix. This process, which is recommended for most compounding situations, will remove but not destroy microorganisms. After filtration has been completed, the sterile solution should be removed immediately, because microorganisms can eventually penetrate the pores of some filters if left on the filter surface for a prolonged period. Also, as bacteria grow on a filter, their byproducts (pyrogenic substances) may pass into the sterile solution. As a general rule, aqueous and organic solvent-based fluids can be filtered with polyvinylidiene fluoride and cellulosic esters; aqueous solutions at extreme pH values, with polyvinylidiene fluoride filters; and organic solvents and gases, with polyvinylidiene fluoride and polytetrafluoroethylene filters. When using filtration, the pharmacist should know whether the drug, preservative, or any other component in the solutions may tend to sorb to the filter material. If so, an alternative filter material should be used. Filtration sterilization is used for drug products that are chemically or physically unstable if sterilized by heat, gas, or radiation sterilization.

Currently, probably more than 80% of all small-volume parenteral products may be sterilized by filtration followed by aseptic processing. Filters suitable for sterilization of pharmaceutical products have a nominal rated pore size of 0.22 μm or less. Membrane filters are available either as flat discs or as cartridges. The cartridges have much larger surface areas and should be used for filtering large volumes of solution or solutions of high viscosity. Filters of different materials are available for a wide variety of solvents and gases; filter compatibility tables should be checked before selecting a filter for each procedure.

Radiation (Ionizing) Sterilization

Radiation, or ionizing, sterilization is a low-temperature method used in situations similar to those in which gaseous sterilization is used—for products or systems that cannot withstand high-temperature sterilization. There are two types of radiation sterilization processes: particulate and electromagnetic. Particulate radiation sterilization commonly uses cobalt-60 or cesium-137. Electromagnetic radiation includes gamma radiation and ultraviolet light.

Sterility Testing

Two common sterility tests are (1) direct inoculation of media and (2) either membrane filtration or incubation with media. Commercial kits and supplies are available to conduct these tests, or samples of the prepared product can be forwarded to a testing laboratory. Sterility testing is a common procedure to document the quality of prepared products.

Depyrogenation

Pyrogens are metabolic products produced by microorganisms. Depyrogenation is the destruction or removal of pyrogens. Endotoxins, the most pathogenic pyrogens, are produced primarily from the lipopolysaccharide constituents of the cell walls of gram-negative bacteria (especially the *Pseudomonas species* and *Escherichia coli*) and secondarily from gram-positive bacteria and fungi. The molecular weight of the endotoxins is in the range of about 20,000 daltons. When injected, these substances can cause fever, chills, pain, and malaise. Although such reactions are rarely fatal, they do cause great discomfort and can even produce shock in seriously ill patients.

Methods of Depyrogenation

Pyrogen removal can be accomplished by any of the following seven methods:

- Heating the equipment or materials at high temperatures ($\geq$170°C for several hours).
- Using charged modified 0.2 and 0.1μm-filter cartridges in a dead-end filtration mode.
- Performing ultrafiltration by size exclusion (using cutoff filters of 10,000 to 100,000 daltons).
- Using reverse osmosis membranes.
- Using activated carbon.
- Using distillation.
- Rinsing with sterile, pyrogen-free water.

The two methods most often used in the pharmacy are heating and rinsing.

Equipment, containers, and stable materials can be depyrogenated using dry heat at a high temperature. At 230°C, the time of exposure is 60 to 90 minutes; at 250°C, the exposure time is 30 to 60 minutes.

Rinsing involves the use of large quantities of sterile water for injection USP to rinse equipment or containers. Because sterile water for injection USP is pyrogen free, using it as a rinse removes pyrogens, which are water soluble, from equipment or supplies.

Pyrogen Testing

Pyrogen testing involves the use of *Limulus* amebocyte lysate (LAL) kits. These kits are generally complete with endotoxin standards and require only sterile water for injection USP for dilutions. All equipment, materials, and supplies used must be depyrogenated, and a strict aseptic technique must be followed. The test involves the manipulation of samples and dilutions and the capability to read a "gel end point." Although pyrogen testing requires some experience and careful technique, compounding pharmacists can do such testing in their facilities.

Validation

Whatever sterilization method is used, the equipment and processes must be validated. Biological indicators are appropriate to use and include *Bacillus subtilis* var *niger* spores for dry heat, *Bacillus stearothermophilus* for moist-heat sterilizers, and *Bacillus pumulis* spores for ionizing radiation.

Standard Operating Procedures (SOPs)

Operation and Validation of Operation of a Dry-Heat Sterilizing Oven

Purpose of SOP

The purpose of this procedure is to provide standardization in the operation of a dry-heat sterilizing oven and to provide a means of validating the oven's operation.

Basic Principles

Personnel involved in dry-heat sterilization should be thoroughly familiar with the sterilization process and the equipment involved. The basic principles and steps involved include the following:

- Establishing that the equipment is capable of operating within the required parameters.
- Conducting replicate cycles employing actual or simulated product and demonstrating the success of the procedure.
- Monitoring the process during routine operation.
- Completing the documentation.

Equipment/Materials

The following equipment is needed to perform this SOP:

- Dry-heat oven capable of attaining and maintaining a temperature of up to approximately 200°C.
- Thermometers that can be placed in the oven and read through the oven window.

Procedure

General Care of the Oven. Keep the exterior of the oven clean by periodic wiping with a cloth dampened with purified water or alcohol, as indicated in the SOP or when needed.

- Keep the oven turned off except when in use.
- If oven is soiled or leakage of a product occurs, clean the oven immediately.

Sterilizing Operation.

1. Before use, turn on the oven to the desired temperature and allow sufficient time for the temperature to be reached, using a thermometer placed in the chamber such that it can be externally read. (Note: Do not depend on the dial used to set the temperature. Adjust dial setting as needed to achieve desired temperature.)
2. When preparing the product for dry-heat sterilization, if a liquid (such as an oil) is being sterilized, prepare a container of the liquid and place in the oven chamber such that the thermometer can be inserted and externally read (generally, the liquid should be in the center of the oven).
3. Place the items to be sterilized evenly distributed in the oven, with ample space for heated airflow between the items.
4. Close the door and observe the temperature on the thermometer placed in the liquid. Start timing for the sterilizing process only after the desired temperature has been reached in the liquid.

5. Continue the sterilization process until the complete time has elapsed.
6. Turn off the heat to the oven and allow the oven to cool. Open the door and remove the items.
7. Clean the oven and close the door.
8. Record the temperature on the log (Figure 8-1).
9. Periodically, transport/ship one of the sterilized units to a contract laboratory for sterility testing.

Validation of Oven Operation. Oven operation should be validated initially and then periodically on the basis of use. Oven temperatures should be checked first with the chamber empty and then with a container of liquid placed in the chamber.

Temperature Consistency of Empty Oven Chamber.

1. Before use, turn on the oven to the desired temperature and allow sufficient time for the temperature to be reached, using a thermometer placed in the chamber such that it can be externally read. (Note: Do not depend on the dial used to set the temperature. Adjust dial setting as needed to achieve desired temperature.)
2. After the temperature has been reached, record the temperature on the log (Figure 8-1) at 15-minute intervals for 2 hours, or other suitable time duration.
3. Turn off the oven and allow it to cool down.
4. Repeat steps 1 through 3.

Temperature Consistency of Filled Chamber (with Liquids).

1. Before use, turn on the oven to the desired temperature and allow sufficient time for the temperature to be reached, using a thermometer placed in the chamber such that it can be externally read. (Note: Do not depend on the dial used to set the temperature. Adjust dial setting as needed to achieve desired temperature.)
2. Prepare containers with a simulated product and seal them. Prepare a container of the liquid and place in the oven chamber such that the thermometer can be inserted and externally read (generally, the liquid should be in the center of the oven).
3. Initiate the process and, after the temperature has been reached in the liquid, record the temperature of the liquid on the log (Figure 8-1) at 15-minute intervals for 2 hours, or other suitable time duration.
4. Turn off the oven and allow it to cool down. Remove the contents and clean the oven chamber.

Temperature Log for Dry-Heat Sterilizing Oven

| Date | Activity | | Time Interval | Temperature | Operator |
	Validation	Sterilization			

Figure 8-1. Sample log for validation and operation of dry-heat sterilizing oven.

Chapter 9

Powders and Granules

Definitions/Types

Powders and granules are not only dosage forms themselves but are also used as a beginning point for other dosage forms. Powders are the fine particles that can result from the comminution of any dry substance. They consist of particles ranging in size from about 0.1 μ to about 10,000 μ, although the most useful pharmaceutical range is approximately 0.1 to 10 μ. To describe particle size, pharmacists generally use the sieve number or mesh fraction terminology. The *United States Pharmacopeia 25/National Formulary 20* uses descriptive terms, such as very coarse, coarse, moderately coarse, fine, and very fine, when referring to the various sieve sizes. Figure 9-1 shows a No. 80-mesh sieve; this number correlates with the USP description standard of "very fine." These terms are defined in Table 9-1.

As dosage forms, *powders* are thorough mixtures of dry, finely divided drugs and excipients that are intended for internal or external use. Powders are easy to administer to pediatric patients or patients of advanced age because the contents of divided powder papers (charts) or bulk powders can be mixed with foods or liquids. One factor that limits their use is the taste of the active drug. Powders are also prepared for use as douches and as tooth powders.

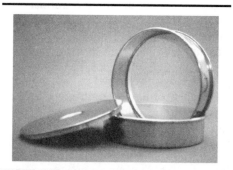

Figure 9-1. Brass sieve (80 mesh).

Granules are dosage forms that consist of particles ranging in size from about No. 4- to No. 10-mesh. The particles are formed when blended powders are moistened and passed through a screen or a special granulator. These moist granules are dried in the air or in an oven. Effervescent granules are especially suitable for products with a salty or bitter taste. The effervescence is provided by mixtures of citric acid and/or tartaric acid combined with sodium biphosphate and/or sodium carbonate. When the mixture is placed in water, it effervesces with the production of carbon dioxide.

Calculations for sample preparations that contain effervescent granules are explained in Chapter 5, "Pharmaceutical Compounding Calculations." A reader who is uncertain about how to determine the required quantities of these granules for a formulation should review Chapter 5.

Table 9-1. Sieve Numbers, Openings, and Descriptive Terms Related to Sieves

Sieve No.	Sieve Opening mm	Sieve Opening μm	Descriptive Standard (USP)	General Applications
2	9.52	9520	Very coarse	Sieve numbers 2 through
3.5	5.66	5660		40 are used to sift granu-
4	4.76	4760		lated effervescent salts
8	2.38	2380		and granulations for com-
10	2.00	2000		pressed tablets.
20	0.84	840	Coarse	
30	0.59	590		
40	0.42	420	Moderately coarse	
50	0.297	297		Sieve numbers 50 through
60	0.250	250	Fine	120 are used to sift pow-
70	0.210	210		dered effervescent salts
80	0.177	177	Very fine	and divided powders.
100	0.149	149		
120	0.125	125		
200	0.074	74		Sieve numbers 200
230	0.063	63		through 400 are used to
270	0.053	53		sift divided powders for
325	0.044	44		dusting, adsorbents,
400	0.037	37		inhalants, and others.

Historical Use

Originally, powders were found to be a convenient mode of administering drugs derived from hard vegetables such as roots (e.g., rhubarb), barks (e.g., cinchona), and woods (e.g., charcoal). As synthetic drugs were introduced, powders were used to administer insoluble drugs such as calomel, bismuth salts, mercury, and chalk.

Historically, powders as a solid dosage form have been used as internal and external medications. Internally, they can be taken orally, administered through the nose as snuffs, or blown into a body cavity as an insufflation. Externally, solid powders can be applied to compromised areas of the body. Powders have also been used to make solutions for topical and oral use and for use as douches. Such traditional applications and modes of administration of the dosage form are still used today. Additional applications have also been developed; for example, powders containing a bioadhesive material can be applied to a specific body area such that the medication will adhere for a prolonged drug effect.

Applications

Powders have qualities that make them an attractive dosage form for certain situations. Unlike a standardized capsule or tablet, powders enable a primary care provider to easily alter the quantity of medication for each dose. Powders can also aid in clinical studies of drug products because the dose can be so readily adjusted. In another example, infants and young children who cannot swallow tablets or capsules will accept powders that can be mixed with a formula or sprinkled in applesauce or some other appropriate food. Also, if a drug is too bulky to be prepared as a capsule or tablet, it may be suitable for a powder dosage form. Powders provide a rapid onset of action because they are readily dispersed, have a large surface area, and generally do not require disintegration but rather just dissolution before absorption.

Composition

Properly prepared, powders will have a uniform, small particle size that has an elegant appearance. Generally, powders are more stable than liquid dosage forms and are rapidly soluble, enabling the drug to be absorbed quickly.

The properties of powders are related to the size and surface area of the particles. For example, large particles that are more dense tend to settle more rapidly than small particles; particles that are more bulky will settle more slowly. This characteristic must be considered when mixing or storing and shipping, when powders of different particle size may become segregated. Another concern stems from the fact that powder dosage forms have a large surface area that is exposed to atmospheric conditions. Thus, powders should be dispensed in tight containers. Further, because powders of small particle size present a greater surface area to the atmosphere, they are more reactive in nature and can adsorb larger quantities of gases, such as carbon dioxide. However, if the powder has a smaller particle size, it can dissolve at a more rapid rate, unless adsorbed gases prevent the water from surrounding the individual particles and wetting them, thereby decreasing their wetting properties. This increase in surface-free energy can increase the absolute solubility of the drug and have a positive effect on its bioequivalence.

This dosage form should not ordinarily be used for drugs with a disagreeable taste or caustic nature. If taste is not a consideration, the powder can simply be prepared as powder papers and packaged in paper, glassine, waxed paper, or small plastic bags, depending on the characteristics of the powder.

Bulk oral powders require the patient to measure the desired quantity of each dose, and thus a measuring device must be provided to ensure accurate measurement. Divided oral powder papers (charts), however, are prepackaged individual doses; the patient simply removes the dose and takes its contents at the appointed time.

Topical powders should have a uniform, small particle size that will not irritate the skin when applied. They should be impalpable and free flowing, should easily adhere to the skin, and should be passed through at least a No. 100-mesh sieve to minimize skin irritation. The powder should be prepared so that it adheres to the skin.

Highly sorptive powders should not be used for topical powders that are to be applied to oozing wounds, as a hard crust may form. A more hydrophobic, water-repellent powder will prevent loss of water from the skin and will not cake on the oozing surfaces. Talc, or any other naturally derived product that is to be used on open wounds, should first be sterilized to avoid an infection in the area.

Topical powders generally consist of a base or vehicle such as cornstarch or talc; an adherent, such as magnesium stearate, calcium stearate, or zinc stearate; and possibly an active ingredient along with an aromatic material. The powder should provide a large surface area, flow easily, and spread uniformly. The large surface area will aid in absorbing perspiration and give a cooling sensation to the skin.

Insufflated powders are finely divided powders that are intended to be applied in a body cavity, such as the ears, nose, vagina, tooth socket, or throat. When using an insufflator, or "puffer," the patient simply "puffs" the desired quantity of powder onto the affected area or into the cavity. This device is particularly appropriate for anti-infectives. Also, a moisture-activated adherent, such as Polyox, can be incorporated into the powder. Polyox is an ethylene oxide polymer with a high molecular weight that forms a viscous, mucoadhesive gel when in contact with moisture. The gel serves to provide a depot for long-term drug delivery spanning several hours.

Preparation

Particle Size Reduction

The first step in preparing powders is to ensure that all the ingredients are in the same particle size range. This task is accomplished through particle size reduction, or comminution. Comminution includes both manual (trituration, levigation, pulverization by intervention) and mechanical methods (ball mills, grinders, coffee mills). The method of particle size reduction chosen depends on the characteristics of the drug. For example, gummy-type materials are best comminuted using pulverization by intervention; insoluble materials for ointments and suspensions by levigation; tough, fibrous materials by coffee grinders or mills with blades; and hard, fracturable powders by trituration. Potent materials and dyestuffs should be comminuted in nonporous mortars, such as glass, so that none of the drug remains in the pores of the mortar to decrease the dose for the current patient or to contaminate the next product to be prepared. For most other purposes, a standard Wedgwood or porcelain mortar and pestle will suffice. Figure 9-2 shows the types of mortars and pestles available from commercial equipment suppliers.

The type of powder that is the starting point and the type of powder that is desired will dictate which technique should be used. For example, if one wants to produce a light, fluffy powder but is starting with a dense powder, light trituration with periodic "fluffing" using a spatula works well. Conversely, if one starts with a fluffy powder and desires to produce a more dense powder, heavy and prolonged trituration with a mortar and pestle is the preferred approach. In any case, all ingredients should be approximately the same particle size for best mixing.

If topical powders are being prepared, the powders are generally passed through a sieve after comminution. It is generally not necessary to sieve these powders for liquid suspensions.

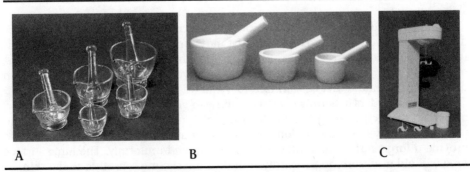

A   B   C

Figure 9-2. Mortars and pestles: *A*, glass mortars and pestles; *B*, ceramic mortars and pestles; *C*, electric mortar and pestle.

Mixing

Pharmaceutical mixing uses a process called geometric dilution; that is, one starts with the ingredient in the smallest quantity, then adds additional ingredients in order of quantity required by approximately "doubling" the portion being mixed with each addition. Mixing can be done in a mortar with a pestle, a bottle, or a plastic bag by shaking (seal bag and include a great deal of air); it can also involve the use of a roller (seal bag and include only a small amount of air), sieve, sifter, or other suitable device. See the box "Hints for Compounding Powders" for other suggestions on mixing powders.

Hints for Compounding Powders

- A coffee grinder will aid in particle size reduction for small amounts of powder. It can be cleaned with a camel's hair brush, and some can be washed with soap and water.
- Mixing powders with similar particle size and density characteristics in a plastic bag using a spatula will lessen the amount of powder floating around the compounding area.
- Dust masks can be used if a powder is excessively light and escapes into the work area.
- Powder that is too fluffy can be compacted slightly by the addition of a few drops of alcohol, water, or mineral oil.
- Magnesium stearate, less than 1% of the total weight of the mix, can be used to enhance the lubrication and flow characteristics of powders.
- Sodium lauryl sulfate, up to 1%, can be added to powders to neutralize electrostatic forces for powders that tend to "fly all over" or are hard to handle.

Physicochemical Considerations

Eutectics

Some powders may become sticky or pasty or they may liquefy when mixed together, such as those listed in Table 9-2. To keep the powders dry, one can mix them with a bulky powder adsorbent such as light magnesium oxide or magnesium carbonate. Also, these powders should be triturated very lightly on a pill tile (Figure 9-3) by using a spatula for mixing rather than a mortar and pestle. The latter will cause compression and make the problem worse. It may also be advisable to double-wrap the papers. Mixing these powders with the bulky powders first and then performing a light blending can minimize the problem.

Another approach is to first make the eutectic and then adsorb the paste or liquid that results onto a bulky powder. One also has the option of dispensing the ingredients separately. After preparation, the charts can be dispensed in a plastic bag.

Table 9-2. Common Substances That Soften or Liquefy When Mixed

Acetanilid	Lidocaine
Acetophenetidin	Menthol
Aminopyrine	Phenacetin
Antipyrine	Phenol
Aspirin	Phenylsalicylate
Benzocaine	Prilocaine
Betanaphthol	Resorcinol
Camphor	Salicylic acid
Chloral hydrate	Thymol

Hygroscopic and Deliquescent Powders

Hygroscopic powders will absorb moisture from the air. Deliquescent powders will absorb moisture from the air to the extent that they will partially or wholly liquefy. These problems must be overcome for the powder to be acceptable to the patient and usable. The best approach is to dispense the ingredients in tight containers and incorporate a desiccant packet or capsule, when necessary. The patient should be instructed to store the powder in a dry place and to keep it tightly closed. To lessen the extent of the problem, the compounding pharmacist, in some situations, can dilute the powder with an inert drying powder to reduce the amount of surface area exposed to the moisture. Common hygroscopic and deliquescent powders are shown in Table 9-3.

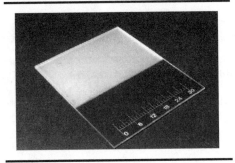

Figure 9-3. Pill tile.

Efflorescent Powders

An *efflorescent powder* (Table 9-4) is a crystalline powder that contains water of hydration or crystallization. This water can be liberated either during manipulations or on exposure to a low-humidity environment. If this occurs, the powder will become sticky and pasty or it may even liquefy. One approach is to use an anhydrous salt form of the drug, keeping in mind the potency differential between its anhydrous form and its hydrated form. Another method is to include a drying bulky powder and to use a light, noncompacting method of mixing the powders.

Table 9-3. Common Hygroscopic and Deliquescent Powders

Ammonium bromide	Pepsin
Ammonium chloride	Phenobarbital sodium
Ammonium iodide	Physostigmine hydrobromide
Calcium bromide	Physostigmine hydrochloride
Calcium chloride	Physostigmine sulfate
Ephedrine sulfate	Pilocarpine alkaloid
Hydrastine hydrochloride	Potassium acetate
Hydrastine sulfate	Potassium citrate
Hyoscyamine hydrobromide	Sodium bromide
Hyoscyamine sulfate	Sodium iodide
Iron and ammonium citrate	Sodium nitrate
Lithium bromide	Zinc chloride

Effervescent Salts

Effervescent salts are usually mixtures of effloresced citric acid and/or tartaric acid combined with sodium biphosphate and/or sodium carbonate. These salts can also be prepared by using uneffloresced citric acid and tartaric acid. After the powders are blended, they are placed in an oven at 95°C to 105°C until a pasty mass is formed. The powders liberate their water of crystallization/hydration, forming a

Table 9-4. Common Efflorescent Powders

Alums	Morphine acetate
Atropine sulfate	Quinine bisulfate
Caffeine	Quinine hydrobromide
Calcium lactate	Quinine hydrochloride
Citric acid	Scopolamine hydrobromide
Cocaine	Sodium acetate
Codeine	Sodium carbonate (decahydrate)
Codeine phosphate	Sodium phosphate
Codeine sulfate	Strychnine sulfate
Ferrous sulfate	Terpin hydrate

moist powder. The mass is then passed through a No. 10-mesh sieve onto a drying tray, where it is dried, broken apart into granules, and packaged. One disadvantage of effervescent powders is their large exposed surface area, which provides for greater reactivity (effervescence) and creates potential stability problems. Granules have the advantage of being able to control the rate of effervescence that occurs when the product is added to water. A powder will rapidly effervesce when added to water and may overflow the container. Because granules expose less surface area, they will hydrate and dissolve slower, resulting in a slower, more controlled effervescence.

Explosive Mixtures

Some combinations of powders (Table 9-5) may react violently when mixed together. Special precautions must be taken if it is necessary to prepare a product containing these mixtures.

Incorporation of Liquids

A liquid that is to be incorporated into a dry powder can be adsorbed onto an inert material (carrier) such as lactose and then geometrically introduced into the bulk of the powder. Pasty material can be added to dry powder by mixing it with increasing quantities of the powder, which will dry out the paste. It is best to add some materials by preparing an alcoholic solution and spraying it evenly on the powder, which has been spread out on a pill tile. The alcohol, or another suitable solvent, should then be allowed to evaporate, leaving the ingredient uniformly dispersed. This method may be especially suitable for high-potency drugs or flavoring agents because it minimizes the possibility that clumps of active drug will develop in the powder blend.

Quality Control

Bulk Powders

The pharmacist should compare the final weight of the product to the theoretical weight. The powder should be examined for uniformity of color, particle size, flowability, and freedom from caking.

Table 9-5. Common Oxidizing and Reducing Agents That May React Violently When Mixed

Oxidizing Agents	Reducing Agents
Bromine	Alcohol
Chlorates	Bisulfites
Chloric acid	Bromides
Chlorine	Charcoal
Chromates	Glycerin
Dichromates	Hydriodic acid
Ethyl nitrite spirit	Hypophosphites
Hydrogen peroxide	Hypophorphorus acid
Hypochlorites	Iodides
Hypochlorous acid	Lactose
Iodine	Nitrites (in some situations)
Nitrates	Organic substances in general
Nitric acid	Phosphorus
Nitrites	Sugar
Nitrohydrochloric acid	Sulfides
Nitrous acid	Sulfites
Perborates	Sulfur
Permanganates	Sulfurous acid
Permanganic acid	Tannic acid
Peroxides	Tannins
Potassium chlorate	Thiosulfates
Potassium dichromate	Volatile oils
Potassium nitrate	
Potassium permanganate	
Sodium peroxide	
Silver nitrate	
Silver oxide	
Silver salts	
Trinitrophenol	

Divided Powders

For divided powders, the pharmacist should individually weigh the divided papers and then compare that weight to the theoretical weight. The packets should be checked to see that they are uniform.

Packaging/Dispensing

The powder mixture is packaged according to its use. Bulk oral powders can be packaged in glass, plastic, metal, or other containers that have a wide mouth to allow use of the powder measure. Divided powders, or powder papers, must be individually folded. Topical powders can be poured into sifter-top containers or powder shakers (Figure 9-4), and insufflations can be filled into plastic puffer units.

Techniques for Preparing Charts

Preparing charts requires placing a specific quantity of powder onto individual papers. A number of methods can be used to determine the correct quantity, including weighing each powder quantity, blocking and dividing, or using a miniature powder measure. The most accurate method is to weigh each powder quantity, a technique that should be used for potent drugs. Blocking and dividing consists of placing the powder in a smooth, even-depth rectangular pile and using a spatula to cut or divide the pile into the desired number of portions. These portions are then placed in the powder paper for folding and dispensing. A miniature powder measure, when full, will contain the correct quantity of drug required for each dose. One approach to making a miniature powder measure is to glue a handle to a base from the appropriate size capsule that, when full, contains the desired quantity of powder. This device can then be used to measure the doses for a chart. After the dose is placed in the paper, the paper is folded and placed in the dispensing package. In the preparation of powder papers, it is common practice to prepare sufficient powder for one extra paper, as some of the powder will be lost during the manipulations.

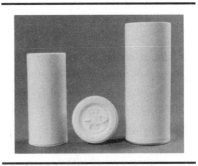

Figure 9-4. Powder shaker.

Methods of dispensing divided powder dosage forms have included such traditional approaches as (1) placing the weighed powder into powder papers, which are then folded and boxed; (2) placing the weighed powder into small zipper storage bags; (3) using a continuous tube of plastic that is then heat sealed to form the bottom of the pouch, after which the weighed powder is introduced and the pouch sealed; and (4) placing self-contained powder papers into a zipper storage bag.

Charts or powder papers can be fashioned from white bond paper, glassine paper, vegetable parchment, waxed paper, or other suitable material. The paper of choice for hygroscopic or deliquescent materials is waxed paper because it is waterproof and its edges can be heat sealed. If limited water resistance is desired, glassine or parchment paper may be satisfactory. Although bond paper has no moisture resistance capability, it has a neat, esthetic, and pleasing appearance. It is common practice to double-wrap hygroscopic powders by using glassine, parchment, or waxed paper as the inner wrap and bond paper as the final or outer wrap. Powders containing volatile ingredients should also be double-wrapped to prevent ingredient loss. Double-wrapping provides ingredient protection and a uniform, pleasing appearance to the final dosage form. After the papers are folded, they are generally packaged in slide-type boxes or shouldered boxes with either hinged or removable lids. The label directions are placed on or, preferably, inside the lid.

Techniques for Folding Powder Papers

The two common methods of preparing folded papers for compounded powder dosage forms are shown in Figures 9-5 and 9-6.[1,2] Directions and diagrams are provided to aid the novice in visualizing the final folded product. These techniques are used to package compounded, individualized powder dosage forms. By following the steps, the pharmacist can, with practice, prepare a neatly folded product.

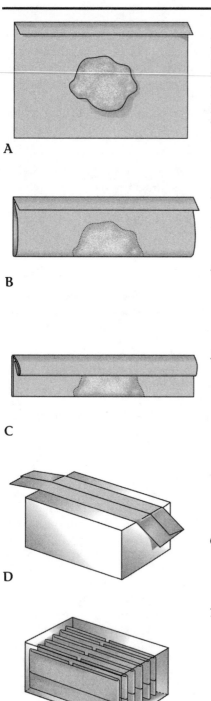

A

B

C

D

E

Fold down the long edge of the paper about ½ in. Several papers may be folded at one time to save time and promote uniformity. A note of caution: Do not try to fold too many papers at one time because the fold on the top piece of paper will be larger than the fold on the bottom piece of paper. The reason is that the paper will not stretch around corners (Figure 9-5A).

1. Place the papers on the counter in a convenient arrangement, out of the way of wind or drafts, with the folded tops away from but facing the pharmacist.

2. Place the weighed individual doses on the center of each paper (Figure 9-5A).

3. Bring up the lower edge of the paper and insert it completely into the top fold of the powder paper (Figure 9-5B).

4. Fold down the top fold toward the pharmacist until the paper fits exactly to the top of the powder box. This can be approximated by folding the paper until the remainder of the paper is divided approximately in half (Figure 9-5C).

5. Center the folded paper lengthwise over an open powder box of the size intended to be used. (Note: The center of the box, as well as the paper, should be marked with a pencil on its edge to remove any guesswork associated with this measurement.) Then fold the equal overhanging ends down while pressing in on the sides of the box. Caution should be used since pressing too hard may bend the box; however, adequate pressure must be applied to allow the powder paper to fit snugly, without bending, when placed into the box (Figure 9-5D).

6. Fold back the ends of the powder paper completely and sharply crease the end folds with a clean spatula to make a permanent fold. All of the ends of the powder papers should lie on a straight line.

7. Place the filled powder papers into the box, with the folds away from the pharmacist (Figure 9-5E). Usually all top folds are up. However, on occasion, they may be alternately up and down. The appearance may not be as neat with this latter procedure, but more folded papers can be placed into the box and there is less tendency for several papers to "pop out" when a single powder is removed.

Figure 9-5. Folding technique for a traditional powder paper.

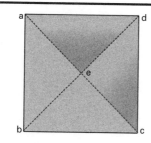

A

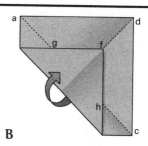

B

1. Use a square piece of powder paper. (Note: If the powder is to be double-wrapped, then both papers must be folded together.) Fold the paper diagonally from point A to point C and then again from point B to point D. When the paper is unfolded, the two diagonal lines will meet at point E. Take point D and fold in to point E to give point F. Unfold the paper to the open position (Figure 9-6A).

2. Bring point B to point F and crease, using a spatula. The fold intersects the AC diagonal line at point G (Figure 9-6B).

3. Bring point C to point G and crease, using a spatula. The fold intersects the AC diagonal line at point H (Figure 9-6C).

4. Bring point A to point H and crease, using a spatula. This fold forms an elongated envelope (Figure 9-6D).

5. Bring the bottom of the envelope up so that it divides it into thirds and leaves the flap to be tucked into the envelope after filling (Figure 9-6E).

6. Place the weighed powder dose into the envelope.

7. Tuck point D into the opening at the bottom, which was previously brought up to form the envelope. This secures the powder packet, which can then be placed into a zipper storage bag and labeled appropriately with the physician's directions (Figure 9-6F).

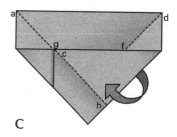

C

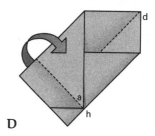

D

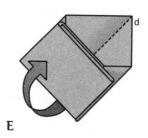

E

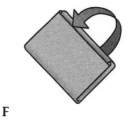

F

Figure 9-6. Folding technique for a self-contained powder paper.

Storage/Labeling

Powder and granule dosage forms should be stored in dry places. They may also require protection from light, depending on the active drug they contain.

Stability

Because powders are dry, they generally provide a stable dosage form as long as they are protected from moisture and heat. According to Chapter <795>, "Pharmacy Compounding,"[3] powders prepared from a manufactured product should have the beyond-use date of 25% of the time remaining on the product's expiration date or 6 months, whichever is earlier. If the product is prepared from USP/NF ingredients, a beyond-use date of 6 months is appropriate, unless evidence is available to support other dating.

Patient Counseling

If bulk oral powders are prescribed, it is critical that the patient be told the exact technique for measuring the dose to be administered and the proper mode of administration. Should the powder be mixed with a liquid? If so, what liquid? Can it be premixed and stored for a day? A week? What happens if some water drops into the package containing the powder? Can the powder be mixed with food(s)? If so, which foods? Hot or cold?

If bulk topical powders are prescribed, the patient should be counseled about the quantity of powder to apply and whether or not rubbing or patting the powder is recommended. What happens if much of the powder falls off the skin? Is it safe to apply it where children will be playing? Does the skin need to be dry? What happens if the skin is sweaty?

Sample Formulations

℞ **Bulk Oral Powder**
_____

Dextrose	25 g
Sodium chloride	2.5 g
Potassium citrate	4.5 g

For electrolyte and rehydration solution

1. Calculate the quantity of each ingredient required for the prescription.
2. Accurately weigh each ingredient.
3. Mix the powders together.
4. Place in container.
5. Label to be diluted to 1000 mL for drinking.

℞ Bulk Topical Powder

Menthol	0.1 g	Zinc oxide	8 g
Camphor	0.2 g	Talc	31 g
Zinc stearate	0.8 g		

M. dusting powder.

1. Calculate the quantity of each ingredient required for the prescription.
2. Accurately weigh each ingredient.
3. Mix the menthol and camphor together to form a liquid (eutectic).
4. Mix the zinc stearate, zinc oxide, and talc by geometric dilution.
5. Incorporate the powders into the liquid geometrically and mix well.
6. Package and label.

℞ Divided Oral Powder

Scopolamine hydrobromide	5 mg
Lactose	2.495 g

Prepare 10 powder papers.

1. Calculate the quantity of each ingredient required for the prescription.
2. Accurately weigh each ingredient. (Note: Depending on the total quantity to be prepared, it may be necessary to prepare a dilution of the scopolamine hydrobromide to accurately obtain the 5 mg.)
3. Geometrically incorporate the lactose into the scopolamine hydrobromide.
4. Place 250 mg of the mixture into each of 10 powder papers.
5. Package and label.

℞ Powdered Dentifrice

Triclosan	1 g	Peppermint oil	0.4 mL
Precipitated calcium carbonate	98 g	Cinnamon oil	0.2 mL
		Wintergreen oil	0.8 mL
Sodium lauryl sulfate	0.4 g		
Saccharin sodium	0.2 g		

Prepare tooth powder.

1. Calculate the quantity of each ingredient required for the prescription.
2. Accurately weigh each ingredient.
3. Mix the triclosan, sodium lauryl sulfate, and saccharin sodium together.
4. Geometrically incorporate the mixture into the precipitated calcium carbonate.
5. Mix the oils together.
6. Incorporate the powder into the oil geometrically and mix until uniform.
7. Package and label.

℞ Powdered Douche

Boric acid	80 g	Thymol	0.3 g
Ammonium aluminum	15 g	Phenol	0.2 g
sulfate		Tannic acid	0.5 g
Menthol	0.5 g		
Sodium lauryl sulfate	0.5 g		

Prepare douche powder.

1. Calculate the quantity of each ingredient for the total quantity to be prepared.
2. Accurately weigh each ingredient.
3. Mix the sodium lauryl sulfate, tannic acid, ammonium aluminum sulfate, and boric acid together (Note: Boric acid powder should be used.)
4. Mix the thymol, phenol, and menthol together to form a liquid.
5. Geometrically incorporate the powder mixture from step 3 into the liquid and mix thoroughly.
6. Package and label.

℞ Misoprostol 0.0027% Mucoadhesive Powder

Misoprostol	400 µg
Polyethylene oxide (Polyox 301)	200 mg
Hydroxypropyl methylcellulose	qs 15 g

1. Calculate the quantity of each ingredient required for the prescription.
2. Obtain two misoprostol 200 µg tablets.
3. Accurately weigh each of the other ingredients.
4. Pulverize the misoprostol tablets to a very fine powder.
5. Add the polyethylene oxide (Polyox 301) followed by the hydroxypropyl methylcellulose (Methocel E4M) and mix well. (Note: It is important to have all the materials of approximately the same particle size.)
6. Package and label.

℞ Adhesive Hydrating Powder

Carboxymethylcellulose sodium	35 g
Polyoxyl WSR-301	15 g
Calcium phosphate	50 g

1. Calculate the quantity of each ingredient required for the prescription.
2. Accurately weigh each of the ingredients.
3. Geometrically, add the carboxymethylcellulose sodium to the Polyoxyl WSR-301 powder using a pill tile/spatula or a mortar and pestle.
4. Incorporate the calcium phosphate geometrically and mix well.
5. Package and label.

References

1. Dittert LW. *Sprowl's American Pharmacy*. 7th ed. Philadelphia: Lippincott; 1974:316–7.
2. Gennaro AR. *Remington: The Science and Practice of Pharmacy*. 20th ed. Baltimore: Lippincott Williams & Wilkins; 2000:697–8.
3. Expert Advisory Panel on Pharmacy Compounding Practices. Pharmacy compounding. In: *United States Pharmacopeia 25/National Formulary 20*. Rockville, Md: United States Pharmacopeial Convention; 2001.

Chapter 10

Capsules

The most versatile of all dosage forms is probably the capsule. Capsules have been used for more than a century and have an important role in drug delivery. In addition to being relatively easy to manufacture, they are amenable to small-scale compounding by the pharmacist, who is able to prepare specific products for individual patient needs. The process of designing and developing products is aided by new excipients that can improve bioavailability and ensure the site-specific release of products, as well as enhance the elegance of this popular dosage form. When a primary care provider prescribes a tablet, the choice is usually, but not always, limited to commercially available products. A capsule, however, can be prepared extemporaneously and provides dosing flexibility for the primary care provider and pharmacist. Capsules can be prepared to be elegant, convenient, and easily identifiable; they are available in many different sizes, shapes, and colors.

Definitions/Types

Dosage forms in which unit doses of powder, semisolid, or liquid drugs are enclosed in either a hard or a soft envelope, or shell, are called capsules. Usually, the shells are composed of gelatin. Capsules are generally of the hard gelatin or soft gelatin type. Hard gelatin capsules can be prepared to release the drug rapidly or over a predetermined time, whereas soft gelatin capsules usually provide standard release.

Hard gelatin capsules consist of two parts: the base or body, which is longer and has a lesser diameter, and the cap, which is shorter and has a slightly larger diameter. The cap is designed to slide over the base portion and form a snug seal.

This dosage form is intended to be swallowed whole. The contents of capsules should be opened and administered in food or liquids only with the concurrence of the pharmacist.

Historical Use

Mothes, a French pharmacist, invented the soft gelatin capsule in 1833; Dublanc made improvements to this invention. Patents were issued to both inventors in 1834. Lehuby developed the hard capsule, for which a patent was issued in 1846, and in 1848 Murdock created a two-piece hard gelatin capsule, which was patented in 1865. Initially, the rate of usage and acceptance of capsules was low. During the 1900s, however, a growing number of drugs became available in solid powder form in dosages that could be easily administered orally, leading to a phenomenal increase in the capsule's popularity. This dosage form was included for the first time in the 12th revision of the *United States Pharmacopeia.*

Because they can be prepared in many colors, capsules are considered elegant and make a nice "presentation" when administered to the patient. They also conceal taste, which is another reason for their popularity. Their increased use can also be attributed to their portability, light weight, and rapid drug release.

Applications

In recent years, pharmacists have been preparing ever greater numbers of capsules extemporaneously. This growth may be due to several marketplace factors. First, low volume has forced some manufacturers to take certain drug products off the market. The pharmacist, who has access to the pure drug chemical or another dosage form of the drug, can easily prepare that product to serve the needs of the individual primary care provider and patient. Second, some patients cannot swallow a tablet but they can swallow a capsule. To aid these individuals, the pharmacist can convert many tablets into a capsule dosage form. Third, capsules enable the primary care provider and pharmacist to combine several drug products into one capsule to minimize the number of prescription products a patient must take. Because patients have to take only one dosage form instead of several, they are more likely to comply with the regimen, which leads to a more positive therapeutic outcome. Finally, the proper formulation of a capsule can affect the release of a drug product; that is, it can slow down or speed up the release.

The primary application of capsules is the oral administration of drugs. The capsule incorporates drugs that might have an unpleasant odor or taste within a practically tasteless shell that dissolves or digests in the stomach after about 10 to 20 minutes.

Capsules can be administered rectally and vaginally by piercing the capsule with a pin or needle to allow the aqueous body fluids to penetrate the capsule and dissolve its contents more easily. Excipients that are very water soluble should be used in these situations because hydrophobic materials may release a smaller quantity of the drug than is desired.

Capsules are not suitable for drugs that are very soluble, such as salts (e.g., potassium chloride, potassium bromide, ammonium chloride). In these situations, the fluid penetrating the capsule rapidly dissolves the salt and creates a highly concentrated solution that may cause nausea and vomiting when it contacts the gastric mucosa.

Capsules are also not appropriate for strongly efflorescent or deliquescent materials. An efflorescent material may cause the capsule to soften when water is lost, whereas a strongly deliquescent powder may make the shell of the capsule brittle when the powder extracts its moisture.

Composition

Hard gelatin capsules are actually cartridges, shells, or "envelopes" that are designed to serve as a carrier for a drug product. Their primary ingredients are gelatin, sugar, and water, but they may contain a dye and/or an opacifying agent. The hard gelatin capsules may also contain about 0.15% sulfur dioxide to prevent decomposition. Soft gelatin, or elastic capsules, are prepared from gelatin, glycerin, and water and can be filled with a liquid, suspension, or powder. The hard and soft gelatin capsules protect the ingredients from direct exposure to the atmosphere before administration and provide a barrier so that the patient will not taste the enclosed contents. After reaching the gastrointestinal tract, capsules may release their contents at different rates based on the physicochemical properties of the active drug and the excipients. Colored capsules are available in almost any form and combination: solid colors (base and cap are the same color) or mixed colors (base and cap are different colors). Special orders of almost any color can be prepared. The pharmacist can also add an approved dye to the powdered material and place the colored powder inside a clear capsule if colored capsules are not available.

Preparation

Source of Equipment and Materials

Materials for the extemporaneous preparation of capsules can be obtained from a variety of sources. Equipment for preparing up to 300 capsules at a time is available at a reasonable cost. Some of the equipment already on hand in a pharmacy can be used for preparing capsules, as well as for carrying out some of the related quality control procedures.

Sources of drugs for capsules include the pure powder, tablets, capsules, and even liquids. The pure powders, which are generally used in their original state, present the fewest complications. Tablets usually must be finely comminuted before they can be incorporated into the capsule powder mix. Obviously, only standard-release tablets should be used, not altered- or controlled-release tablets. Capsules can be a source of the drug if one opens the capsule shell and uses the contents. "Closed capsules," which have gelatin bands, seals, or locking mechanisms, provide a greater challenge. They should be cut into two pieces with a clean razor blade to remove the powder. Some pharmacists, however, break up the capsules in a mortar and then separate the powder from the shell fragments by passing it through a sieve. Liquids can be evaporated to dryness by using appropriate means, or they may be soaked up with an adsorbent before their incorporation into the capsule powder mix. Injectable products can be reconstituted and used, but they may be somewhat more expensive as a source of the active ingredient.

The section "Standard Operating Procedures (SOPs)" provides calculations involved in preparing a formula for the first time. (See the SOP "Developing a Capsule Formulation.")

Preparation of the Powder

To prepare the powder, one must first weigh or measure the individual ingredients. It is best to prepare enough quantity to produce an extra capsule or an additional 5% to 10% of the preparation, which will allow for any loss of powder during manipulations. Preparing excess quantity does not apply to controlled drug substances, however. The particle sizes of solid ingredients should be reduced by comminution to approximately the same size range. The powders should then be passed through a sieve (No. 60 to 100 mesh, depending on the powders). Then the preparation should be mixed by geometric dilution to ensure that the active drugs are distributed uniformly throughout the mix. If the powders are light and fluffy and difficult to manage, one may add a few drops of alcohol, water, or mineral oil to improve workability. The choice of material to add depends on the powders involved; usually only one or two drops of liquid are sufficient. Many pharmacists now mix powders in plastic bags. (See the section "Mixing" in Chapter 9, "Powders and Granules.") If done properly, this method will decrease the amount of powder floating in the air and minimize contamination of the ingredients. Personal safety may dictate that a mask or other protective gear be worn. Whichever method is used, the primary goal when mixing ingredients is homogeneity.

Selection of the Right Capsule Size

Eight different sizes of gelatin capsules are generally used for human consumption, ranging from the smallest, No. 5, through the largest, No. 000 (Table 10-1). The numerical designations are arbitrary and do not indicate a capsule's capacity. The capacity of a capsule depends on the density and characteristics of the powders it contains. The capsule size offers only a relative volume designation. Examples of the weights of materials that can be held by capsules are shown in Table 10-2. Selected physicochemical properties of some capsule diluents are shown in Table 10-3.

Table 10-1. Approximate Capacities of Capsules (in milliliters)

Human Sizes	Capacity
5	0.12
4	0.21
3	0.30
2	0.37
1	0.50
0	0.67
00	0.95
000	1.36
Veterinary Sizes	**Capacity**
10	30
11	15
12	7.5

Veterinary compounding has been increasing dramatically in recent years. Capsules for veterinary use are available in sizes designated as No. 10, No. 11, and No. 12, with capacities of 1 oz, ½ oz, and ¼ oz, respectively.

Generally, capsules can be used to encapsulate between 65 and 1000 mg of powdered material. Capsule selection is usually a simple matter. Some patients may have difficulty swallowing the larger capsules (No. 00, No. 000), but others, especially patients of advanced age, may find the smaller capsules (No. 5, No. 4) hard to handle. The capsule size selected should be slightly larger than is needed to hold the powder because additional powder will be added to produce a full capsule. Ways exist to compensate for the handling and swallowing problems. If the active drug powder bulk is small, more diluent can be added to increase the size of a capsule for handling convenience. If the powder bulk is too large, the total amount can be divided into two smaller capsules that are easier to swallow.

Table 10-2. Different Powder Weights (in milligrams) for Various Sizes of Capsules[a]

Powder Material	Capsule Size							
	5	4	3	2	1	0	00	000
Acetaminophen	130	180	240	310	420	540	750	1100
Aluminum hydroxide	180	270	360	470	640	820	1140	1710
Ascorbic acid	130	220	310	400	520	700	980	1420
Aspirin	65	130	195	260	325	490	650	975
Bismuth subnitrate	120	250	400	550	650	800	1200	1750
Calcium carbonate	120	200	280	350	460	600	790	1140
Calcium lactate	110	160	210	260	330	460	570	800
Cornstarch	130	200	270	340	440	580	800	1150
Lactose	140	210	280	350	460	600	850	1250
Quinine sulfate	65	97	130	195	227	325	390	650
Sodium bicarbonate	130	260	325	390	510	715	975	1430

[a]Depending on the actual powder density.

The "Rule of Sixes" is an interesting technique for the extemporaneous filling of conventional hard gelatin capsules. The method is as follows:

1. Set up six "6s."   6   6   6   6   6   6
2. List the capsule size.   0   1   2   3   4   5
3. Subtract values in step 2 from those in step 1 to determine the average fill weight in grains.   6   5   4   3   2   1
4. Convert fill weight to grams (1 grain = 0.065 g).
   0.390   0.325   0.260   0.195   0.130   0.065
5. Determine fill volume in milliliters (see Table 10-4).
   0.67   0.50   0.37   0.30   0.21   0.12
6. Calculate and list average capsule fill density (divide weight values in step 4 by volume values in step 5).
   0.58   0.65   0.70   0.65   0.62   0.54

As can be seen, the average fill density of the capsules is about 0.62 g/mL.

Table 10-4 gives the bulk densities of typical active drugs and excipients. The bulk densities for these materials range between 0.4 and 0.8 g/mL, with an average of 0.6 g/mL, which is close to the fill density of empty, two-piece, hard gelatin capsules; therefore, the fill density forms the basis for the Rule of Sixes.

The bulk density of a powder is determined by adding a known weight of powder mix to a 100-mL graduated cylinder and measuring the volume. For example, if 75 g of powder is added to a 100-mL graduated cylinder and occupies 100 mL volume, the powder's bulk density is 75 g/100 mL, or 0.75 g/mL. However, if the cylinder is gently tapped on a padded counter surface 100 to 200 times, the powder will settle and occupy less volume. If the weight is divided by this new volume, a new measurement, known as the "tapped density" or "packed bulk density," is obtained. If the new volume is now 85 mL, then the tapped density is 75 g/85 mL, or 0.88 g/mL. The difference between the bulk density and the tapped density is used to determine the approximate compressibility of the powder mix in percentages.

The percentage of compressibility is determined by subtracting the ratio of the bulk density divided by the tapped bulk density from 1 and multiplying by 100,

Table 10-3. Selected Physicochemical Characteristics of Capsule/Tablet Diluents

Diluent	Density (g/mL)	Bulk Density	Tapped Density	Melting Point (°C)	pH	Hygroscopic	Stable	Container
Calcium carbonate	2.70	0.80	1.2	825^a	—	—	Yes	W
Calcium phosphate, dibasic								
Anhydrous	2.89	0.78	0.82	—	7.3 (20%)	No	Yes	W
Hydrate	2.39	0.92	1.17	—	7.4 (20%)	No	Yes	W
Calcium phosphate, tribasic	3.14	0.80	0.95	1670	6.8 (20%)	—	Yes	W
Calcium sulfate								
Anhydrous	2.96	0.70	1.28	1450	10.4 (10%)	Yes	Yes	W
Dihydrate	2.32	0.67	1.12	—	7.3 (10%)	No	Yes	W
Cellulose, microcrystalline	1.59	0.34	0.48	260–270 (chars)	5–7	Yes	Yes	W
Cellulose, powdered	1.50	0.14–0.39	0.21–0.48	—	4–7.5 (10%)	Little	Yes	W
Dextrates	1.54	0.68	0.72	141	3.8–5.8 (20%)	—	Yes	W
Dextrin	1.50–1.59	0.80	0.91	178^a	—	—	Yes	W
Dextrose excipient	1.54	0.83	1.00	83	3.5–5.5 (20%)	No	Yes	W
Fructose	1.58	—	—	102–105	5.35 (9%)	Yes	Yes	W
Kaolin	2.60	—	—	—	—	—	Yes	W
Lactitol	1.54	—	—	—	4.5–7 (10%)	No	Yes	W
Lactose	1.55	0.62	0.94	202	—	No	Yes	T
Mannitol	1.51	0.43	0.73	166–168	—	No	Yes	W
Sorbitol	1.50	0.45	0.40	110–112	4.5–7 (10%)	Yes	Yes	T
Starch	1.48	0.46	0.66	—	5.5–6.5 (2%)	Yes	Yes	W
Starch, pregelatinized	1.52	0.59	0.88	—	4.5–7.0 (10%)	Yes	Yes	W
Sucrose	1.6	0.60	0.82	160–186^a	—	Yes	Yes	W
Sugar, compressible	—	0.49	0.60	—	—	Yes	Yes	W
Sugar, confectioner's	—	0.47	0.83	—	—	Yes	Yes	W

^{a}Melts with some decomposition.

Table 10-4. Bulk Densities of Typical Active Drugs and Excipients

Material	Bulk Density (g/mL)
Activated charcoal	0.32
Aluminum magnesium silicate	0.34
Ascorbic acid	0.51, 0.72
Barium sulfate	0.96
Bentonite	0.8, 0.96
Cab-O-Sil	0.03
Calcium carbonate	0.7
Calcium phosphate	0.77
Calcium sulfate	0.72
Cellulose derivatives	0.41, 0.43, 0.45, 0.72
Citric acid	0.77
Cornstarch	0.64, 0.67, 0.69
Dextrose	0.58, 0.62
FDC dye mixes	0.62
Kaolin	0.80
Magnesium carbonate	0.19
Magnesium oxide	1.04
Magnesium stearate	0.33
Maltodextrin	0.48
Mannitol	0.61
Meprobamate	0.56
Pentaerythritol	0.7
Sodium bicarbonate	0.80, 0.99
Sodium chloride	1.28
Sodium phosphate	1.28
Sodium sulfate	1.36
Sucrose	0.56, 0.85
Talc	0.56
Thiamine hydrochloride	0.75
Titanium dioxide	0.77
Urea	0.62
Vitamin mixes	0.56, 0.67, 0.70
Zinc oxide	0.88

Source: Dry Materials Feeding Handbook. *Accurate Bulk Solids Metering, Whitewater, Wisc.*

as shown here using the values in the previous example: $1 - (0.75/0.88) \times 100 = 14.8\%$ compressibility. This information can be used to estimate the quantity of powder that can be placed into the overfill capacity of empty, two-piece, hard gelatin capsules. As the percentage of compressibility increases, more powder mix can be placed inside the empty capsule. This information should aid in calculating the size of capsules to be used for various powder mixes.[1]

Another general rule that can be used in selecting capsule size is the "Rule of Seven." This rule has several easy steps: (1) convert the weight of the powder per capsule to grains, (2) subtract the number of grains from 7, and (3) match the result with the following listing:

If the resulting number is	Then choose capsule size
−3	000
−2	00
−1 or 0	0
+1	1
+2	2
+3	3
+4	4
+5	5

If, for example, the weight of powder per capsule is 325 mg (5 grains), then $7 - 5 = 2$. The capsule size is 2.

This method does not work if the resulting number is higher than +5 or lower than −3. Nevertheless, because it is quick and easy, it serves as a good starting point for the preparation of hard gelatin capsules.[2]

When selecting the size of a capsule, one should be aware that the required quantity of powder is to be held in the base of the capsule, with the cap simply ensuring powder retention. After the cap is in place, the capsule can be tapped to spread the contents throughout the entire capsule if a clear capsule is used.

Once the proper capsule size has been selected, the entire quantity of capsules required for the specific prescription should be removed from bulk stock. The container should then be closed to reduce any risk of contamination.

Encapsulation Process

Two general methods of encapsulation of powders are commonly used today: individual hand filling and capsule machine filling. Each approach for encapsulating powders and methods for encapsulating semisolids and liquids are described in the following sections.

Individual Hand Filling

When hand filling, the pharmacist should arrange the powder on a suitable surface using a spatula so that the thickness of the pile is about one third the length of the capsule body. The hands should not touch the powder when punching the capsules. Wearing gloves or fingercots will minimize contact with the powder and prevent fingerprints from appearing on the capsules. Another option is to slip the cap from a second capsule over the base of the capsule to be filled (the filling capsule). The second cap thus acts as a holder. Using this technique, the compounding pharmacist does not touch the capsules directly.

As the capsule is pressed into the powder on the working surface, the pharmacist should rotate it slightly to pack the powder in the capsule. When the capsule is full, the pharmacist will feel a slight resistance as the capsule is pressed through the powder. After a few capsules are filled and weighed, the pharmacist will usually develop a feel for how much resistance is required for the capsule to be full.

After the capsule has been filled by using this method, the pharmacist should check its weight and then add or remove powder to obtain the weight desired. Weighing should be performed on a pharmaceutical or electronic laboratory balance by using an empty gelatin capsule of the same size as a tare.

An alternative method involves "blocking and dividing" the powder into individual portions for each capsule. This approach results in an approximation, which is not always accurate and thus not recommended.

Some powders will not stick in the capsules when they are punched out. One way to solve this problem is to place the capsule base on its side and use a spatula to guide or fill the powder. Care must be taken to ensure that the capsule is not scraped or scratched.

Granular materials are particularly difficult to punch into capsules because they are not adequately cohesive. Reducing the particle size to the point at which the powders become more cohesive may alleviate the problem.

Capsule Machine Filling

A number of manually operated capsule filling devices are commercially available for filling up to 50, 100, or 300 capsules at a time (Figure 10-1). These machines can be used for preparing smaller quantities by blocking off unused holes with an index card or self-sticking note.

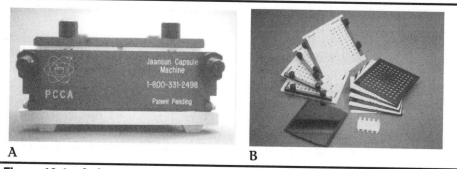

Figure 10-1. *A,* Jaansun capsule machine; *B,* base unit for capsule sizes 00, 0, 1, and 3.

Using these machines requires a careful determination of the capsule formulation. The powder is blended as previously discussed. Empty gelatin capsules are placed into the device so that the cap is on top. The machine is worked to separate the base from the cap, and the portion of the machine holding the caps is removed and set aside. The capsule bases are allowed to drop into place so that the top of the base is flush with the working surface. The powder mix is then spread over the working surface. A plastic spatula can be used to spread the powder evenly into the capsule bases. Alternatively, the machine can be tapped to spread the powder and drop it down into the capsule bases. A small device consisting of several pegs can be used to tamp the powder into the capsule bases gently and evenly. Any remaining powder is then spread evenly over and into the capsule bases, followed by additional tamping. These procedures are repeated until all of the powder is in the capsules. The portion of the machine holding the capsule caps is then fitted over the machine and fixed in place. The filled capsules are capped, removed, dusted with a clean cloth, and packaged.

Filling Capsules with a Semisolid Mass

Producing a capsule containing a semisolid material requires a different approach. Two methods are used to place semisolid materials into hard gelatin capsules: forming a pipe or pouring a melt.

Material that is sufficiently plastic can be rolled into a pipe with a diameter slightly less than that of the inner diameter of the capsule in which it will be enclosed. The quantity of material desired is cut with a spatula or knife, with the length removed determining the weight of the material to be enclosed in the capsule shell. The pieces can be dusted with cornstarch and then inserted individually into the capsules.

If a material is too fluid, cornstarch or a similar material can be added to achieve a firmer consistency. The quantity to add can be determined empirically.

If the material is too firm to roll into a pipe but its melting point is in a satisfactory temperature range, it can be melted until it is fluid and then poured into the bases of the gelatin capsules. After the capsules have cooled, the caps are replaced. When this technique is used, it is helpful to have a stand to hold the capsule bodies. This stand can be made by drilling holes into a block of wood or plastic that are the same size as the diameter of the caps. Caps are inserted into the holes and glued in place to prevent any scratching of the capsule bodies. The bases and caps of the required quantity of capsules are separated. The capsule bases are then inserted into the stationary caps, and the melt is poured into the bases and allowed to cool. The separated caps are placed on the bases, and the completed capsules are removed from the holder.

This method can also be used to enhance the bioavailability of drugs that are poorly soluble and exhibit bioavailability problems. In these cases, the drug is added to a melt of a material such as polyethylene glycol (PEG). The mixture is heated and stirred until the powder is either melted or thoroughly mixed in the PEG. After the melt is cooled to just above the melting point of the PEG, it is poured into the capsule shells as described. When this method is used, the desired quantities can be measured using a pipet, syringe, or calibrated dropper to deliver the volume to the individual capsules. Excipients useful in formulating these products are shown in Table 10-5.

Filling Capsules with Liquids

Occasionally, pharmacists must prepare hard gelatin capsules containing liquid materials. This task can be accomplished easily as long as the liquid material does not dissolve the gelatin. The method should work with alcoholic solutions, fixed oils, or volatile oils because gelatin is not soluble in these materials. A partially hydrogenated cottonseed oil can be used as a vehicle as it has a low melting point, oil-soluble drugs are soluble in it, and it is a solid at room temperature. Experimentation may be required, however, to determine the solubility of the gelatin in the liquid.

This approach calls for the liquid to be measured accurately using a pipet (micropipet) or a calibrated dropper and then dropped into the capsule base, taking care not to touch the opening. To soften the gelatin at the opening of the caps, one can either touch the gelatin cap, open end down, to a moist towel or dip a cotton swab in warm water and then rub it around the edge of the cap. The cap is placed over the base containing the liquid with a slight twist, enabling the softened edge of the cap to form a seal with the base to prevent leakage. Before the capsules are packaged, they should be placed on a clean, dry sheet of paper to check for leakage. Table 10-1 lists the volumes of the various capsules. Sealing can also be accomplished by painting a warm gelatin solution around the capsule, as well as along the inside of the cap, before placing the cap on the base.

Table 10-5. Excipients Used As Matrices for Semisolid Capsules

Vegetable oils
- Cotton seed
- Maize
- Nut
- Olive
- Soya

Hydrogenated vegetable oils
- Castor
- Coconut
- Cotton seed
- Palm
- Soya

Vegetable fats
- Carnauba wax
- Cocoa butter

Animal fats
- Beeswax
- Lanolin
- Speraceti

Hydrocarbons
- Paraffin

Fatty alcohols
- Cetyl
- Lauryl
- Stearyl

Fatty acids
- Lauryl
- Myristic
- Palmitic
- Stearic

Esters
- Ethyl oleate
- Glycol stearates
- Isopropyl myristate

Mixed esters
Liquid
- Labrafil
- Miglyol 812

Solid
- Suppocire
- Witepsol

Cleaning Capsules

The compounding pharmacist must take every precaution to minimize traces of moisture or body oils on capsules because moisture causes powders to stick to the surface, creating an unsightly appearance and a disagreeable taste. Cleaning the capsules will be difficult if they become moist or sticky. The use of gloves ensures that the working environment is hygienic and helps preserve the capsule's dry, shiny appearance.

If gloves are not available, the pharmacist should (1) wash and dry hands thoroughly, (2) keep the fingers dry by stripping a towel through tightly clenched fingers until friction develops and a clearly perceptible heat is generated, and (3) prepare four or five capsules before repeating the hand-cleaning procedure.

If the capsules have been kept dry, clinging surface powder can be removed by rolling the capsules between the folds of a cloth or shaking them in a cloth that has been formed into a bag or hammock. Another method of cleaning capsules is to place them in a container filled with sodium bicarbonate, sugar, or salt and then gently roll the container. The contents are next poured into a No. 10—mesh sieve, which allows the cleaning salt to pass through but retains the capsules.

It must be emphasized that these cleaning methods are effective only if the capsules have been kept clean and dry. Once capsules have become soiled and dull, they cannot be effectively cleaned.

The box "Hints for Compounding Capsules" contains additional suggestions for preparing this versatile dosage form.

Hints for Compounding Capsules

- Sodium lauryl sulfate, up to 1%, can be added to powders to neutralize electrostatic forces.
- Capsules may be colored by adding a dye to the powder before it is placed in a clear capsule. This helps to distinguish various strengths of powders and capsules. Also, mixing bases and caps of different colored capsules customizes the colors. It is best to use two capsule machines for this process.
- Liquids can be incorporated into capsules by mixing with melted polyethylene glycol 6000 or 8000 or a related concentration of this substance. The mixture can be poured into capsules, where it will solidify. The capsule can then be closed and dispensed.
- Liquids can be dispensed in capsules by using a syringe to drop the liquid into the capsule base. Oils can be mixed with a fat or fatty acid, including cocoa butter, and slightly heated. The mixture can then be poured into capsules.
- The locking-type capsules available today minimize the loss of their contents, whether powder, liquid, or semisolid; they also work well with hand-operated capsule-filling machines.

Physicochemical Considerations

Physical and chemical interactions between active drugs, between active drug(s) and excipients, and between active drugs and excipients and the gelatin shell must be considered. For example, hard gelatin capsules normally contain about 10% to 15% moisture, yet gelatin can absorb up to 10 times its weight in water. Capsules stored in high humidity absorb moisture and can become misshapen. If stored in low humidity, they become dry and brittle and can crack. A relative humidity range of 30% to 45% is best for good encapsulation. If the drug to be encapsulated requires a drier environment, such an environment should be provided.

Various agents can be added to improve the characteristics of the material used in the preparation or administration of a capsule. Magnesium stearate is sometimes used to enhance the flowability of particles, which makes it easier to fill capsules. Although it is usually present at concentrations less than 1%, it is hydrophobic and can affect the bioavailability of drug. Thus, up to 1% sodium lauryl sulfate can be incorporated to enhance the bioavailability of drugs contained within capsules.

Incompatibilities

Deliquescent powders can be prepared by the addition of a finely powdered bulking material such as starch or magnesium oxide. This practice lessens the tendency of the powders to absorb moisture.

Table 10-6. Useful Excipients in Capsule Preparation

Excipients That Enhance Compatibility of Eutectic Mixtures
Effective
  Magnesium carbonate
  Kaolin
  Light magnesium oxide
Less effective
  Heavy magnesium oxide
  Tribasic calcium phosphate
  Silica gel
Relatively ineffective
  Talc
  Lactose
  Starch

Excipients Used as Diluents for Other Purposes in Capsules
Bentonite
Calcium carbonate
Lactose
Mannitol
Magnesium carbonate
Magnesium oxide
Silica gel
Starch
Talc
Tapioca powder

Eutectic mixtures can be incorporated into capsules by keeping the problematic ingredients separate, adding an inert powder, and mixing lightly before encapsulating the ingredients. Also, using the next larger size capsule will decrease the contact of the powder particles with each other and hence minimize their tendency to liquefy. Materials that help to prevent or correct eutectics are included in Table 10-6, along with other excipients that are useful in capsule preparation. An alternative technique is to first form the eutectic and subsequently absorb the liquid into a powder, which is then encapsulated.

Capsules within Capsules

If one ingredient must be separated from the others in a formulation, it may be necessary to fill a small capsule, such as a No. 5, with one powder and then place that capsule, along with the remaining ingredients, within a larger capsule. For elegance, the inside capsule should not be visible through the larger capsule.

Tablets within Capsules

If a small tablet containing a necessary ingredient is commercially available, it can be placed inside the capsule. A small quantity of the additional powder should be deposited in the base before and after adding the tablet. The inside tablet should not be visible through the filled capsule.

Altered-Release Capsules

The rate of release of a capsule's contents will vary according to the nature of the drug and the capsule's excipients. If the drug is water soluble and a fast release is desired, the excipients should be hydrophilic and neutral. If a slow release of a water-soluble drug is desired, the excipients should be hydrophobic to delay the rate at which the drug dissolves. If the drug is insoluble in water and a fast release is desired, hydrophilic excipients should be used. Release of a drug may be slowed by adding hydrophobic and neutral excipients or gel-forming excipients.

Rapid-Release Capsules

A more rapid/immediate release of the capsule contents can be accomplished by piercing holes in the capsule to allow faster penetration of fluids in the gastrointestinal tract, or by adding a small quantity of sodium bicarbonate and citric acid to help open the capsule by the production of carbon dioxide. Adding 0.1% to 1% of sodium lauryl sulfate can allow water to penetrate the capsule more quickly and speed dissolution.

Slow Release

If a slower release of the active drug is desired, the active drug powder can be mixed with various excipients, such as cellulose polymers (methylcellulose) or sodium alginate. In general, the rate of release is delayed as the proportion of polymer or alginate is increased relative to water-soluble ingredients, such as lactose. Because it is difficult to predict the exact release profile for a drug and to obtain consistent results from batch to batch, attempts to alter release rates to this extent should be used only in special circumstances.

Delayed-Release Capsules

Capsules can be coated to delay the release of the active drug until it reaches a selected portion of the gastrointestinal tract. Materials that have been found to be suitable include stearic acid, shellac, casein, cellulose acetate phthalate, and natural and synthetic waxes; the basis of their suitability is that they have acid insolubility but are soluble in alkaline environments. Many of the newer coating materials depend on time:erosion rather than acid:base factors; that is, rather than being pH dependent, their coating erodes over timed exposure to gastrointestinal contents. A number of newer materials have predictable pH solubility profiles. The dispensing pharmacist should avoid coatings applied to modify the release of a drug, but he or she can add a coating to conceal taste, which can enhance patient compliance.

The application of a coating requires skill and additional equipment. A general coating can be applied, but it should be used only in medications that are not critical in nature. In many cases, the pharmacist must develop experience in preparing specific formulations, depending on the requests of the primary care providers and the needs of the individual patients.

Three methods are used to coat capsules: beaker-flask coating, dipping, and spraying.

> ▸ *Beaker-flask coating.* Place a small quantity of the coating material in the flask and gently heat until it has melted. Add a few capsules, remove from the heat, and rotate the flask to start applying the coating. Periodically add

a few more drops of melted coating while continuing to rotate. The addition of small quantities of coating material keeps the capsules from sticking together and clumping.

▸ *Dipping.* Heat the coating material in a beaker at the lowest feasible temperature. Dip the individual capsules, using tweezers. Allow the coating to cool and repeat the process until a sufficient layer has been applied to the capsule.

▸ *Spraying.* Prepare an alcoholic or ethereal solution of the coating material. Place solution in a small sprayer (a model airplane paint sprayer works well). Place the capsules on a screen in a well-ventilated area. Apply the solution of the coating material in thin coats, allowing sufficient time for drying between coats. (A hair dryer may be used for this step if care is taken.) Repeat the process until a sufficient layer has been developed.

Quality Control

Because the pharmacist is responsible for the quality of the capsules prepared, it is important to keep the work area clean and neat and to conduct quality control checks to ensure that the products contain the correct material in the right quantity. One check is to routinely read the label on the bottle at least three times and to record the necessary information (e.g., source, lot number) on the compounding formulation record.

The only reliable method of filling capsules accurately is to weigh each individual capsule. Because such an approach is generally not feasible, the pharmacist can instead weigh representative samples. It is good practice to weigh some capsules individually and to weigh others in groups of 10 capsules. The two methods together provide data that document the accuracy of the capsule fill, which can be included in the formulation record. Weighing groups of at least 10 capsules at a time is advised because empty gelatin capsules can vary by as much as 15% in their weight. Although 15% seems like a large number, the capsule shell is light and represents little of the total weight of a filled capsule. Composite weighings will average out any small variations in the weight of the empty capsules. (See the SOPs "Quality Assessment for Powder-Filled, Hard Gelatin Capsules" and "Quality Assessment of Special Hard Gelatin Capsules.")

Packaging/Storage

Empty gelatin capsules should be stored at room temperature at constant humidity. High humidity can cause the capsules to soften, and low humidity can cause them to dry and crack. It is best to store capsules in glass containers, which protect against both extreme humidity and dust.

Storage of filled capsules depends on the characteristics of the drug they contain. For example, hard gelatin capsules filled with semisolids should be stored away from excessive heat, which can cause the contents to soften or melt.

Stability

Capsules are dry or, if they are filled with liquids or semisolids, they contain nonaqueous liquids. For this reason, they generally provide a stable dosage form as long as they are protected from moisture and heat. According to Chapter <795>,

"Pharmacy Compounding,"[3] powders prepared from a manufactured product should have a beyond-use date of 25% of the time remaining on the product's expiration date or 6 months, whichever is earlier. If the product is prepared from USP/NF ingredients, a beyond-use date of 6 months is appropriate, unless evidence is available to support other dating.

Patient Counseling

Capsule sizes Nos. 5 through 0 are generally not too difficult to swallow; however, many patients can have difficulty swallowing the No. 00 and No. 000 capsules. If this is the case, the patient may be advised to place the capsule on the back of the tongue before drinking a liquid, or to place the capsule in warm water for a few seconds before taking it, which makes it slide over the mucous membranes more easily. Also, a teaspoonful of a flavored candy gel can be placed in the mouth and swished around; the capsule is then placed into the mouth and easily swallowed. The pharmacist can also suggest alternatives such as smaller capsules or even a liquid preparation.

Sample Formulations

Capsules with Dry Powder Fill

R̲x̲ **Morphine Sulfate 10 mg and Dextromethorphan Hydrobromide 30 mg**

Morphine sulfate	1 g
Dextromethorphan hydrobromide	3 g
Lactose	35.5 g

1. Calculate the quantity of each ingredient required for the prescription.
2. Accurately weigh the morphine sulfate, dextromethorphan hydrobromide, and lactose.
3. Reduce the particle size, if necessary, and mix well.
4. Fill 100 No. 1 capsules with 395 mg of the powder mix. (Note: It may be necessary to alter the quantity of lactose per capsule, depending upon the bulk density of the lactose being used.)
5. Check the weights of the capsules.
6. Package and label.

Capsules with Semisolid Fill

R𝑥 **Tri-Estrogen Capsules**

Estriol	200 mg
Estrone	25 mg
Estradiol	25 mg
Polyethylene glycol 1450	20 g
Polyethylene glycol 3350	20 g

1. Calculate the quantity of each ingredient required for the prescription.
2. Accurately weigh each ingredient.
3. Using geometric dilution, mix the estrogen powders.
4. Using low heat to about 65°C, melt the polyethylene glycols.
5. Sprinkle on the estrogen powders and thoroughly mix.
6. Load a capsule machine, if available, with 100 No. 1 capsules and remove the caps.
7. To determine the volume of mixture to place in each capsule, perform the following steps:
    - Using a micropipet, place 330 µL of the estrogen:polyethylene glycol melt into each of three capsule bases.
    - Weigh the three capsules and obtain the average weight for each.
    - Adjust the volume delivered, if necessary, to obtain capsules with a tared weight of 403 mg.
8. Place the required volume in each of the capsules, according to step 7.
9. Allow the mixture to harden and replace the caps on the capsules.
10. Check the weights of about 10 capsules for uniformity and accuracy.
11. Package and label.

℞ Progesterone 100 mg Semisolid-Fill, Hard Gelatin Capsules (#100)

Progesterone	10 g
Polyethylene glycol 1450	20 g
Polyethylene glycol 3350	20 g

1. Calculate the required quantity of each ingredient for the total amount to be prepared.
2. Accurately weigh/measure each ingredient.
3. Using low heat (60°C–65°C) melt the PEGs.
4. Sprinkle on the progesterone powder and thoroughly mix.
5. Load a capsule machine with 100 capsules (No. 1) and remove the caps.
6. Using a micropipet, place 330 µL of the progesterone:PEG melt into each of three capsule bases. Weigh the three capsules and obtain the average weight for each. Adjust the volume delivered, if necessary, to obtain capsules that weigh 500 mg each.
7. Fill all the capsules with the drug:melt mixture.
8. Allow the mixture to harden and replace the caps on the capsules.
9. Check the weights of 10 capsules for uniformity and accuracy.
10. Package and label.

Capsules with Liquid Fill

℞ Progesterone 100 mg in Peanut Oil Capsules

Micronized progesterone		10 g
Peanut oil	qs	30 mL

M. progesterone 100 mg capsules.

1. Calculate the quantity of each ingredient required for the prescription.
2. Accurately weigh the progesterone.
3. Mix the progesterone with about 20 mL of peanut oil, in small portions.
4. Add sufficient peanut oil to make 30 mL and mix well.
5. Load a capsule machine with 100 No. 1 empty gelatin capsules.
6. Using a micropipet, add 300 µL of the mixture to each of the 100 capsules.
7. Remove the filled capsules from the capsule machine.
8. Package and label.

Standard Operating Procedures (SOPs)

Determining Volume of Capsule Ingredients and Diluents

Purpose of SOP

The purpose of this procedure is to establish appropriate guidelines and documentation for determining the percentage of capsule volume occupied by active ingredients to determine the quantity of diluent required per capsule.

Compounding Principle

When many dosage forms are prepared, the volume occupied by the various ingredients must be determined. Some examples are fixed-volume dosage forms such as capsules, molded suppositories, molded troches/lozenges, and molded tablets. Because of the differences in densities of the ingredients, different substances will occupy different volumes in the dosage form, especially capsules. For example, a No. 1 capsule can hold from approximately 225 mg of quinine sulfate to approximately 650 mg of bismuth subnitrate, almost a 3-fold difference. When the actual densities of the ingredients are not known, the percentage of the capsule volume occupied by each ingredient can be determined to calculate the quantities of diluent needed. Figure 10-2 provides a method of documenting the calculations involved in compounding capsule formulations; the form is easily applied to multi-ingredient capsules. It is necessary to have the packing statistics for capsules or to determine them. To experimentally determine the packing statistics for each ingredient, the pharmacist can fill five tared capsules with each of the respective ingredients and obtain the individual capsule weights. The pharmacist can average these five weights to obtain the packing statistics for the individual ingredients.

Physical Quality Assessment of Powder-Filled, Hard Gelatin Capsules

Purpose of SOP

The purpose of this procedure is to provide a method of documenting physical quality assessment tests of and observations on powder-filled, hard gelatin capsules.

Equipment/Materials

The following items are used in one or more of the quality assessment tests:

- Balance
- Hot plate/stirrer
- 100-mL beaker
- Thermometer

Procedure

The necessary tests should be conducted, and the results/observations recorded on the worksheet "Physical Quality Assessment of Powder-Filled, Hard Gelatin Capsules" (Figure 10-3).

Capsule Formulation Development Using
Percent of Volume Occupied

Ingredient	Quantity Required per Capsule (A)	Weight of Filled Capsule (B)	A/B = % Filled (C)
_____	_____	_____	_____
_____	_____	_____	_____
_____	_____	_____	_____
_____	_____	_____	_____
_____	_____	_____	_____
_____	_____	_____	_____
_____	_____	_____	_____
_____	_____	_____	_____
_____	_____	_____	_____

% of Capsule Filled = _____ (D)

% Diluent Required = 100% − (D) = _____ (E)

Weight of Capsule Filled with Diluent = _____ (F)

Quantity of Diluent Required per Capsule = (F) × (E) = _____ (G)

(Note: Change percentage (E) to decimal (E) by dividing by 100.)

Quantity of Diluent Required for the Prescription =

Number of Capsules × (G) = _____

Notes:

Column (A) is from the prescription.

Column (B) is obtained by averaging the weight of at least five tared capsules that have been filled with the respective ingredient(s).

Column (C) is obtained by dividing Column (A) by Column (B) and multiplying by 100 to obtain percentage.

Value (D) is obtained by adding the "percentage" values in Column (C).

Value (E) is obtained by subtracting Value (D) from 100% to obtain the percentage of the capsule that is vacant.

Value (F) is obtained by averaging the weight of at least five tared capsules that have been filled with the diluent.

Value (G) is obtained by multiplying Value (E) by Value (F). Value (G) is the quantity of diluent that will be required per capsule.

Multiplying (G) by the number of capsules to be prepared will give the total quantity of diluent required for the prescription.

Figure 10-2. Worksheet for determining packing statistics for capsules.

Average Weight of Filled Capsules.

1. Tare the balance with 10 empty capsules.
2. Select 10 filled capsules at random.
3. Place all 10 filled capsules on the balance and record the weight on the worksheet.
4. Calculate the average weight of each capsule by dividing the weight of the 10 filled capsules by 10.

Individual Weight Variation of Capsule Contents and Active Ingredient.[1]

1. Tare the balance with a single empty capsule.
2. Weigh individually each of the 10 filled capsules used in the average weight test, and record the results on the worksheet (Figure 10-3).
3. Calculate the actual weight of the active ingredient in each capsule using the following proportional equation:

   Actual weight of filled capsule/Theoretical weight of filled capsule = Actual weight of active ingredient/Theoretical weight of active ingredient

   For example, a filled capsule is supposed to weigh 400 mg and contain 25 mg of active drug, but the actual weight of the filled capsule is 380 mg. The actual quantity of active drug per capsule is calculated as follows:

   $$380 \text{ mg}/400 \text{ mg} = x/25 \text{ mg}$$
   $$x = 23.75 \text{ mg of active drug}$$

4. To calculate the lower value for the theoretical weight of the active ingredient, multiply the theoretical weight by 85%. Calculate the upper value by multiplying the theoretical weight by 115%. Record the results on the worksheet (Figure 10-3).
5. To calculate the lower limit of the theoretical weight of the active ingredient, multiply the theoretical weight by 75%. Calculate the upper limit by multiplying the theoretical weight by 125%. Record the results on the worksheet (Figure 10-3).
6. Determine whether the weight variation of the active ingredient is within the range of 85.0% to 115.0% of label claim and whether any capsule is outside the range of 75.0% to 125.0% of label claim. If 2 or 3 capsules are outside the range of 85.0% to 115.0% of label claim, but not outside the range of 75.0% to 125.0% of label claim, test an additional 20 capsules. If more than 3 capsules are outside the range, discard the batch. The requirements are met if not more than 3 capsules of the 30 are outside the range of 85.0 to 115.0% of label claim and no capsule is outside the range of 75.0% to 125.0% of label claim. If any capsule is outside the range of 75.0% to 125.0% of label claim, the batch should be rejected.

Dissolution of Powder-Filled Capsule Shells.

‣ Place one capsule in a beaker of purified water USP maintained at 37°C with a stir bar rotating at about 30 revolutions per minute. The gelatin shell should be disrupted within about 20 to 30 minutes.

Disintegration of Powder-Filled Capsule Contents.

‣ Place one immediate-release capsule in a beaker of purified water USP maintained at 37°C with a stir bar rotating at about 30 revolutions per minute.

Physical Quality Assessment of Powder-Filled, Hard Gelatin Capsules

Product_____   Strength _____

Lot/Rx Number _____   Date _____

A. Weight–Overall Average Weight
   I. Weight of 10 filled capsules   _____ g
   II. Average weight of each filled capsule   _____ g
       (Divide weight of 10 filled capsules by 10.)

B. Weight–Individual Weight Variation
   I. Record the weight of each capsule in Column I.

Column I (Actual Capsule Weight)	Column II (Actual Active Ingredient Weight)
1. _____	_____
2. _____	_____
3. _____	_____
4. _____	_____
5. _____	_____
6. _____	_____
7. _____	_____
8. _____	_____
9. _____	_____
10. _____	_____

   II. Calculate the actual active ingredient weight per capsule and record it in Column II, as follows:

       Based on the *theoretical active ingredient weight* per *theoretical capsule weight,* calculate the *actual active ingredient weight per capsule.* For this calculation, use the actual capsule weight from part A, step II, above:
       _____ g

       Example: If the total theoretical capsule weight was 400 mg and was to contain 25 mg of active drug (actual active ingredient weight), but the actual capsule weight was 380 mg, the actual quantity of active drug per capsule (actual active ingredient weight) would be as follows:

        Actual capsule weight/Theoretical capsule weight =
    Actual active ingredient weight/Theoretical active ingredient weight
$$380/400 = x/25$$

       Thus, $x = 23.75$ mg, so 23.75 mg is the actual active ingredient weight per capsule.

   III. Multiply the *theoretical active ingredient weight* per capsule by 85.0% and 115.0% and record the results:
      Lower value (85%): _____ g   Upper value (115%): _____ g

(continued)

IV. Multiple the *theoretical active ingredient weight* per capsule by 75.0% and 125.0% and record the results:
Lower limit (75%): _____ g   Upper limit (125%): _____ g

V. Do any of the 10 individual active drug weights fall outside the lower and upper values in part B, step III?   Yes _____ No _____
If yes, how many?   _____ (If 2 or 3, repeat the test.)

VI. If yes, do any of the 10 individual active drug weights fall outside the upper and lower limits in part B, step IV?   Yes _____ No _____
If yes, discard the batch.

C. Dissolution of Capsule Shell   Yes _____ No _____

D. Disintegration of Capsule Contents   Yes _____ No _____

E. Active Drug Assay Results _____
Initial Assay _____
After Storage No. 1 _____
After Storage No. 2 _____

F. Physical Observation:
Color of Product _____
Uniformity_____Yes _____ No _____
Extent of Fill _____Yes _____ No _____
Locked_____Yes _____ No _____

G. Was sample set aside for physical observation?   Yes _____ No _____
If yes, record results.

Date   Observation
_____   _____
_____   _____
_____   _____
_____   _____
_____   _____
_____   _____
_____   _____
_____   _____
_____   _____
_____   _____
_____   _____
_____   _____
_____   _____

Figure 10-3. Sample worksheet for physical quality assessment of powder-filled, hard gelatin capsules.

The contents of the capsule should be broken apart or dispersed within 30 minutes.

Assay of Active Drug. As appropriate, depending on how many capsules are compounded, have representative samples of the capsules assayed for active drug content by a contract analytical laboratory. The initial assay is performed soon after preparation of the formulation. Stability can be assessed by storing the product at room temperature and having the assay repeated on the stored samples.

Physical Appearance Tests. The following tests are important in ensuring that each capsule contains the desired quantity of ingredients:

- *Product color check:* Check the description on the master record formula. It may be advisable to use a color chart for determining the actual color of the product.
- *Uniformity test.* Check capsules for uniformity of appearance.
- *Extent of fill test.* Check capsules for uniformity of extent of fill for assurance all capsules have been filled.
- *Locked-capsule test.* Check capsules for assurance they have all been tightly closed and locked.

Physical Stability Tests.

1. Prepare an additional quantity of capsules; package and label (for physical stability observations).
2. Weekly, observe the product for signs of discoloration or change.
3. Record a descriptive observation on the form at each observation interval.

Physical Quality Assessment of Special Hard Gelatin Capsules

Purpose of SOP

The purpose of this procedure is to provide a method of documenting basic physical quality assessment tests and observations of liquid-filled, semisolid-filled, solid-filled, altered-release, and coated hard gelatin capsules. Results and observations should be recorded on the worksheet "Physical Quality Assessment of Special Hard Gelatin Capsules" (Figure 10-4).

Equipment/Materials

The following items are used in one or more of the quality assessment tests:

- Balance
- Hot plate/stirrer
- 100-mL beaker
- Thermometer
- Color chart

Procedure

The procedure described in the SOP "Physical Quality Assessment of Powder-Filled, Hard Gelatin Capsules" applies to special hard gelatin capsules except for the sections "Dissolution of Powder-Filled Capsule Shells" and "Disintegration of Powder-Filled Capsule Contents." Only procedures for these two tests on special hard gelatin capsules are discussed in this section.

Physical Quality Assessment of Special Hard Gelatin Capsules

Product_____   Strength_____

Lot/Rx Number _____   Date _____

A. Weight–Overall Average Weight
  I.   Weight of 10 filled capsules   _____ g
  II. Average weight of each filled capsule   _____ g
       (Divide weight of 10 filled capsules by 10.)

B. Weight–Individual Weight Variation
  I.   Record the weight of each capsule in Column I.

     Column I   Column II
     (Actual Capsule Weight)   (Actual Active Ingredient Weight)
        1. _____   _____
        2. _____   _____
        3. _____   _____
        4. _____   _____
        5. _____   _____
        6. _____   _____
        7. _____   _____
        8. _____   _____
        9. _____   _____
       10. _____   _____

  II. Calculate the actual active ingredient weight per capsule and record it in Column II, as follows:

       Based on the *theoretical active ingredient weight* per *theoretical capsule weight,* calculate the *actual active ingredient weight per capsule.* For this calculation, use the actual capsule weight from part A, step II: _____ g

       Example: If the total theoretical capsule weight was 400 mg and was to contain 25 mg of active drug (actual active ingredient weight), but the actual capsule weight was 380 mg, the actual quantity of active drug per capsule (actual active ingredient weight) would be as follows:

       Actual capsule weight/Theoretical capsule weight =
       Actual active ingredient weight/Theoretical active ingredient weight
       $$380/400 = x/25$$

       Thus, x = 23.75 mg, so 23.75 mg is the actual active ingredient weight per capsule.

  III. Multiply the *theoretical active ingredient weight* per capsule by 85.0% and 115.0% and record the results:
       Lower value (85%): _____ g   Upper value (115%): _____ g

(continued)

IV. Multiply the *theoretical active ingredient weight* per capsule by 75.0% and 125.0% and record the results:
Lower limit (75%): _____ g   Upper limit (125%): _____ g

V. Do any of the 10 individual active drug weights fall outside the lower and upper values in part B, step III?   Yes _____ No _____
If yes, how many? _____ (If 2 or 3, repeat the test.)

VI. If yes, do any of the 10 individual active drug weights fall outside the upper and lower limits in part B, step IV?   Yes _____ No _____
If yes, discard the batch.

C. Dissolution of Capsule Shell Yes _____ No _____
   Immediate-Release   Yes _____ No _____
   Coated-Capsule:
      0.1 N HCl   Yes _____ No _____
      0.1 N NaOH   Yes _____ No _____

D. Disintegration of Capsule Contents:
   Immediate-Release Yes _____ No _____
   Altered-Release   Yes _____ No _____

E. Active Drug Assay Results
   Initial Assay _____
   After Storage No. 1 _____
   After Storage No. 2 _____

F. Physical Observation:
   Color of Product _____
   Uniformity   Yes _____ No _____
   Extent of Fill Yes _____ No _____
   Locked   Yes _____ No _____

G. Was sample set aside for physical observation? Yes _____ No _____
   If yes, record results.
   Date   Observation
   _____   _____
   _____   _____
   _____   _____
   _____   _____
   _____   _____
   _____   _____
   _____   _____
   _____   _____
   _____   _____
   _____   _____

Figure 10-4. Sample worksheet for physical quality assessment of special hard gelatin capsules.

Dissolution of Special Hard Gelatin Capsules.

- *Immediate-release (rapid-release) capsules:* Place one capsule in a beaker of purified water USP maintained at 37°C with a stir bar rotating at about 30 rpm. The gelatin shell should be disrupted within about 20 to 30 minutes.
- *Capsules with acid-resistant coating:* Place one capsule in a beaker of 0.1 N hydrochloric acid maintained at 37°C for 30 minutes. The shell should not disrupt. Place the capsule in a beaker of 0.1 N sodium hydroxide maintained at 37°C for 30 minutes, the shell should disrupt.

Disintegration of Contents of Special Hard Gelatin Capsules.

- *Immediate-release (rapid-release) capsules:* Place one capsule in a beaker of purified water USP maintained at 37°C with a stir bar rotating at about 30 rpm. The contents of the capsule should be broken apart or dispersed within 30 minutes.
- *Altered-release (slow-release) capsules:* Place one capsule in a beaker of purified water USP maintained at 37°C with a stir bar rotating at about 30 rpm. The contents of the capsule should not be broken apart but appear as a swollen gel plug remaining intact for at least 2 hours, even though it may decrease in size.

References

1. Nash RA. The "Rule of Sixes" for filling hard-shell gelatin capsules. *Int J Pharm Compound.* 1997;1(1):40–1.
2. Al-Achi A, Greenwood RB. The "Rule of Seven" for determining capsule size. *Int J Pharm Compound.* 1997;1(3):191.
3. Expert Advisory Panel on Pharmacy Compounding Practices. Pharmacy compounding. In: *United States Pharmacopeia 25/National Formulary 20.* Rockville, Md: United States Pharmacopeial Convention; 2000.

Chapter 11

Tablets

The tablet is the most frequently prescribed commercial dosage form. This dosage form is stable, elegant, and effective. It provides the patient with a convenient product for handling, identification, and administration. Commercially available tablets can be made at a rate of thousands per minute, but they are available only in fixed dosage strengths and combinations. In many instances, the available products do not match the requirements of specific patients. Until recently, tablets were beyond the scope of the compounding pharmacist. Today, however, some pharmacists extemporaneously prepare molded and compressed tablets for their patients. Pellet presses and single-punch tableting machines now make compounding tablets feasible. In the near future, preblended powders may be available that will make it easier to incorporate small quantities of active drugs into the tablet preparation, taking into consideration the tablet's hardness, friability, and disintegration rates.

Definitions/Types

Sublingual molded tablets are placed under the tongue. They dissolve rapidly, releasing the medication for absorption sublingually, or they can be swallowed. Generally, sublingual tablets contain lactose and other ingredients that are quite water soluble and dissolve quickly.

Buccal molded tablets are administered in the cheek pouch. They dissolve rather quickly, and the released medication can be absorbed or swallowed. The excipients can be manipulated between hydrophilicity and hydrophobicity based on the desired release rate.

Sintered tablets can be prepared either to dissolve in the mouth, if they are flavored, or to be swallowed. They generally contain the active drug, a diluent, and a meltable binder such as polyethylene glycol (PEG) 3350.

Compressed tablets are designed to be swallowed. Although they are generally prepared by using large, expensive tableting machines, they can be extemporaneously prepared by using pellet punches or single-punch tableting machines.

Chewable tablets must be chewed and swallowed. Formulated to be pleasant tasting, they should not leave a bitter or unpleasant aftertaste. Chewable tablets are typically prepared by compression and usually contain sugars (mannitol, sorbitol, or sucrose) and flavoring agents.

Soluble effervescent tablets are prepared by compression and contain mixtures of acids and sodium bicarbonate, which release carbon dioxide when dissolved in water. Citric acid or tartaric acid may be used. These tablets are intended to be dispersed in water before they are administered and should not be swallowed whole.

Implants or pellets are small, sterile, solid masses containing a drug with or without excipients. They can be prepared by compression or molding. Implants are intended for implantation in the body, usually subcutaneously, and provide continuous release of the drug over time. These preparations must be sterile, free of pyrogens, and prepared in a clean environment. They can be implanted by means of a special injector or a superficial incision. Testosterone and estradiol are two agents that have been prepared as implants or pellets.

Historical Use

The tablet originated in England in the 1800s as a compressed pill. In 1878, Burroughs Wellcome and Company applied the term *tablet* to this dosage form. John Wyeth and his brother introduced compressed tablets into the United States in 1882 in the form of compressed hypodermic tablets and compressed tablet triturates. In 1892, a British manufacturer was granted use of the term *tablet* for biconvex discs. Today, tablets make up most of the drug dosage forms on the market because of their economy, ease of preparation, accuracy of dosage, and ease of administration.

Applications

With the exception of molded tablets, few tableted dosage forms have been compounded in recent years. This situation may soon change, as new methods and techniques are developed and new equipment becomes available. It is likely that tablets will be compounded in greater numbers in the future by using single-punch tableting machines and preblended excipients. Compounding pharmacists would simply weigh the required ingredients, mix the powders, punch out the tablets, check them for hardness and disintegration, and dispense them to the patient.

Composition

Tablets are generally composed of the active drug, diluents, binders, disintegrants, lubricants, coloring agents, and flavoring agents. Diluents include lactose, sucrose, mannitol, and starch. (See Chapter 10, "Capsules," Table 10-3.) Binders are adhesive materials used to hold the powders together and include water, alcohol, starch paste, sucrose syrup, gelatin solutions, acacia mucilage, glucose solutions, and polymer solutions (PEG, polyvinylpyrolidone) in water, alcohol, or hydroalcoholic mixtures. Disintegrants include cellulose derivatives, starch, and some commercially available superdisintegrants (Table 11-1). Lubricants are commonly used for high-speed tableting machines, but they can be used for extemporaneously preparing tablets if a punch and die system is available to minimize tablet sticking. Lubricants include calcium stearate, magnesium stearate, zinc stearate, starch, talc, PEG, and numerous other waxes or waxlike materials (Table 11-2). The actual composition of a tablet will depend on the method of preparation and the characteristics desired.

Table 11-1. Some Physicochemical Characteristics and Packaging Requirements of Capsule and Tablet Disintegrating Agents

Item	Solubility		pH of Aqueous Dispersion (concentration)	Container Specifications
	Water	**Alcohol**		
Alginic acid	IS	—	1.5–3.5 (3%)	W
Microcrystalline cellulose	IS	—	5.0–7.0 (supernatent)	T
Croscarmellose sodium	PartSol	—	5.0–7.0 (1%)	T
Crospovidone	IS	—	5.0–8.0 (1%)	T
Polacrilin potassium	IS	—	—	W
Sodium starch glycolate	—	—	3.0–5.0 (3.3%)	W
Starch (potato)	IS	IS	4.5–7.0 (20%) 5.0–8.0 (20%)	W
Pregelatinized starch	SlS	IS	4.5–7.0 (10%)	W

Preparation

Tablets that can be compounded include those that are molded, sintered, and even compressed. A compounding pharmacist can prepare compressed tablets, but only in unique situations.

Molded Tablets

Molded tablets are generally prepared by mixing the active drug with lactose, dextrose, sucrose, mannitol, or some other appropriate diluent that can serve as the base. This base must be readily soluble and should not degrade during the tablet's preparation. Lactose is the preferred base, but mannitol adds a pleasant, cooling sensation and additional sweetness in the mouth. Combinations of sugars can also be used.

Molded tablet triturate molds can be made from plastic or metal, with the latter more commonly used today (Figure 11-1). A formula must be developed to determine the capacity of the mold based on the respective tablet base. Because different bases will have different densities, the capacity must be determined for each base. This determination is made by first preparing tablets that consist of the base alone, then weighing the entire batch, dividing the weight by the number of tablets to obtain the average weight per tablet for that base.

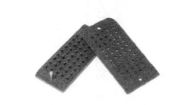

Figure 11-1. Tablet triturate molds.

Table 11-2. Physicochemical Characteristics of Capsule/Tablet Lubricants

	True Density (g/cm³)	Bulk Density (g/cm³)	Tapped Density (g/cm³)	Melting Point (°C)	Container Specifications
Calcium stearate	1.064–1.096	0.16–0.38	0.20–0.48	149–160	W
Glyceryl behenate	—	—	—	70	T
Glyceryl palmitostearate	—	—	—	52–55	T
Magnesium stearate	1.092	0.159	0.286	117–159	T
Mineral oil, light	0.818–0.880	—	—	—	T
Polyethylene glycol	1.15–1.21	—	—	Varies	W
Sodium stearyl fumarate	1.107	0.2–0.35	0.3–0.5	224–245	W
Stearic acid	0.980	0.537	0.571	≥54	W
Stearic acid, purified	0.847 (70°C)	—	—	66–69	W
Talc	2.7–2.8	—	—	—	W
Vegetable oil, hydrogenated, type I	—	—	0.57	61–66	W
Zinc stearate	1.09	—	0.26	120–122	W

The preparation of molded tablets involves forcing a dampened mass into the cavities of a tablet mold. Generally, these molds are made from plastic or metal and are designed as two plates, one containing pegs and the other containing matching holes or cavities. The mass is moistened and pressed into the plate containing the holes. While the mass remains moist, the cavity plate is situated on the peg plate with the pegs or pins aligned. The cavity plate is then allowed to drop, causing the pegs to push out the moist tablets. The tablets are left undisturbed as they dry, after which they are removed and packaged.

If the active drug used weighs more than a few milligrams, the drug's density factor should be determined. This determination involves moistening a portion of the active drug with 50% ethanol in water, filling some of the mold cavities, drying the tablets, and then weighing them. Dividing the total weight by the number of tablets prepared will give the average weight of the tablet consisting of the active drug. The quantity of drug that will be required in the prescription per tablet can then be divided by the weight of the pure drug tablet to obtain a percentage of the tablet cavity that will be occupied by the active drug. This percentage subtracted from 100 will give the percentage of the tablet cavity that will be occupied by the tablet base. Multiplying this percentage by the weight of the pure base tablet will give the quantity of base that is required per tablet. (See Chapter 5, "Pharmaceutical Compounding Calculations," for a sample calculation and step-by-step instructions for its solution.)

Sintered Tablets

Sintered tablets are modified molded tablets. They are prepared by blending the active drug with a diluent, which together make up approximately 65% of the tablet weight. The remaining 35% will consist of PEG 3350 or a mixture of PEGs with various molecular weights. The powder mixture is then pressed firmly into the cavity portion of a tablet triturate mold, which rests on a flat surface. The mold should be lubricated with a vegetable oil spray before use. The cavity portion of the mold containing the tableting materials is placed on a sieve or similar device and set in an oven at about 90°C for about 10 to 12 minutes. The mold is removed from the oven and allowed to cool. The cavity mold is then placed on top of the matching peg mold so that the individual tablets can be worked free.

Alternatively, a small quantity of 50% ethanol in water can be used to form a mass to aid in filling the cavities. The cavity portion of the mold is placed on the peg portion and allowed to slide down, exposing the individual tablets. The entire unit is placed inside an oven at around 90°C for about 12 minutes. After the unit is removed and allowed to cool, the tablets can be taken out and packaged. In general, sintered-molded tablets are more robust than other molded tablets and can better withstand handling.

Chewable Tablets

Chewable tablets can be prepared with a single-punch press or a single-punch tableting machine. The matrix consists largely of mannitol, a sugar that has a sweet, cooling taste and is easy to manipulate. Other ingredients can include binders, lubricants, colors, and flavors. The mixture is prepared and the required quantity weighed. The powder is then placed into the cavity of a press, where the tablet is compressed. If a tableting machine is used to punch out the tablets, the powder blend is placed in the hopper, and the tablet size and hardness are adjusted before the operation begins.

Effervescent Tablets

Effervescent tablets can be prepared by compressing mixtures of sodium bicarbonate with either citric acid or tartaric acid. A formulation is given as follows:

℞ Effervescent Tablets	
Active drug	** g
Effervescent mixture	qs
Citric acid	15.6%
Tartaric acid	31.3%
Sodium bicarbonate	53.1%

These tablets must be packaged in tight containers to prevent moisture from causing premature effervescence. They are prepared with either a single-punch press or a single-punch tableting machine.

Compressed Tablets

If the occasion arises, small quantities of compressed tablets can be prepared with a pellet press (Figure 11-2). If the quantity of tablets is large enough to justify the expense, a small tableting machine can be used. Generally, the active drug is mixed with a diluent (e.g., lactose), a disintegrant (e.g., starch), and a lubricant (about 1% magnesium stearate) to form a powder blend. Ingredients can be modified on the basis of the desired qualities of the tablets.

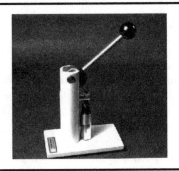

Figure 11-2. Pellet press.

Quality Control

Routine quality control tests for tablets should include tablet weight, weight variation, appearance, and disintegration. To test for disintegration, tablets (except chewable tablets) can be dropped into a beaker containing a No. 10—mesh screen situated about 2 in. from the bottom of the beaker. The screen should be supported by hooks attached to the top of the beaker. A stir bar is placed in the bottom of the beaker, and the entire apparatus is set on a magnetic stirrer. A total of 1 L of water is placed in the beaker, and the stirrer is turned on at a moderate speed. The pharmacist should note and record the time that it takes for the tablet to break apart. Although the disintegration time depends on the product, it generally should be within 15 to 30 minutes. Although dissolution is the determining test, most compounding pharmacies lack that capability because analytical instruments are required to determine the actual quantity of drug that has gone into solution.

Storage/Labeling

Tablets should be stored at room temperature, unless directions indicate otherwise. Tablets should be labeled as to the proper mode of administration, that is, swallowable, sublingual, buccal, or chewable.

Stability

Tablets are a solid dosage form that should be relatively stable in the dry state. Because they are dry, they generally constitute a stable dosage form as long as they are protected from moisture and heat. According to Chapter <795>, "Pharmacy Compounding,"[1] tablets prepared from a manufactured product should have a beyond-use date of 25% of the time remaining on the product's expiration date or 6 months, whichever is earlier. If the product is prepared from USP/NF ingredients, a beyond-use date of 6 months is appropriate, unless evidence is available to support other dating.

Patient Counseling

The patient should be counseled about the proper mode of administration. If chewable, the tablet should be thoroughly chewed before it is swallowed. Sublingual tablets should be placed under the tongue, whereas buccal tablets should be placed in the cheek pouch between the cheek and gum. After these types of tablets dissolve, the medication should still be held in the mouth for a brief time to allow absorption of the medication. Patients should be informed that the buccal and sublingual routes of administration are used when rapid action is desired or when the prescribed drugs might degrade in the stomach if swallowed. Instructions about proper storage in a cool, dry place and away from children should be included.

Sample Formulations

℞ Sodium Fluoride 2.2 mg Tablet Triturates (#100, using a 60-mg mold)

Sodium fluoride	220 mg
Sucrose, powdered	1.150 g
Lactose, hydrous	4.630 g

M. sodium fluoride tablets.

1. Calculate the quantity of each ingredient required for the prescription.
2. Accurately weigh each ingredient.
3. Mix the powders together geometrically, starting with the sodium fluoride and the sucrose, then the lactose, until thoroughly mixed.
4. Prepare about 10 mL of a solution containing 7.5 mL ethanol (95%) in water.
5. Add the alcohol solution to the powder a drop at a time and mix well until the mixture attains the consistency of a playing dough or modeling clay.
6. Fill the holes of a tablet triturate mold plate with the mixture until all holes are uniformly filled.
7. Place this portion of the mold plate onto the portion containing the pegs and gently push down until the tablets are sitting on top of the pegs.
8. Allow to air dry.
9. Gently remove the tablets.
10. Package and label.

℞ Ibuprofen 200 mg Compressed Tablets (#100)

Ibuprofen	20 g
Caffeine	10 g
Avicel PH 101	14 g
Stearic acid	200 mg

1. Calculate the quantity of each ingredient required for the prescription.
2. Accurately weigh each ingredient.
3. Using geometric dilution, mix the powders, starting with the ibuprofen and caffeine. Then incorporate the Avicel PH 101 and, finally, the stearic acid. (Note: The stearic acid is used as a lubricant to prevent the powder from sticking to the tablet press; therefore, it should be added last so that it is distributed uniformly on the other powders.)
4. Weigh 442 mg of the mixture, place it in a tablet press, and then prepare the tablet, ensuring that the amount of pressure used is consistent and that the tablet will disintegrate within 10 minutes when placed in water.
5. Package and label.

Reference

1. Expert Advisory Panel on Pharmacy Compounding Practices. Pharmacy compounding. In: *United States Pharmacopeia 25/National Formulary 20*. Rockville, Md: United States Pharmacopeial Convention; 2001.

Chapter 12

Lozenges/Troches

Dosage forms that dissolve slowly in the mouth, or that can be easily chewed and swallowed, are gaining in popularity, especially among pediatric patients. Hard (compressed or molded) preparations of this dosage form are called lozenges, troches, or drops. Soft (molded) lozenges/troches are often called pastilles, and chewable, gelatin-based lozenges/troches are often called gummy, novelty-shaped products. The term *lozenge* will be used in this chapter to refer to all variations of the dosage form.

Definitions/Types

Lozenges are various-shaped, solid dosage forms, usually containing a medicinal agent and a flavoring substance, that are intended to be dissolved slowly in the oral cavity for localized or systemic effects. Molded lozenges have a softer texture because they contain a high percentage of sugar or a combination of a gelatin and sugar.

Hard lozenges have hard candy bases made of sugar and syrup and often incorporate an adhesive substance such as acacia. Commercial lozenges are made on a tableting machine using high compression pressures. Ingredients should be heat stable if they are to be incorporated into compounded lozenges.

Recently, soft lozenges and chewable lozenges have been reintroduced into pharmacy and are enjoying increased popularity. *Soft lozenges* generally have a polyethylene glycol (PEG) base, whereas *chewable lozenges* have a glycerinated gelatin base. These dosage forms usually are chewed and are a means of delivering the product to the gastrointestinal tract for systemic absorption.

Historical Use

Lozenges have long been used to deliver topical anesthetics and antibacterials for the relief of minor sore throat pain and irritation. Today, they are used for analgesics, anesthetics, antimicrobials, antiseptics, antitussives, aromatics, astringents, corticosteroids, decongestants, demulcents, and other classes and combinations of drugs.

Soft lozenges are similar to a historical form of medication that is now making a comeback—the "confection." *Confections* are defined as heavily saccharinated, soft masses containing medicinal agents. Their growing popularity is largely due to the use of polymers (PEGs) as the matrix for the dosage form. Confections are easy to use, convenient to carry, easy to store (i.e., at room temperature), and generally pleasant tasting. PEG-based lozenges have a tendency to be hygroscopic and may soften if exposed to high temperatures. Consequently, storage in a cool, dry place is recommended for these lozenges.

Today, a popular lozenge for pediatric use is the chewable lozenge, or "gummy-type" candy product. The gelatin base for these chewable lozenges is similar to the historical glycerin suppositories, or glycerinated gelatin suppositories that consisted of 70% glycerin, 20% gelatin, and 10% purified water. Some of the earlier soft lozenges consisted of a gelatin or a glycerogelatin base. These lozenges were prepared by pouring the melt either into molds or out on a sheet of uniform thickness. The dosage forms were then punched out using various-shaped punches. The last step often included dusting of the product with cornstarch or powdered sugar to decrease tackiness.

Applications

Lozenges are experiencing renewed popularity as a means of delivering different drug products, especially for patients who cannot swallow solid oral dosage forms. Lozenges are also used for medications designed for slow release. This dosage form maintains a constant level of the drug in the oral cavity or bathes the throat tissues in a solution of the drug. Medicated lozenges are usually intended for local treatment of infections of the mouth or throat; however, they may contain active medications that produce a systemic effect.

The lozenge dosage form has a number of advantages. It is easy to administer to both pediatric patients and patients of advanced age, it has a pleasant taste, and it extends the time that a quantity of drug remains in the oral cavity to elicit a therapeutic effect. Also, pharmacists can prepare lozenges extemporaneously with minimal equipment and time.

One disadvantage of the lozenge is that children can mistake it for candy. Parents should be cautioned not to refer to medications as candy and to keep the product out of the reach of children.

Composition

Hard Lozenges

Hard candy lozenges are mixtures of sugar and other carbohydrates in an amorphous (noncrystalline) or glassy condition. These lozenges can be considered solid syrups of sugars and usually have a moisture content of 0.5% to 1.5%. Hard lozenges should not disintegrate but instead provide a slow, uniform dissolution or erosion over 5 to 10 minutes. They should have a smooth surface texture and a pleasant flavor that masks the drug taste. Their primary disadvantage is the high temperature required for preparation. Hard candy lozenges generally weigh between 1.5 and 4.5 g.

Excipients such as sorbitol and sugar have demulcent effects, which relieve the discomfort of abraded tissue caused by coughs and sore throat. A portion of the active drug product may actually be absorbed through the buccal mucosa, thereby escaping the first-pass metabolism that occurs when a drug is swallowed and absorbed through the gastrointestinal tract.

Soft Lozenges

Soft lozenges have become popular because of the ease with which they can be extemporaneously prepared and their applicability to a wide variety of drugs. The bases usually consist of a mixture of various PEGs, acacia, or similar materials. An alternative and older form of soft lozenges is the pastille, which is a soft lozenge, is usually transparent, and consists of a medication in a gelatin, a glycerogelatin, or an acacia:sucrose base. These lozenges may be colored and flavored, and they can be either slowly dissolved in the mouth or chewed, depending on the intended effect of the incorporated drug.

Chewable Lozenges (Gummy, Novelty-Shaped Products)

Chewable lozenges have been on the market for a number of years. They are highly flavored and frequently have a slightly acidic taste. Because their fruit flavor often masks the taste of the drug, they are an excellent way of administering drug products. These lozenges are relatively easy to prepare extemporaneously. The most difficult part involves preparing the gelatin base. Chewable lozenges are especially useful for pediatric patients and are an effective means of administering medications for gastrointestinal absorption and systemic use.

Preparation

Lozenges are prepared by molding a mixture of carbohydrates to form hard candies, by molding a matrix to form a soft lozenge, or by molding a gelatin base into a chewable mass. Each approach is described.

Hard lozenges are usually prepared by heating sugar and other components to a proper temperature and then pouring the mixture into a mold or by pulling the mass out into a ribbon while it cools and then cutting the ribbon to

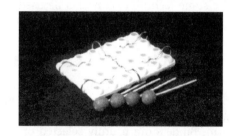

Figure 12-1. Sucker mold.

the desired length. A commercial method is to compress the materials into a very hard tablet. The mold shown in Figure 12-1 can be used to make suckers.

Both soft lozenges and chewable lozenges are usually prepared by pouring a melted mass into molds (Figure 12-2). Another method, which depends on the ingredients, involves pouring the mass out to form a sheet of uniform thickness and then punching out the lozenges by using a punch of the desired shape and size.

If molds are unavailable, the plastic snap cap from a plastic vial can be used as a mold. A vegetable spray can be applied to the cap, if needed, and the preparation can be poured into the cap. After solidification, the cap can be peeled away from the lozenge. Alternatively, the melt can be dropped onto a heavy sheet of aluminum foil that

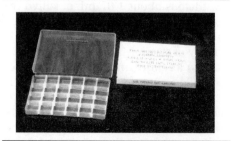

Figure 12-2. Troche mold.

is sitting on a bed of ice cubes. The drops will immediately solidify, usually in a circular form, on contact with the cold foil.

Molds used in the preparation of lozenges must be calibrated to determine the weight of the lozenge using the applicable base. The calibration can be done as follows:

1. Prepare the lozenge mold, and confirm that the cavities are clean and dry.
2. Obtain and melt sufficient lozenge base to fill 6 to 12 molds.
3. Pour the molds, cool, and trim if necessary.
4. Remove the blank lozenges and weigh.
5. Divide the total weight by the number of blank lozenges to obtain the average weight of each lozenge for this particular base. Use this weight as the calibrated value for that specific mold when using that specific lot of lozenge base.

The powders contained in the lozenges may also occupy a specific volume, and an adjustment may be required in the quantity of the base used. These "dosage replacement calculations" are analogous to those used with suppositories. (See Chapter 5, "Pharmaceutical Compounding Calculations," for sample calculations.)

In general, the quantity of flavoring agent added to medicated lozenges is about 5 to 10 times that used in candy lozenges to compensate for the flavor of the medication. If the flavoring agent (an oil) is immiscible with the base, it can be dissolved in glycerin; the glycerin solution is then incorporated into the product. The same technique can also be used to incorporate an oily drug into a lozenge. The solvent technique often uses a ratio of 1 part solvent to 3 to 5 parts drug.

Physicochemical Considerations

A binder is used in most lozenges. *Binders* are substances added to tablet or lozenge formulations to add cohesiveness to powders, providing the necessary bonding that contributes to the maintenance of the integrity of the final dosage form. Binders are usually selected on the basis of previous experience of the formulator, particular product needs, literature or vendor information, and individual preferences. Binders can be added at any of several steps in the process, depending on the specific procedure being used and the speed at which the lozenge should disintegrate. Table 12-1 lists the official binding agents and provides a description of their physicochemical characteristics.

Dosage forms are removed from the mouth at various rates. Generally, the rate of removal, going from the most rapid to the slowest, is as follows: tablets/capsules, solutions, suspensions, chewable tablets, and lozenges. According to salivary kinetics, there is about 1.07 mL of saliva resident in the mouth before swallowing and about 0.71 mL after swallowing. The baseline flow rate for saliva of about 0.3 mL/minute may be increased to about 10.6 mL/minute when stimulated. The frequency of swallowing is about 0.6 to 2.3 times per minute. Based on these calculations, a lozenge can increase the residence time of a drug in the oral cavity.

If flavors and preservatives are included in the product formulation, their characteristics should be considered. For example, the odor of a 0.08% solution of methylparaben has been described as "floral," "gauze pad," or "face powder" sweet. A 0.015% solution of propylparaben has a tongue-numbing effect, producing a slight sting and minimal aroma. A 0.125% butylparaben solution has the least aroma of all. Preservatives have a tendency to partition into flavors, because they are not always water soluble, and most flavors are oily in nature.

Table 12-1. Some Physicochemical Characteristics and Packaging Requirements of Binding Agents

Item	Usual Concentration (%)	Solubility		pH of Aqueous Dispersion (concentration)	Container Specifications
		Water	Alcohol		
Acacia NF	2–5	FS	—	4.5–5.0 (5%)	T
Alginic acid NF	2–5	IS	—	1.5–3.5 (3%)	W
Carboxymethylcellulose sodium USP	1–5	—	IS	6.5–8.5 (1%)	T
Cellulose microcrystalline NF	1–90	IS	—	5.0–7.0 (12.5%)	T
Dextrin NF	—	VS	—	—	W
Ethylcellulose NF	1–5	IS	FS	5.0–7.5 (2%)	W
Gelatin NF					
Type A	1–5	Sol	IS	3.8–6.0 (1%)	W
Type B	1–5	Sol	IS	5.0–7.4 (1%)	W
Glucose, liquid NF	—	Misc	SpS	—	T
Guar gum NF	1–10	Disp	—	5.0–7.0 (1%)	W
Hydroxypropyl methylcellulose USP	1–5	Swells	IS	5.5–8.0 (1%)	W
Methylcellulose USP	1–5	Swells	IS	5.5–8.0 (1%)	W
Polyethylene glycol NF	5–50	FS	Sol	4.5–7.5 (5%)	T
Polyethylene oxide NF	—	Sol	—	—	T, LR
Povidone USP	2–5	FS	FS	3.0–7.0 (5%)	T
Starch, pregelatinized NF	—	SIS	IS	4.5–7.0 (10%)	—
Syrup NF	2–25	Misc	Misc	—	T

The type of medication prepared as a lozenge is limited only by flavor, dose restrictions, and/or chemical compatibility. Some materials are so unpalatable or irritating that they are unsuitable for this type of administration. The following are examples of different active ingredients used in lozenges:

▸ *Benzocaine.* The usual dose of benzocaine is in the range of 5 to 10 mg per lozenge. It is extremely reactive with the aldehydic components of candy base and flavor components. As much as 90% to 95% of available benzocaine may be lost when added to a candy base, but a PEG base is compatible.

▸ *Hexylresorcinol.* The dose of hexylresorcinol is about 2.4 mg per lozenge. It is somewhat susceptible to reaction with aldehydic components. No flavoring or "mouth-feel" problems are associated with this material because of its low dose and lack of appreciable flavor.

▸ *Dextromethorphan.* The dose of dextromethorphan hydrobromide is about 7.5 mg per lozenge. It is easy to incorporate into a candy base because of its melting point (122°C–124°C) and solubility (1.5 g in 1000 mL of purified water). It is compatible with most flavors, and it is stable over a wide pH range. Conversely, it does have a bitter taste, an anesthetic mouth feel, and an unpleasant aftertaste. Masking doses greater than about 2 mg per lozenge requires special considerations.

Quality Control

The weight and uniformity of individual lozenges can be easily determined. Appearance, odor, and hardness can be observed and recorded. (See the Standard Operating Procedure (SOP) "Performing Quality Assessment of Lozenges and Lollipops.")

Storage/Labeling

Lozenges (hard, soft, and chewable) should be stored either at room temperature or in a refrigerator, depending on the active drug incorporated and the type of vehicle used. These products should be kept in tight containers to prevent drying. This measure is especially needed for chewable lozenges, which can dry out and become difficult to chew. If a disposable mold with a cardboard sleeve is used, it is best to slip this unit into a properly labeled, sealable plastic bag.

Stability

Completed products are dry and, thus, generally provide a stable dosage form, as long as they are protected from moisture and heat. According to Chapter <795>, "Pharmacy Compounding,"[1] lozenges prepared from a manufactured product should have a beyond-use date of 25% of the time remaining on the product's expiration date or 6 months, whichever is earlier. If the product is prepared from USP/NF ingredients, a beyond-use date of 6 months is appropriate, unless evidence is available to support other dating. Other considerations follow.

Hard candies are hygroscopic and are usually prone to absorption of atmospheric moisture. Considerations must, therefore, include the hygroscopic nature of the candy base, the storage conditions of the lozenges, the length of time they will be stored, and the potential for drug interactions.

Lozenges should be stored away from heat and out of the reach of children. They should be protected from extremes of humidity. Depending on the storage requirement of both the drug and the base, either room temperature or refrigerated temperature is usually indicated.

Because lozenges are solid dosage forms, preservatives are generally not needed. However, hard candy lozenges are hygroscopic; therefore, their water content may increase, and bacterial growth can occur if they are not packaged properly. Because any water present would dissolve some sucrose, the highly concentrated sucrose solution that results can be bacteriostatic in nature and will not support bacterial growth. The paraben preservatives were discussed earlier in this chapter.

All hard candy lozenges eventually become grainy, but the speed at which this tendency occurs depends on the ingredients that are used. When the concentration of corn syrup solids is greater than 50%, the graining tendencies decrease, but moisture absorption tendencies can increase. Increased moisture absorption increases product stickiness and causes the medications to interact. Sucrose solids in concentrations greater than 70% tend to increase graining tendencies and the speed of crystallization. Formulations that contain between 55% and 65% sucrose or 35% and 45% corn syrup solids generally offer the best compromise in dealing with problems related to graining, moisture absorption, and preparation time.

Acidulents, such as citric, tartaric, fumaric, and malic acids, can be added to a candy base to strengthen the flavor characteristics of the finished product and to control pH to preserve the stability of the incorporated medication. Regular hard candy has a pH of about 5 to 6, but it may be as low as 2.5 to 3 when acidulents are added. Calcium carbonate, sodium bicarbonate, and magnesium trisilicate can be added to increase the lozenge pH to as high as 7.5 to 8.5.

Patient Counseling

The patient should be counseled about the purpose of a hard lozenge, which is to provide a slow, continual release of the drug over a prolonged period of time. Hard lozenges should not be chewed. Soft and chewable lozenges are to be taken only as directed and should not be considered candy. They should be kept out of the reach of children.

Because the hard lozenges are designed to provide a slow, uniform release of the medication directly onto the affected mucous membrane, the compounding pharmacist is faced with the challenge of developing flavor blends that mask any unpleasant taste produced by the medication, while maintaining a smooth surface texture as the lozenge slowly dissolves. If the medication has no significant taste, flavoring will not be a problem. If the medication has a strong, disagreeable taste, however, that taste should be minimized to enhance patient compliance.

Sample Formulations

Lozenge Vehicles

For the following vehicles, the gelatin is dissolved in a hot mixture of the glycerin/water/sorbitol solution in which the parabens have been previously dissolved. It is advisable to use a tared vessel to determine water loss during heating, so that an appropriate amount can be replaced. The amount of flavor oil can be determined by trial-and-error taste tests. One can start at about 9% and make adjustments as needed.[2]

| | | | Vehicle | | | | |
Ingredients	A	B	C	D	E	F	G
Sodium saccharin	0.1 g	—	0.1 g	0.05 g	0.05 g	0.05 g	0.05 g
Gelatin	20 g	20 g	20 g	30 g	30 g	30 g	20 g
Glycerin	70 mL	20 mL	40 mL	30 mL	30 mL	30 mL	40 mL
Sorbitol 70% solution	—	50 mL	30 mL	30 mL	25 mL	26 mL	26 mL
Polyethylene glycol 6000	—	—	—	—	5 g	4 g	4 g
Methylparaben	0.15 g	0.15 g	0.15 g	0.15 g	0.15 g	0.15 g	0.15 g
Propylparaben	0.05 g	0.05 g	0.05 g	0.05 g	0.05 g	0.05 g	0.05 g
Flavor oil	qs mL	qs mL	qs mL	qs mL	qs mL	qs mL	qs mL
Purified water USP	qs 100 mL	100 mL	100 mL	100 mL	100 mL	100 mL	100 mL

Ingredient-Specific Formulations

Sample formulations are presented to illustrate the differences in the types of lozenges and their applications. These formulas can be adjusted according to the quantity of active drug to be used.

Hard Lozenges

 Hard Sugar Lozenges

Powdered sugar	42 g
Light corn syrup	16 mL
Distilled water	24 mL
Active drug, example	1.0 g
Mint extract	1.2 mL
Food coloring, green	qs

1. Calculate the quantity of each ingredient required for the prescription.
2. Accurately weigh or measure each ingredient.
3. Combine the sugar, corn syrup, and water in a beaker and stir until well mixed.
4. Cover the mixture and heat on a hot plate at a high setting until the mixture boils; continue boiling for 2 minutes.
5. Uncover and remove from heat at 61°C. Do not stir the mixture until the temperature drops to 55°C.
6. Quickly add the active drug, mint extract, and food coloring and stir until well mixed.
7. Coat the mold to be used with a vegetable spray.
8. Pour the melt into the molds.
9. Cool, package, and label.

℞ **Anti-Gag Lollipops (36 lollipops)**

Sodium chloride	46.56 g
Potassium chloride	3 g
Calcium lactate	6.12 g
Magnesium citrate	2.04 g
Sodium bicarbonate	22.44 g
Sodium phosphate monobasic	3.84 g
Silica gel	3.60 g
Polyethylene glycol 1450	qs

1. Calculate the quantity of each ingredient required for the prescription.
2. Calibrate the lollipop mold for the formula.
3. Accurately weigh each ingredient.
4. Triturate all the powders together to obtain a small, uniform particle size.
5. Melt the PEG 1450 at a temperature in the range of 50°C to 55°C in a suitable beaker or other container.
6. Slowly add the powders with thorough mixing.
7. Cool to approximately 45°C.
8. Pour into a mold that has been previously sprayed with a vegetable-based oil, wiping off the excess.
9. Cool for approximately 90 minutes and remove from the molds.
10. Package and label.

℞ **Pediatric Chocolate Troche Base**

Chocolate (good quality)	60 g
Vegetable oil (bland)	40 g

1. Calculate the quantity of each ingredient required for the prescription.
2. Weigh or measure each of the ingredients.
3. Heat the vegetable oil by using low heat or a double boiler/water bath.
4. Add the chocolate and stir until melted. Cool.
5. Package and use for compounding.

R℞ Sildenafil Citrate 25 mg Sublingual Troches (#24)

Sildenafil citrate	600 mg
Aspartame	500 mg
Silica gel	480 mg
Acacia	360 mg
Flavor	qs
Polyethylene glycol 1450	22 g (will vary depending on mold and size of tablet used as the source of the drug)

1. Calculate the quantity of each ingredient required for the prescription.
2. Accurately weigh each ingredient and obtain the required number of sildenafil citrate tablets (24 of the 25 mg, 12 of the 50 mg, 6 of the 100 mg tablets).
3. In a mortar, triturate the sildenafil citrate tablets to a very fine powder.
4. Add the aspartame, silica gel, and acacia and triturate further to a fine powder.
5. Melt the PEG 1450 to about 55°C to 60°C.
6. Add the powders from step 4 and mix well.
7. Cool a few degrees, add the flavor(s), and pour into troche molds.
8. Allow to solidify.
9. Package and label.

Soft Lozenges

R℞ Steroid Linguets *** mg

Fattibase/cocoa butter	76 g
Steroid powder	** g
Acacia	3 g
Cinnamon oil	5 gtts
Artificial sweetener	14 gtts

1. Calculate the quantity of each ingredient required for the prescription.
2. Accurately weigh or measure each ingredient.
3. Melt the Fattibase/cocoa butter at about 40°C/35°C.
4. Add the acacia powder followed by the steroid and mix well.
5. Add the artificial sweetener and the cinnamon oil and mix well.
6. Pour into 1-g molds and place in a refrigerator to cool and harden.
7. Package and label. Store in a refrigerator.

R̶x̶ Polyethelene Glycol Troches

Polyethylene glycol 1000	10 g
Active drug, example	1 g
Aspartame sweetener	20 packets
Mint extract	1 mL
Food color	2 drops

1. Calculate the quantity of each ingredient required for the prescription.
2. Accurately weigh or measure each ingredient.
3. Melt the polyethylene glycol 1000 on a hot plate to about 70°C and gradually add the active drug powder and the aspartame sweetener by stirring.
4. Add the coloring and flavoring and pour into troche molds.
5. Allow to cool at room temperature.
6. Package and label.

R̶x̶ Polyethelene Glycol Troches with Suspending Agent

Polyethylene glycol 1000	34.5 g
Active drug, example	4.8 g
Silica gel	0.37 g
Acacia	0.61 g
Flavor	5 drops

1. Calculate the quantity of each ingredient required for the prescription.
2. Accurately weigh or measure each ingredient.
3. Blend the powders together until uniformly mixed.
4. Heat the polyethylene glycol 1000 until melted at approximately 70°C.
5. Add the powder mix to the melted base and blend thoroughly.
6. Cool to less than 55°C, add the flavor, and mix well.
7. Pour into troche or cough drop molds.
8. Cool, package, and label.

(Note: This formulation is based on a mold that weighs approximately 1.8 g. The formula can be adjusted to other mold weights.)

R_x **Powdered Sugar Troches**

Powdered sugar	10 g
Active drug, example	1 g
Acacia	0.7 g
Purified water	qs

1. Calculate the quantity of each ingredient required for the prescription.
2. Accurately weigh or measure each ingredient.
3. Mix the acacia and purified water together in a mortar to form a mucilage.
4. Sift the powdered sugar and active drug together and gradually add sufficient mucilage to make a mass of the proper consistency.
5. Roll the mass into the shape of a cylinder and cut into 10 even sections (approximately twice the length of the diameter).
6. Allow to air dry, package, and label.

Chewable Lozenges

 Gelatin Base

Glycerin	155 mL
Gelatin	3.4 g
Purified water	21.6 mL
Methylparaben	0.44 g

1. Calculate the quantity of each ingredient required for the prescription.
2. Accurately weigh or measure each ingredient.
3. Heat a water bath to boiling.
4. In a beaker, add the purified water, glycerin, and methylparaben; stir and heat for 5 minutes.
5. Over a 3-minute period, add the gelatin very slowly while stirring until it is thoroughly dispersed and free of lumps.
6. Continue to heat for 45 minutes.
7. Remove from heat, cool, and refrigerate until used.

℞ Drug Product in Gelatin Base

Gelatin base	43 g
Bentonite	800 mg
Aspartame	900 mg
Acacia powder	720 mg
Citric acid monohydrate	1.08 g
Flavor	14–18 drops
Active ingredient	—

1. Calculate the quantity of each ingredient required for the prescription.
2. Accurately weigh or measure each ingredient.
3. Calibrate the particular mold to be used for this product.
4. Melt the gelatin base using a water bath.
5. Triturate the powders together and add to the gelatin base melt; thoroughly mix until evenly dispersed.
6. Add the desired flavor and mix.
7. Continuously mix and pour the melt into the pediatric chewable lozenge molds and allow to cool. If the mixture congeals while pouring, it may be necessary to reheat and then continue pouring.
8. Package and label.

℞ Morphine 10 mg Troches (#24)

Morphine sulfate	240 mg
Aspartame	250 mg
Flavor	qs
Polybase	24 g

1. Calculate the quantity of each ingredient required for the prescription.
2. Accurately weigh or measure each ingredient.
3. Melt the Polybase using gentle heat to about 60°C.
4. Add the morphine sulfate and the aspartame powders and mix well.
5. Cool a few minutes and add flavor while the mixture is still fluid.
6. Mix thoroughly and pour into 1-g molds.
7. Cool, package, and label.

℞ **Fentanyl 50 µg Chewable Gummy Gels (24 chewable gels)**

Fentanyl citrate	1.884 mg
Chewable gummy gel base	23.35 g
Bentonite	0.5 g
Aspartame	0.5 g
Acacia powder	0.5 g
Citric acid monohydrate	0.65 g
Flavor concentrate	10–12 drops

1. Calculate the quantity of each ingredient required for the prescription.
2. Accurately weigh or measure the ingredients.
3. Blend the fentanyl citrate, bentonite, aspartame, acacia powder, and citric acid monohydrate together.
4. Heat the chewable gummy gel base on a water bath until fluid.
5. Incorporate the dry powder from step 3 into the base and stir until evenly dispersed.
6. Add the flavor concentrate and mix well.
7. Pour into suitable molds and allow to cool.
8. Package and label.

(Note: Because mold capacities vary, it may be necessary to calibrate the specific mold being used and to adjust the formula before actual preparation.)

Standard Operating Procedure (SOP)

Performing Quality Assessment of Lozenges and Lollipops

Purpose of SOP

The purpose of this procedure is to provide a method of documenting uniformity between batches and of conducting quality assessment tests of and observations on lozenges and lollipops.

Equipment/Materials

The following items are used in one or more of the quality assessment tests:

- Balance
- Graduates
- Beaker
- Weight

Procedure

The appropriate tests should be conducted and the results/observations recorded on the worksheet "Quality Assessment Form for Lozenges and Lollipops" (Figure 12-3).

Weight.

- Accurately weigh the product on a balance.

Specific Gravity.

1. To calculate the specific gravity, identify the weight and volume of the product.
2. Record the weight of the individual dosage form or a strip/tube/package of the dosage forms (tared weight).

To determine the volume of water displaced, do the following:

Single Unit.

1. Place 5 mL of water in a 10-mL graduate.
2. Add the dosage form and read the water level.
3. Subtract 5 mL from the level in step 2 to determine the volume of water occupied by the dosage form.
4. If the dosage form floats, place a weight attached to a paper clip in the graduate before adding the water to the 5-mL mark. Then, wrap one end of the paper clip around the dosage form to hold it below the water surface and place it in the graduate. Proceed as in step 3.

Multiple Unit Packages (Lozenge Boxes).

1. Place the empty package in a beaker that will hold it with minimal extra space.
2. Add an exact known quantity of water to cover the product. It may be necessary to add a weight to the package; this same weight should be used for the actual product.
3. With a fine-line marker and with the beaker sitting on a level surface, mark the water level on the outside of the beaker.
4. Remove the beaker contents, empty, and dry the beaker.
5. Place the dosage form (and the weight if used) into the beaker.
6. Measure the same volume of water as in step 2 into a graduate.
7. Pour the water into the beaker only to the mark from step 3.
   (Note: Do quickly before the dosage form dissolves.)
8. Measure the volume of water remaining in the beaker.

Calculations. Now that the weight and volume of the product are obtained, the specific gravity can be calculated by dividing the weight (grams) by the volume (milliliters).

Active Drug Assay Results. As appropriate, have representative samples of the product assayed for active drug content by a contract analytical laboratory. Stability can be assessed by storing the product at room, refrigerated, and/or frozen temperatures and having the assay repeated on the stored samples.

Color of Product. It may be advisable to use a color chart for determining the actual color of the product.

Clarity. Clarity is evaluated by visual inspection. On the worksheet, 1 is the clearest and 5 is the least clear on the scale provided.

Surface Texture.

▸ Observe the product to determine smoothness of the surface.

Appearance.

▸ Determine whether the product appears dry or oily/moist.

Feel.

> ▸ Touch the product to determine whether it is sticky (tacky) or hard (plastic) or bounces back (elastic).

Melting Test. This test is performed on some soft lozenge/troche products.

1. Heat a 200-mL beaker of water to 37°C on a magnetic stirring unit that is set at about 50 rpm.
2. Add a dosage unit to the water. (Note: It may be necessary to add a weight to the dosage unit to pull it below the water surface.)
3. After 30 minutes, record your observations as Yes, No, or the appropriate number with 1 being the most melted on the scale provided.

Dissolution Test. This test is performed on PEG as well as gelatin and water-soluble products.

1. Proceed as in the melting test.
2. After 30 minutes, record your observations as Yes, No, or the appropriate number with 1 being the most dissolved on the scale provided.

Physical Observation.

> ▸ Describe the appearance and organoleptic qualities of the product.

Physical Stability.

1. Prepare a few additional dosage forms, package, and label "For Physical Stability Observations."
2. Weekly, observe the product for signs of discoloration, dryness, cracking, mottling, mold growth, and so forth.
3. Record a descriptive observation on the form (Figure 12-3) at each observation interval. (Sufficient lines are provided for observations for 8 weeks or approximately 60 days.)

References

1. Expert Advisory Panel on Pharmacy Compounding Practices. Pharmacy compounding. In: *United States Pharmacopeia 25/National Formulary 20*. Rockville, Md: United States Pharmacopeial Convention; 2001.
2. Palmer HA, Semprebon M. Extemporaneous lozenge formulations. *Int J Pharm Compound*. 1998;2(1):71–72.

Quality Assessment Form for Lozenges and Lollipops

Product _____   Date _____

Lot/Rx number _____   Form   Lozenge _____   Lollipop _____

Characteristic	Theoretical	Actual	Normal Range
Weight/volume	_____	_____	_____
Specific gravity	_____	_____	_____
Active drug assay results	_____	_____	_____
Initial assay	_____	_____	_____
After storage No. 1	_____	_____	_____
After storage No. 2	_____	_____	_____
Color of product	_____	_____	_____

Characteristic							
Clarity	Clear	1	2	3	4	5	Opaque
Texture-surface	Smooth	1	2	3	4	5	Rough
Appears dry	Yes	1	2	3	4	5	No
Appearance	Dry	1	2	3	4	5	Oily/moist
Feels tacky	Yes	1	2	3	4	5	No
Feels plastic	Yes	1	2	3	4	5	No
Feels elastic	Yes	1	2	3	4	5	No
Melting test	Yes	1	2	3	4	5	No
Dissolution test	Yes	1	2	3	4	5	No

Sample set aside for physical stability observation: Yes   No

If yes, results: Date   Observation

_____   _____

_____   _____

_____   _____

_____   _____

_____   _____

_____   _____

_____   _____

_____   _____

_____   _____

_____   _____

_____   _____

_____   _____

Figure 12-3. Sample worksheet for assessment of lozenges and lollipops.

Suppositories

Definitions/Types

Suppositories are solid dosage forms that are used to administer medicine through the rectum, vagina, or urethra. Suppositories melt, soften, or dissolve in the body cavity.

Rectal suppositories are cylindrical or conical and are tapered or pointed at one end. They generally weigh approximately 2 g and are about 1 to 1.5 in. long. Infant rectal suppositories weigh about half that of adult suppositories.

Vaginal suppositories, formerly called pessaries, are available in ovoid, globular, or other shapes and weigh about 3 to 5 g each. Compounded vaginal suppositories that use water-soluble bases, such as polyethylene glycol (PEG) or glycerinated gelatin, are the preferred form because they minimize leakage. Some vaginal suppositories are actually compressed tablets and are often called inserts.

Urethral suppositories, formerly called bougies, vary in their dimensions, depending on the sex of the patient. Suppositories for females are about 5 mm in diameter, 50 mm in length, and 2 g in weight. Suppositories for males are 5 mm in diameter, 125 mm in length, and 4 g in weight.

Historical Use

Suppositories have been used for several thousand years and were cited in the early writings of the Egyptians, Greeks, and Romans. Suppositories at that time consisted of pieces of cloth, plants, wood, or other material that were used plain or soaked in a solution of a "medication" and administered. Cocoa butter revolutionized the preparation of suppositories and has served as a suppository base for many years.

Applications

Suppositories can be used to administer drugs to infants and small children, to severely debilitated patients, to those who cannot take medications orally, and to those for whom the parenteral route might be unsuitable. The drugs contained in this dosage form have either local or systemic application. Local applications include the treatment of hemorrhoids, itching, and infections. Systemic applications involve a variety of drugs, including antinauseants, antiasthmatics, analgesics, and hormones.

This dosage form could be used more often in compounded formulations. For example, compounded suppositories that contain metoclopramide, haloperidol, dexamethasone, diphenhydramine, and benztropine can be administered prophylactically to control severe nausea and vomiting; salbutamol can be administered rectally for long-term prophylactic treatment of asthma; and a prolonged-release, morphine alkaloid suppository has been introduced for chronic pain.

Types/Composition of Bases

A suppository base should be stable, nonirritating, chemically and physiologically inert, compatible with a variety of drugs, stable during storage, and esthetically acceptable. It should not melt or dissolve in rectal fluids and should not bind or otherwise interfere with the release or absorption of drug substances. Other desirable characteristics depend on the drugs to be added. For example, bases with higher melting points can be used to incorporate drugs that generally lower the melting points of the base (e.g., camphor, chloral hydrate, menthol, phenol, thymol, and volatile oils) or to formulate suppositories for use in tropical climates. Bases with lower melting points can be used when adding materials that will raise the melting points or when adding large amounts of solids. Examples of suppository bases are shown in Table 13-1.

Table 13-1. Sample Bases, Primarily of U.S. Origin/Availability

Base	Composition	Melting Range/ Point (°C)
Cocoa butter	Mixed triglycerides of oleic, palmitic, stearic acids	34–35
Cotomar	Partially hydrogenated cottonseed oil	35
Dehydag	Hydrogenated fatty alcohols and esters	
Base I		33–36
Base II		37–39
Base III	Also contains glycerides of saturated fatty acids C12–C16	9 ranges
Fattibase	Triglycerides from palm, palm kernel, and coconut oils with self-emulsifying glyceryl monostearate and polyoxyl stearate	35.5–37
Hexaride Base 95		33–35
Hydrokote 25	Higher melting fractions of coconut and palm kernel oil	33.6–36.3
Hydrokote 711	Same as above	39.5–44.5
Hydrokote SP	Same as above	31.1–32.3
Polybase	A homogeneous blend of PEGs and polysorbate 80	60–71

Table 13-1. Sample Bases, Primarily of U.S. Origin/Availability (cont.)

Base	Composition	Melting Range/ Point (°C)
S-70-XX95	Rearranged hydrogenated vegetable oils	34.4–35.6
S-070-XXA	Same as above	38.2–39.3
Suppocire OSI	Eutectec mixtures of mono-, di-, tri-glycerides derived from natural	33–35
Suppocire OSIX	vegetable oils; each type having slightly different properties	33–35
Suppocire A	Same as above	35–36.5
Suppocire B	Same as above	36–37.5
Suppocire C	Same as above	38–40
Suppocire D	Same as above	42–45
Suppocire DM	Same as above	42–45
Suppocire H	Same as above but with the addition of polyoxyethylated glycerides	36–37.5
Suppocire L	Same composition as Suppocire H	38–40
Tegester Triglycerides	Specially prepared triglyceride bases	
TG-95		32.2–34.5
TG-MA		34.5–36.0
TG-57		34.0–36.5
Tween 61	Used alone or in combination with PEG sorbitan monostearate	35–49
Wecobee FS	Triglycerides derived from coconut oil	39.4–40.5
Wecobee M	Same as above	33.3–36
Wecobee R	Same as above	33.9–35
Wecobee S	Same as above	38–40.5
Wecobee SS	Same as above	40–43
Wecobee W	Same as above	31.7–32.8
Witepsol (Selected examples)	Triglycerides of saturated fatty acids C12-C18 with varied portions of the corresponding partial glycerides	
H-5		35.2
H-12		32–33
H-15		33–35
H-19		34.8
H-85		42–48

Oil-Soluble Bases

Cocoa butter, or theobroma oil, is an oleaginous base that softens at 30°C and melts at 34°C. It is a mixture of liquid triglycerides entrapped in a network of crystalline, solid triglycerides. Palmitic and stearic acids make up about half of the saturated fatty acids, and oleic acid makes up the one unsaturated fatty acid. Cocoa butter has four different forms—α, β, β', and γ—with melting points of 22°C, 34°C to 35°C, 28°C, and 18°C, respectively. The β form, which is the most stable, is preferable for suppositories. Cocoa butter will melt to form a nonviscous, bland oil. Because it is immiscible with body fluids, it may leak from the body orifice. Polymorphs with lower melting points will eventually convert to a more stable form over time. Chloral hydrate will decrease the melting point of cocoa butter. To avoid problems with the cocoa butter suppositories sticking when released from the molds, the pharmacist must not overheat the cocoa butter and must make sure the molds are clean and dry before using.

Hydrogenated Vegetable Oil Bases

Fattibase is a preblended suppository base that offers the advantages of a cocoa butter base with few of the drawbacks. It is composed of triglycerides derived from palm, palm kernel, and coconut oils, with self-emulsifying glyceryl monostearate and polyoxyl stearate used as emulsifying and suspending agents. This base is stable with a low irritation profile, needs no special storage conditions, is uniform in composition, and has a bland taste and controlled melting range. It exhibits excellent mold release characteristics and does not require mold lubrication. Fattibase is a solid with a melting point of 35°C to 37°C, has a specific gravity of 0.890 at 37°C, is opaque-white, and is free of suspended matter.

Wecobee bases are derived from palm kernel and coconut oils; they are rendered emulsifiable by the incorporation of glyceryl monostearate and propylene glycolmonostearate. These bases also exhibit most of cocoa butter's desirable features but few of its shortcomings. They are stable and exhibit excellent mold release characteristics.

Witepsol bases number about 12 and are nearly white and almost odorless. Witepsol H 15's melting range and release characteristics are similar to those of cocoa butter. These bases solidify rapidly in the mold, and lubrication is not necessary, as the suppositories contract nicely. Witepsol bases with a high melting point can be mixed with those with a low melting point to provide a wide array of possible melting ranges (i.e., 34°C to 44°C). Because the Witepsol bases contain emulsifiers, they will absorb limited quantities of water.

Water-Soluble Bases

When a water-soluble base is used, the drug dissolves and mixes with the aqueous body fluids. Water-soluble bases may cause some irritation, however, because they may produce slight dehydration of the rectal mucosa by taking up water and dissolving. Nevertheless, they are a widely used base for suppository formulation.

PEG suppository bases are the most popular water-soluble bases. Their advantage is that the ratios of the low to the high molecular weight individual PEGs can be altered to prepare a base with a specific melting point or one that will overcome any problems that result from having to add excess powder or liquid to a suppository. Table 13-2 lists the pertinent characteristics of various PEGs. PEG bases are incompatible with silver salts, tannic acid, aminopyrine, quinine, ichthammol, aspirin, benzocaine, clioquinol, and sulfonamides. Sodium barbital, salicylic acid, and camphor will crystallize out of PEG suppositories. High concentrations of salicylic acid will soften PEGs, and aspirin will complex with PEGs. PEG-based suppositories may be irritating to some patients. Suppositories prepared with PEG should not be stored or dispensed in a polystyrene prescription vial because PEG interacts adversely with polystyrene. All PEG suppositories should be dispensed in glass or cardboard containers.

Table 13-2. Characteristics of Selected PEGs

Molecular Average Weight	Molecular Range Weight	Melting Range (°C)	Water Solubility (approx. % by weight)
300	285–315	–15 to –8	100
400	380–420	4–8	100
600	570–630	20–25	100
1000	950–1050	37–40	80
1450	1300–1600	43–46	72
3350	3000–3700	54–58	67
4600	4400–4800	57–61	65
8000	7000–9000	60–63	63

Polybase is a preblended suppository base. A white solid, it consists of a homogeneous mixture of PEGs and polysorbate 80. It is a water-miscible base that is stable at room temperature, has a specific gravity of 1.177 at 25°C with an average molecular weight of 3440, and does not require mold lubrication.

Glycerinated gelatin suppositories, composed of 70% glycerin, 20% gelatin, and 10% water, should be packaged in tight containers because they are hygroscopic. They are not recommended as a rectal suppository base because they can exert an osmotic effect and a defecation reflex. A glycerin base is composed of glycerin (87%), sodium stearate (8%), and purified water (5%). These bases have occasionally been used for the preparation of vaginal suppositories.

Preparation

Three methods are used to prepare a suppository: hand molding, fusion, and compression. Compounding suppositories generally involves hand molding and fusion, but compression can be used in some instances. Powders to be incorporated into suppositories should be in an impalpable form.

Hand molding requires considerable skill but enables one to avoid using heat while preparing the suppository, because this technique generally uses cocoa butter, which can easily be manipulated, shaped, and handled at room temperature. Hand molding involves grating the cocoa butter, adding the active ingredient, mixing thoroughly by using either a mortar and pestle or a pill tile and spatula, pressing the mix together until it resolidifies, shaping the mixture into a long cylinder with a diameter the size of the suppository to be prepared, cutting it into the desired length, rounding the tips, packaging, and labeling. Plastic gloves can be worn when forming the suppository; it is also advisable to work through a filter paper or to use cornstarch or talc to decrease the tackiness of the cocoa butter.

When using the fusion method, the pharmacist gently heats the base material and then mixes in the active ingredients and any excipients. The melt is then poured into the molds and allowed to cool. After cooling, the suppositories are trimmed, packaged, and labeled. Disposable molds, such as the suppository strips and shells shown in Figure 13-1, can be used for molding and dispensing suppository products.

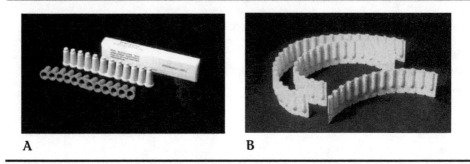

A   B

Figure 13-1. Disposable suppository molds: *A*, shells; *B*, strips.

A straw or thin glass tube can be used as the mold when preparing urethral suppositories. A 1-mL tuberculin syringe can also be used if the lower portion of the barrel is cut off (a pencil sharpener can be used). A large-diameter needle, attached to the syringe filled with the suppository melt, will aid in transferring the product into the 1-mL tuberculin syringe. The urethral suppository can be removed from the 1-mL syringe barrel by inserting the plunger and forcing out the suppository after slight warming. Also, the syringe can be used as an aid for administering the urethral suppository by pressing on the plunger and forcing the suppository directly into the urethra. Commercial reusable molds for urethral suppositories are also available (Figure 13-2).

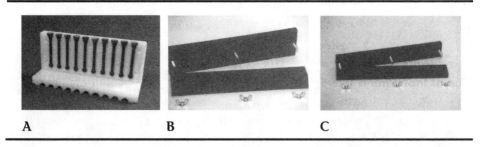

A   B   C

Figure 13-2. Urethral suppository molds: *A*, ball end; *B*, male; *C*, female.

Cold compression is suitable for bases that can be formed into suppositories under pressure. It is especially appropriate for ingredients that are heat labile. Cold compression can be used for such bases as a mixture of 6% hexanetriol-1,2,6 with PEG 1450 and 12% polyethylene oxide polymer 4000.

If fusion or cold compression is used, blanks must be prepared to calibrate the molds. These steps should be followed when performing this calibration.

1. Prepare the suppository molds and confirm that the cavities are clean and dry.
2. Obtain and melt sufficient suppository base to fill 6 to 12 molds.
3. Pour the base into the molds, cool, and trim.
4. Remove the suppositories and weigh.
5. Divide the total weight by the number of blank suppositories prepared to obtain the average weight of each suppository for this particular base.
6. Use this weight as the calibrated value for that specific mold using that specific lot of suppository base.

The following five steps are involved in the preparation of suppositories: (1) preparing the mold, (2) preparing the base, (3) preparing the active drug, (4) mixing and pouring, and (5) cooling and finishing.

Preparing the Mold

Molds should be clean and dry at the start. If prepared and heated properly, good suppository bases should require no lubricants; however, if a lubricant is needed, the choice depends on the properties of the base. If a water-soluble base is used, light mineral oil is a good lubricant. However, glycerin and propylene glycol are good lubricants for oil-soluble bases. Only enough lubricant should be used to provide a thin layer on the walls of the mold. Excessive lubricant will pool at the tip of the mold and produce misshapen suppositories, whereas inadequate lubricant will make it difficult to remove the suppositories. The lubricant can be applied either by spraying or by using a lubricant-treated cloth to wipe the molds. Some pharmacists have also used a commercial vegetable spray as a lubricant. The mold should be equilibrated at room temperature for the pouring procedure.

Preparing the Base

The method of preparation will determine the type of base. If hand molding is used, the pharmacist must grate the cocoa butter. The pharmacist can also grate it for the fusion method. If fusion is used, one must take care not to exceed a temperature of about 34° to 35° to prevent the formation of an unstable polymorph of the cocoa butter base. In such a case, an α form might result, which would produce a suppository with a low melting point that would melt at room temperature and might stick to the mold. Cocoa butter should be melted to form a mixable, pourable liquid that is creamy but hazy in appearance; it should not be melted to a clear yellow state.

For cold compression, the desired base is obtained in grated or granular form and mixed with the active drug. The required quantity of the mix is placed in the chamber/barrel and the piston/plunger is moved into place, forcing the material into the attached mold unit. Pressure is then released and the molded, compressed suppositories are removed.

PEG bases can be melted by using either a water bath or direct heat to a temperature of approximately 60°C. Even though PEG bases are very heat stable, they should not be heated excessively. Rather, they should be heated gently to just a few degrees above their melting range.

Preparing the Active Drug

The active drug should be comminuted to a uniform, small particle size to ensure that it is distributed evenly throughout the base and to minimize settling in the melt. The best source of ingredients for the extemporaneous compounding of suppositories is the pure drug powder. If pure powder is unavailable, commercial dosage forms such as injections, tablets, or capsules can be used. If any excipients are present in these dosage forms, however, they may affect the physicochemical properties and stability of the finished product. In many cases, depending on the solubility of the drug and the excipients, it may be possible to first mix the dosage form with a solvent (alcohol 95%) and then filter, collect the filtrate, dry, and use the resulting active drug powder.

In general, the maximum quantity of excipient that can be incorporated is about 30% of the blank weight of the suppository. For example, for a 2-mL disposable mold, the maximum excipient would be about 600 mg.

Liquids may occupy too much volume to be easily incorporated, and the vehicles may not be compatible with selected suppository bases. Tablets and capsules may contain excessive powder, which could produce suppositories that are too brittle. Adding a large quantity of liquid to an oily suppository base may require the preparation of a water-in-oil emulsion. This preparation can be done by incorporating 10% wool fat or 2% cholesterol in up to 15% aqueous solutions in cocoa butter, or by using one of the modern triglyceride vegetable oil bases such as Fattibase, Wecobee, or Witepsol. In the case of PEG bases, a higher percentage of the higher molecular weight PEGs can be used to accommodate the liquid.

Mixing and Pouring

The drug is either mixed directly into the base or "wetted" before incorporation. A stirring rod or a magnetic stirring setup can be used for mixing. The mixing process should be long enough to distribute the drug uniformly but not so long as to lead to drug or base deterioration. As soon as the melt is ready, it can be poured into the mold, which has been brought to room temperature and is situated with the openings on top. A cold or frozen mold should never be used because it can cause fractures and fissures throughout the suppository. The pharmacist should fill each cavity slowly and carefully, starting at one end of the mold, ensuring that no air bubbles are incorporated into the suppository. A slight excess of material may be allowed to build up on the top of the mold as the next cavity is filled, and so on. To prevent layering in the suppositories, the pouring process should not be stopped until all the molds have been filled. The pharmacist can use a 10-mL syringe, or other suitable size, filled with melt to fill the molds as long as the melt does not cool too rapidly. The mold should be at room temperature so that the melt does not solidify prematurely as it is poured down the sides of the mold cavity. Premature solidification could result in unfilled mold tips and deformed suppositories. If disposable molds are used, PEG melts should be poured at a minimum temperature, because some molds may collapse at about 70°C. If the melt is poured at around 60°C, such a collapse should not occur. Other bases should be kept near their respective melting temperatures.

Cooling and Finishing

The molds should be allowed to set for 15 to 30 minutes at room temperature and then refrigerated for 30 minutes, if necessary. Any excess material can be removed from the top of the mold (the back of the suppository) with the blade of a stainless steel spatula, which has first been dipped in a beaker of warm water. Removing this excess will also give the backside of the suppository a nice smooth surface. A razor blade also works well. The suppositories should then be carefully removed from the molds, packaged, and labeled. If the mold is still cool from refrigeration, the suppositories should be slightly contracted, which will make removal easier. Wrapping the individual suppositories with foil wrappers, although not necessary, presents an elegant product to the patient.

Additional suggestions for preparing suppositories are provided in the box "Hints for Compounding Suppositories."

Hints for Compounding Suppositories

- A 10% overage of materials should be calculated to allow for loss during preparation and overpouring.
- If disposable molds are not marked with lines for reproducible filling, the extent of fill should be determined from the blank.
- If using plastic disposable molds, the temperature of the melt must be lower than that which will melt or soften the mold.
- A constant temperature dry bath filled with sand set at 37°C provides the proper temperature for softening and melting fatty acid and cocoa butter bases in a short time.
- Vegetable extracts, moistened by levigation with a small quantity of melted base, will more readily distribute the active drug throughout the base.
- A large quantity of powder, dampened with a few drops of a bland oil, such as mineral oil, or a water-miscible liquid, such as glycerin, will be easier to incorporate into some bases.
- Liquid ingredients, mixed with a powder such as starch, will be less fluid and easier to incorporate into a base.

Physicochemical Considerations

A number of factors affect the decisions the pharmacist must make when preparing a suppository. Questions the pharmacist should ask before formulating this dosage form include the following:

- Is the desired effect to result from systemic or local use?
- Is the route of administration rectal, vaginal, or urethral?
- Is a rapid or a slow and prolonged release of the medication desired?

The rate of drug release is an important factor in the selection of a suppository base. If a drug does not release its medication within 6 hours, the patient may not receive its full benefit, as the drug may be expelled. Thus, among the factors that must be considered in the selection of a suppository base is the drug's solubility. One way to ensure maximum release of the drug from the base is to apply the principle of "opposite characteristics." This principle means that water-soluble drugs should be placed in oil-soluble bases, and oil-soluble drugs should be placed in water-soluble bases. Oil-soluble bases (e.g., cocoa butter) melt quickly in the rectum to release the drug, whereas PEG bases must dissolve in mucosal fluids, a process that can take longer. If PEGs with a higher molecular weight are used, the dissolution time is extended. Moistening the suppositories with warm water immediately before insertion facilitates not only insertion but also dissolution.

The release of the drug and the onset of drug action thus depend on the liquefaction of the suppository base, the dissolution of the active drug, and the diffusion of the drug through the mucosal layers. For example, the time for liquefaction of a hydrogenated vegetable oil—or cocoa butter—based suppository is approximately 3 to 7 minutes; for a glycerinated gelatin suppository, about 30 to 40 minutes; and for a PEG suppository, about 30 to 50 minutes. Table 13-3 gives a general summary of the relationship of drug release, the drug, and the suppository base.

Other factors must also be considered when preparing a suppository. They include the presence of water, hygroscopicity, viscosity, brittleness, density, volume contraction, special problems, incompatibilities, pharmacokinetics, and bioequivalence.

Table 13-3. Drug Release Rates of Various Suppository Formulations

Drug:Base Characteristics	Approximate Drug Release Rate
Oil-soluble drug:Oily base	Slow release; poor escaping tendency
Water-soluble drug:Oily base	Rapid release
Oil-soluble drug:Water-miscible base	Moderate release
Water-miscible drug:Water-miscible base	Moderate release; based on diffusion; all water soluble

Presence of Water

When preparing suppositories, the pharmacist should avoid using water to incorporate an active drug. Water may accelerate the oxidation of fat, increase the degradation rate of many drugs, enhance reactions between the drug and other components in the suppository, support bacterial/fungal growth, and require the addition of bacteriostatic agents. Furthermore, if the water evaporates, the dissolved substances may crystallize.

Hygroscopicity

Glycerin and PEG-containing suppositories are hygroscopic. The rate of moisture change depends on the chain length of the molecule as well as the temperature and humidity of the environment. PEGs with molecular weights greater than 4000 have less tendency to be hygroscopic than do the lower-weight PEGs.

Viscosity

Viscosity considerations are also important in the preparation of the suppositories and the release of the drug. If the viscosity of a base is low, it may be necessary to add a suspending agent such as silica gel to ensure that the drug is uniformly dispersed until solidification occurs. When preparing the suppository, the pharmacist should stir the melt constantly and keep it at the lowest possible temperature to maintain high viscosity. After the suppository has been administered, the release rate of the drug may be slowed if the viscosity of the base is very high. The increased viscosity causes the drug to diffuse more slowly through the base to reach the mucosal membrane for absorption.

To increase the viscosity of a fatty base, the pharmacist can increase the fatty acid chain length of compounds in the base. For example, increased C-16 and C-18 monoglycerides and diglycerides can be added to the base. Other approaches involve adding cetyl, stearyl, and myristyl alcohols and stearic acid in concentrations of about 5% or adding about 2% aluminum monostearate to the base.

Brittleness

Brittle suppositories can be difficult to handle, wrap, and use. Cocoa butter suppositories are usually not brittle unless the percentage of solids present is high. In general, brittleness results when the percentage of nonbase materials exceeds about 30%. Synthetic fat bases with high stearate concentrations or those that are highly hydrogenated are typically more brittle. *Shock cooling* occurs when the melted base is chilled too rapidly, possibly causing fat and cocoa butter suppositories to crack. This condition can be prevented by ensuring that the temperature of the mold is as close to the temperature of the melted base as possible. Suppositories should not be placed in a freezer, which also causes shock cooling. The addition of a small quantity (usually less than 2%) of Tween 80, Tween 85, fatty acid monoglycerides, castor oil, glycerin, or propylene glycol will make these bases more pliable and less brittle.

Density

To determine the weight of the individual suppositories, it is important to know the density of the incorporated materials. For example, if the density of the insoluble powders is too great, the suspended materials will have a tendency to settle and stratify in the molds, resulting in a poor appearance and possibly a brittle suppository.

It has been stated that if the quantity of the active drug is less than 100 mg, the volume occupied by the powder is insignificant and need not be considered. This principle is usually based on a 2 g suppository weight. Obviously, if a suppository mold weighing less than 2 g is used, or if the quantity of the active drug to be added is greater than 100 mg, the powder volume should be considered. The pharmacist should know the density factors of various bases and drugs to determine the proper weights of the ingredients to be used.

The density factors of cocoa butter are known. For other bases, the density factor can be calculated as the ratio of the blank weight of the base and the cocoa butter. Density factors for a number of ingredients are shown in Table 13-4.

Two methods of calculating the quantity of base that will be occupied by the active medication are the Dosage Replacement Factor Method and the Density Factor:Paddock Method. The following equation is used to determine the dosage replacement factor:[1]

$$f = \frac{100\,(E - G)}{(G)(x)} + 1$$

where f equals the dosage replacement factor, E equals the weight of the pure base suppositories, and G equals the weight of suppositories with x% of the active ingredient.

This equation can be used both for calculating the dosage replacement factor (Table 13-5) and for calculating the weight of the prepared suppositories. A sample calculation for each method is given in Chapter 5, "Pharmaceutical Compounding Calculations."

Volume Contraction

Bases, excipients, and active ingredients generally occupy less space at lower temperatures than at higher temperatures. When preparing a suppository, the pharmacist pours hot melt into a mold and allows the melt to cool. During this cooling process, the melt has a tendency to contract in size. This contraction makes

Table 13-4. Density Factors for Cocoa Butter Suppositories

Active Drug	Density Factor
Aloin	1.3
Alum	1.7
Aminophylline	1.1
Aminopyrine	1.3
Aspirin	1.1
Barbital sodium	1.2
Belladonna extract	1.3
Benzoic acid	1.5
Bismuth carbonate	4.5
Bismuth salicylate	4.5
Bismuth subgallate	2.7
Bismuth subnitrate	6.0
Boric acid	1.5
Castor oil	1.0
Chloral hydrate	1.3
Cocaine hydrochloride	1.3
Codeine phosphate	1.1
Digitalis leaf	1.6
Dimenhydrinate	1.3
Diphenhydramine hydrochloride	1.3
Gallic acid	2.0
Glycerin	1.6
Ichthammol	1.1
Iodoform	4.0
Menthol	0.7
Morphine hydrochloride	1.6
Opium	1.4
Paraffin	1.0
Pentobarbital sodium	1.2
Peruvian balsam	1.1
Phenobarbital	1.2
Phenol	0.9
Potassium bromide	2.2
Potassium iodide	4.5
Procaine	1.2
Quinine hydrochloride	1.2
Resorcinol	1.4
Salicylic acid	1.3
Secobarbital sodium	1.2
Sodium bromide	2.3
Spermaceti	1.0
Sulfathiazole	1.6
Tannic acid	1.6
White wax	1.0
Witch hazel fluid extract	1.1
Zinc oxide	4.0
Zinc sulfate	2.8

it easier to release the suppository from the mold, but it may also produce a cavity at the back, or open end, of the mold. Such a cavity is undesirable and can be prevented if the melt is permitted to approach its congealing temperature immediately before it is poured into the mold. It is advisable to pour a small amount of excess melt at the open end of the mold to allow for the slight contraction during cooling. Scraping with a blade or spatula dipped in warm water will remove the excess after solidification, but care must be taken not to remove the metal from the mold. The heated instrument can also be used to smooth out the back of the suppository.

Table 13-5. Dosage Replacement Factors for Selected Drugs[a]

Active Drug	Dosage Replacement Factor
Balsam peru	0.87
Bismuth subgallate	0.37
Bismuth subnitrate	0.33
Boric acid	0.67
Camphor	1.49
Castor oil	1.0
Chloral hydrate	1.67
Icthammol	0.91
Mild silver protein	0.61
Phenobarbital	0.81
Phenol	0.9
Procaine hydrochloride	0.8
Quinine hydrochloride	0.83
Resorcinol	0.71
Silver protein, mild	0.61
Spermaceti	1.0
Wax, white/yellow	1.0
Zinc oxide	0.15–0.25

[a]Cocoa butter is arbitrarily assigned a value of 1 as the standard base.

Special Problems

Some active drugs are more difficult to incorporate into a base and require additional preparation steps. Before vegetable extracts are added, they can be moistened by levigation with a small amount of melted base. This step makes it easier to distribute the active drug throughout the base.

Hard, crystalline materials can be incorporated either by pulverizing them to a fine state or by dissolving them in a small quantity of solvent, which is then taken up into the base. An aqueous solvent and a PEG base are appropriate for water-soluble materials. Alternatively, if the material is water soluble and an oily base must be used, wool fat could be used to take up the solution for incorporation into the suppository base.

When liquid ingredients are mixed with an inert powder such as starch, they become less fluid, which makes them easier to handle. The suppository produced will thus hold together better.

Several ways are used to incorporate excess powder into a suppository base, depending on the base used. If the base is oil miscible, one can add a few drops of a bland oil like sesame oil or mineral oil. When excess powder is incorporated into water-soluble bases, the pharmacist can vary the ratio of low to high melting point ingredients. For example, because additional powders will make the suppository harder, using a higher percentage of a PEG having a low molecular weight would result in a suppository of the proper character.

Incompatibilities

A number of ingredients are incompatible with PEG bases. They include benzocaine, clioquinol, sulfonamides, ichthammol, aspirin, silver salts, and tannic acid. Other materials reported to have a tendency to crystallize out of PEG include sodium barbital, salicylic acid, and camphor.

Pharmacokinetics

Factors affecting absorption include anorectal or vaginal physiology, suppository vehicle, absorption site pH, drug pKa, degree of ionization, and lipid solubility. In some instances, suppositories have been proven to have better absorption than orally administered medications.

Bioequivalence Examples

Both rectal and oral routes of administration can be bioequivalent. The rectal route, however, should be considered as an alternative administration route for some drugs, such as etodolac. Some prodrugs may degrade before they are absorbed through the gastrointestinal tract. The use of cyclodextrins to improve the pharmaceutical properties of drugs has been well documented. When a cyclodextrin is incorporated with a prodrug in a suppository dosage form, the rectal bioavailability of the selected prodrug may be enhanced.

Single dosing of fluconazole orally has been demonstrated to be equivalent to once-daily dosing for 3 days of terconazole (80 mg each). The terconazole was contained in a vaginal suppository with a cocoa butter base. In the case of late evaluation of the infection, the cure rates for the oral and vaginal administration were 75% and 100%, respectively.

Bioavailability of solids can be maximized by using the smallest particle size available. Also, drugs that are available as water-soluble salt forms will generally go into solution easier in the mucosal fluids, followed by migration to the rectal wall and absorption. The addition of sodium caprate increases the bioavailability of penicillins and cephalosporins, and the addition of bile salts and fatty acids can increase the permeability of some other drugs.

Quality Control

Quality control of suppositories can include uniformity of weight and uniformity of texture and physical appearance. The uniformity of texture can be assessed by sectioning a suppository longitudinally and laterally and then ensuring that each section presents a smooth, uniform surface. (See the Standard Operating Procedure (SOP) titled "Performing Quality Assessment of Suppositories.")

Patient Counseling

Patients should be instructed on how to properly store the suppository, unwrap a wrapped suppository, and resolidify a melted suppository. The proper method of disposing of unused suppositories should also be discussed. Patients should also be counseled on the proper insertion of the suppository: whether to moisten it before insertion, how far to insert it, and how long to remain inactive after insertion, as follows: (1) position the patient on the left side with the upper leg flexed; (2) lubricate the suppository with a water-soluble lubricant or a small amount of water, if needed; (3) gently insert the suppository in the rectum a finger's depth at an angle toward the umbilicus so the suppository is placed against the rectal wall for absorption, rather than being left in the canal or pushed into a mass of stool; and (4) after the finger is withdrawn, hold the buttocks together until the urge to expel has ceased.

Packaging

It is best to wrap suppositories individually or to dispense them in the disposable molds in which they are prepared. If suppositories are not packaged properly, they may become deformed, stained, broken, or chipped. Foil suppository wrappers are available in various colors. Wrapped suppositories are usually placed in wide-mouthed containers or in slide, folding, or partitioned boxes (Figure 13-3) for dispensation to the patient. Suppositories that are dispensed in disposable molds are often placed in cardboard sleeves or plastic bags, labeled, and dispensed.

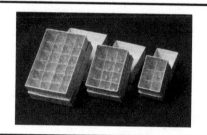

Figure 13-3. Suppository boxes.

Storage/Labeling

Suppositories must be protected from heat and can be stored in a refrigerator. They should not be frozen. Glycerin and PEG-based suppositories should be protected from moisture, as they tend to be hygroscopic.

If the suppositories are wrapped, it is usually a good idea to include the instruction, "Unwrap, Moisten, and Insert" or "Unwrap and Insert," on the label.

Stability

The completed products are generally considered dry or nonaqueous and thus provide a stable dosage form as long as they are protected from moisture and heat. According to Chapter <795>, "Pharmacy Compounding,"[2] these products should have a beyond-use date of 25% of the time remaining on the expiration date, if the product is prepared with a manufactured product, or 6 months, whichever is earlier. If the product is prepared from USP/NF ingredients, a beyond-use date of 6 months is appropriate, unless evidence is available to support other dating.

The USP description of stability considerations for suppositories includes observations for excessive softening and evidence of oil stains on packaging materials.

The pharmacist may have to remove the wrappings of individual suppositories to check for evidence of instability.

According to the *United States Pharmacopeia 25/National Formulary 20*, the major indication of instability in suppositories is excessive softening. In some cases, suppositories may dry out, harden, or shrivel. As a general rule, the guidelines recommend storage in a refrigerator, unless otherwise indicated.

The formation of polymorphs is evidence of cocoa butter instability during preparation. These polymorphs may be liquid at room temperature. To avoid this situation, the pharmacist may substitute an appropriate hydrogenated vegetable oil base for the cocoa butter. If necessary, fatty materials with higher melting points, such as white wax or paraffin, can be added to fatty bases or cocoa butter, with low melting points, to increase the melting point of the formulation. However, the suppository must be able to melt when administered. To check the melting point, the pharmacist can place a sample suppository in a beaker of water that has been heated to 37°C. If the suppository does not melt, the formulation should not be used for patient therapy.

If water is incorporated into an oily base with the use of an emulsifying agent (nonionic surfactant, wool fat, and the like), the product may become rancid. In this case the suppository usually will not be as stable as if the same drug were added to a PEG-based suppository containing water.

Most suppository formulations do not contain preservatives or antioxidants because water is usually excluded from the formulations, nonoxidizing bases are generally used, and the drug is generally stable in a solid dosage form.

Sample Formulations

Suppository Bases

These bases are prepared according to the instructions given in the section "Preparing the Base."

General Purpose #1 Base

Polyethylene glycol 8000	50%
Polyethylene glycol 1540	30%
Polyethylene glycol 300	20%

General Purpose Soft Base

Polyethylene glycol 3350	60%
Polyethylene glycol 1000	30%
Polyethylene glycol 300	10%

General Purpose Firm Base

Polyethylene glycol 8000	30%
Polyethylene glycol 1540	70%

Polyethylene Glycol Bases for Progesterone Suppositories

	Formula 1	Formula 2
Polyethylene glycol 8000	40%	20%
Polyethylene glycol 300	60%	80%

 Base for Water-Soluble Drugs

Polyethylene glycol 8000	60%
Polyethylene glycol 1540	25%
Cetyl alcohol	5%
Purified water	10%

Ingredient-Specific Formulations

R͓ **Estradiol Suppositories**

Estradiol	1 mg
Silica gel	20 mg
Fatty acid base	qs

1. Calculate the quantity of each ingredient required for the prescription.
2. Accurately weigh each ingredient.
3. Carefully heat the fatty acid base to about 35°C to 37°C, being careful not to overheat.
4. Sprinkle the estradiol powder and silica gel onto the melted base and mix thoroughly.
5. Remove from heat and pour into molds that are at room temperature, not chilled. Once the pouring has started, do not stop. If reusable molds are used, allow a small quantity of the melt to "bead up" on the back of the suppository to allow for contraction.
6. Place in a refrigerator to harden.
7. Remove from refrigerator and allow to set at room temperature for a few minutes.
8. Trim the suppositories and package. If reusable molds are used, trim the suppositories, remove from molds, wrap if desired, and package.
9. Label.

℞ Morphine Sulfate Slow Release Suppositories

Morphine sulfate	50 mg
Alginic acid	25%
Fatty acid base	qs

1. Calculate the quantity of each ingredient required for the prescription.
2. Accurately weigh each ingredient.
3. Pass the alginic acid through a No. 200 mesh sieve.
4. Melt the fatty acid base in a glass beaker to about 50°C.
5. Sprinkle the alginic acid on the fatty acid base and mix well.
6. Sprinkle the morphine sulfate on the mixture and stir until well mixed.
7. Place the mixture on an ultrasonic bath for 10 minutes for thorough and complete mixing.
8. Cool slightly, then pour continuously into molds held at room temperature.
9. Cool and trim.
10. Package and label.

℞ Ondansetron Hydrochloride Suppositories

Ondansetron hydrochloride	8 mg
Micronized silica gel	25 mg
Fatty acid base	qs

1. Calculate the quantity of each ingredient required for the prescription.
2. Accurately weigh each ingredient.
3. Triturate the ondansetron hydrochloride with the micronized silica gel.
4. Melt the fatty acid base and heat to approximately 50°C.
5. Sprinkle the powder on the melt and mix thoroughly.
6. Remove from heat for a few minutes.
7. Pour into molds (equilibrated at room temperature).
8. Place in refrigerator to harden.
9. Trim, package, and label.

℞ Antiemetic Suppositories

Haloperidol	5 mg
Diphenhydramine hydrochloride	25 mg
Lorazepam	2 mg
Silicon dioxide	30 mg
Polyethylene glycol base	qs

1. Calculate the quantity of each ingredient required for the prescription.
2. Accurately weigh each ingredient.
3. Mix the powders together.
4. Heat the PEG base to about 60°C.
5. Sprinkle the powders onto the melted PEG base and mix well.
6. Pour the melt into molds (maintained at room temperature) slowly and smoothly; stir intermittently to ensure the powders remain well mixed.
7. Allow the suppositories to solidify (refrigerate if necessary).
8. Remove from molds and trim.
9. Package and label.

℞ Fluconazole 200 mg Suppositories

| Fluconazole | 200 mg |
| Polyethylene glycol base | qs |

1. Calculate the quantity of each ingredient required for the prescription.
2. Accurately weigh each ingredient and/or count the required number of fluconazole tablets.
3. Pulverize the fluconazole tablets to provide the fluconazole powder.
4. Melt the PEG base at about 60°C.
5. Sprinkle the powder onto the melted base and stir.
6. Cool slightly, then pour into molds.
7. Cool, trim, package, and label.

℞ **Nifedipine, Lidocaine, and Nitroglycerin Suppositories (#30)**

Nifedipine		200 mg
Lidocaine HCl		1.5 g
Nitroglycerin 0.4 mg tablets		#25
Polybase or fatty acid base	qs	75 g

1. Calculate the quantity of each ingredient required for the prescription.
2. Calibrate the suppository mold, using the Polybase or the fatty acid base.
3. Accurately weigh each ingredient. Count out the nitroglycerin tablets.
4. Mix nifedipine and lidocaine powders together.
5. Levigate the nitroglycerin tablets with a small quantity of ethyl alcohol.
6. Gently melt the selected base.
7. Add the powders and the nitroglycerin to the melted base and mix well.
8. Pour into molds and allow to cool.
9. Cool, trim, package, and label.

(Note: This preparation should be prepared in a room with subdued light because of the light sensitivity of the nifedipine.)

Standard Operating Procedure (SOP)

Performing Quality Assessment of Suppositories

Purpose of SOP

The purpose of this procedure is to provide a method of documenting uniformity between batches and to conduct quality assessment tests of and observations on suppositories.

Materials

The following items are used in one or more of the assessment tests:

- Balance
- Graduated cylinders
- Beaker
- Set of weights

Procedure

The appropriate tests should be conducted and the results/observations recorded on the worksheet "Quality Assessment Form for Suppositories" (Figure 13-4).

Weight.

- Accurately weigh the product on a balance.

Specific Gravity.

1. To calculate the specific gravity, identify the weight and volume of the product.
2. Record the weight of the individual dosage form or a strip/package of the dosage forms (tared weight).

To determine the volume of water displaced, do the following:

Single Unit.

1. Place 5 mL of water in a 10-mL graduate.
2. Add the dosage form and read the water level.
3. Subtract 5 mL from the water level measurement in step 2 to determine the volume of water occupied by the dosage form.
4. If the dosage form floats, place a weight attached to a paper clip in the graduate before adding the water to the 5-mL mark. Then wrap one end of the paper clip around the dosage form to hold it below the water surface and place it in the graduate. Proceed as in step 3.

Multiple Unit Packages (Suppository Strip).

1. Place the empty package in a beaker that will hold it with minimal extra space.
2. Add an exact known quantity of water to cover the product. It may be necessary to add a weight to the package; this same weight should be used for the actual product.
3. With a fine-line marker and with the beaker sitting on a level surface, mark the water level on the outside of the beaker.
4. Remove the beaker contents and dry the beaker.
5. Place the dosage form (and the weight if used) into the beaker.
6. Measure the same volume of water as in step 2 into a graduate.
7. Pour the water into the beaker only to the mark from step 3. (Note: Do quickly before the dosage form dissolves.)
8. Measure the volume of water remaining in the beaker.

Calculations. Now that the weight and volume of the product are obtained, the specific gravity can be calculated by dividing the weight (grams) by the volume (milliliters).

Active Drug Assay Results. As appropriate, have representative samples of the product assayed for active drug content by a contract analytical laboratory. Stability can be assessed by storing the product at room, refrigerated, and/or frozen temperatures and having the assay repeated on the stored samples.

Color of Product. It may be advisable to use a color chart for determining the actual color of the product.

Clarity. Clarity is evaluated by visual inspection. On the worksheet, 1 is the clearest and 5 is the least clear on the scale provided.

Surface Texture.

‣ Observe the product to determine smoothness of the surface.

Appearance.

‣ Determine whether the product appears dry or oily/moist.

Feel.

‣ Touch the product to determine whether it is sticky (tacky) or hard (plastic) or bounces back (elastic).

Melting Test. This test is performed on fatty acid and cocoa butter products, as well as on oil-based products.

1. Heat a 200-mL beaker of water to 37°C on a magnetic stirring unit that is set at about 50 rpm.
2. Add a dosage unit to the water. (Note: It may be necessary to add a weight to these dosage units to pull them below the water surface.)
3. After 30 minutes, record your observations as Yes, No, or the appropriate number with 1 being the most melted on the scale provided on the form (Figure 13-4).

Dissolution Test (for PEG and gelatin and water-soluble products)

1. Proceed as in the melting test.
2. After 30 minutes, record your observations as Yes, No, or the appropriate number with 1 being the most dissolved on the scale provided on the form (Figure 13-4).

Physical Observation.

▸ Describe the appearance and organoleptic qualities of the product.

Physical Stability.

1. Prepare a few additional dosage forms, package, and label "For Physical Stability Observations."
2. Weekly, observe the product for signs of discoloration, dryness, cracking, mottling, mold growth, and so forth.
3. Record a descriptive observation on the form (Figure 13-4) at each observation interval. (Sufficient lines are provided for observations for 8 weeks or approximately 60 days.)

References

1. Coben LJ, Lieberman HA. Suppositories. In: Lachman L, Lieberman HA, Kanig JL. *The Theory and Practice of Industrial Pharmacy.* 3rd ed. Philadelphia: Lea and Febiger; 1986:564–88.
2. Expert Advisory Panel on Pharmacy Compounding Practices. Pharmacy compounding. *United States Pharmacopeia 25/National Formulary 20.* Rockville, Md: United States Pharmacopeial Convention; 2000.

Quality Assessment Form for Suppositories

Product _____   Date _____

Lot/Rx number _____   Dosage form: Suppository _____

Characteristic	Theoretical						Actual	Normal Range
Weight/volume							_____	_____
Specific gravity							_____	_____
Active drug assay results							_____	_____
Initial assay							_____	_____
After storage No. 1							_____	_____
After storage No. 2							_____	_____
Color of product							_____	_____
Clarity	Clear	1	2	3	4	5		Opaque
Texture-surface	Smooth	1	2	3	4	5		Rough
Appears dry	Yes	1	2	3	4	5		No
Appearance	Dry	1	2	3	4	5		Oily/moist
Feels tacky	Yes	1	2	3	4	5		No
Feels plastic	Yes	1	2	3	4	5		No
Feels elastic	Yes	1	2	3	4	5		No
Melting test	Yes	1	2	3	4	5		No
Dissolution test	Yes	1	2	3	4	5		No

Sample set aside for physical stability observation: Yes   No

If yes, results: Date   Observation

_____   _____

_____   _____

_____   _____

_____   _____

_____   _____

_____   _____

_____   _____

_____   _____

_____   _____

_____   _____

_____   _____

_____   _____

_____   _____

Figure 13-4. Sample worksheet for quality assessment of suppositories.

Chapter 14

Sticks

Medication sticks are a convenient form for administering topical drugs; they are not limited to applications to the lips. Their development is interesting because it involves the history of cosmetics, which parallels human history. Although cosmetics are viewed as preparations aimed at improving a person's appearance, many cosmetic products also serve as either medications or drug vehicle bases. The medication stick is a recent product that is being used for both cosmetic and medical purposes. Today, medication sticks provide pharmacists, patients, and primary care providers with a unique, convenient, relatively stable, easy-to-prepare dosage form for the topical delivery of drugs. Their use will probably continue to increase in the future.

Definitions/Types

On the basis of their characteristics, sticks can be grouped in three main categories: soft opaque, soft clear, and hard.

Soft opaque sticks can contain petrolatum, cocoa butter, and polyethylene glycol (PEG) bases. Most medication sticks are of this type.

Soft clear sticks usually contain the bases sodium stearate and propylene glycol. Water or alcohol is also added.

Hard sticks consist of crystalline powders either fused by heat or held together with a binder such as cocoa butter or petrolatum.

Because sticks are a cosmetic form, a brief review of cosmetic formulations is appropriate. Lipstick is the prototype of all cosmetic sticks, including poured mascara and deodorant sticks. Lipsticks vary greatly in their physical properties. They can be quite hard, soft, greasy or sticky, brittle and crumbly, or smooth and velvety. All lipsticks, however, have a definite mechanical function, which is to provide a vehicle to facilitate easy, uniform application of color to the lips. Thus, the consistency of this cosmetic is of vital importance. If the stick is too hard, it is difficult to apply. If it crumbles or is too sticky, it will smear, which generates consumer complaints. The same principles apply to the formulation of medication sticks.

The materials that give body to sticks are waxes, polymers, resins, dry solids fused into a firm mass, and fused crystals. An example of a fused stick is a styptic pencil. Resin is used in connection with epilating wax. The resin and pitch or waxes are melted and poured into appropriate molds in which they solidify in stick form.

Historical Use

The science of cosmetic preparations is as old as recorded history, perhaps older. In the earliest times, cosmetics were associated with religious practices; for example, aromatic incense, oils, and ointments were used to anoint the living and the dead. In late fifth century BC, Hippocrates advanced the study of dermatology and advocated correct diet, exercise, sunlight, special baths, and massage as aids to good health and beauty. Cosmetic literature in the 15th to 17th centuries was limited to the "books of secrets," which were devoted not only to bodily embellishment, home, and other topics but also to medicine. Over the years, formulas were written down in various published books, but it was not until the 1940s that actual cosmetic compendia were published in English.

Beginning about 1000 AD, cosmetics, when not made in the home, were usually prepared by pharmacists. During the period 1200 to 1500, cosmetics began to be viewed as a separate specialty, distinct from medicine. Later, cosmetics split into two branches: those used for routine beautification of the skin and those used for the correction of various disorders of the skin, hair, nails, and teeth. The latter drew on the disciplines of dermatology, pharmacology, dentistry, ophthalmology, dietetics, and other accepted medical arts.

The first *Pharmacopoeia of London*, published in 1618, showed that the pharmacists had all the necessary equipment and skills to make and sell cosmetic products, but the stringent regulations governing their work kept most of them exclusively occupied with the compounding of medications. This situation changed little as the 17th and 18th centuries progressed. Cosmetic products of all kinds continued to be made principally in the home, although the number of shops selling many items slowly increased. Pharmacists and "druggists" (a new term of German origin) sold the raw materials, but few professional apothecaries sold any cosmetics other than assorted essences and "perfumed waters."

The period preceding World War I saw the introduction of sticks made from a base of oil and wax generally colored with carmine. These sticks, which came to be known as lipsticks, applied a colored layer to the lips that, when removed, left them their natural color. Although most dyes were water insoluble, it was discovered that adding water-soluble dye to the stick could actually dye the lips, provided they had been moistened before applying the lipstick. The use of these lipsticks was an early approach to the use of sticks containing a material that interacted with the skin. Some of these water-soluble dyes would develop an intense red color as the pH was lowered.

In recent years cosmetic scientists have introduced and improved cosmetic products for different applications. Some of these products are still widely used in the pharmaceutical sciences, including powders, sticks, gels, solutions, suspensions, pastes, ointments, and oils. Examples would include styptic pencils and products such as Chap Stick lip balm, which became available in the early 1940s.

Applications

Medication sticks are a convenient form for administering topical medications. They come in different sizes and shapes, are readily transportable, and can be applied directly to the affected site of the body. Sticks can be easily compounded by using different materials to produce topical or systemic effects. Medications and ingredients that have been incorporated into sticks include local anesthetics, sunscreens, oncology drugs, antivirals, and antibiotics. Sticks containing antibiotics, antivirals, and oncology agents are usually packaged in 5-g tubes, whereas sticks containing local anesthetics are usually packaged in 1- or 2-oz tubes.

The medication in a soft stick is applied by raising the stick above the tube level and simply rubbing it onto the skin, where it softens and flows easily onto the affected area. The medication usually cannot be seen on the skin. When a hard stick is applied, the tip of the stick is moistened and then touched to the affected area. The crystalline powder used to prepare the stick can leave a white residue on the skin.

Composition

Preparing sticks requires different bases depending on the application. There are two types of bases: melting bases and moistening bases.

Melting Bases

Melting bases include the bases used to prepare soft opaque and soft clear sticks. These bases, which will soften and melt at body temperatures, include cocoa butter, petrolatum, waxes, PEGs, and the like. Active drugs can include any agent that can be applied directly to a specific skin site or over a larger area of skin to relieve such discomforts as muscle sprains and arthritis. Penetration enhancers (e.g., glycerin, propylene glycol, alcohol, and surfactants) can increase the amount of transdermal drug delivery. Using waxes, oils, or plain polymers such as PEGs alone achieves a topical effect. Melting bases can be further divided into opaque and clear. Opaque bases include waxes, oils, PEGs, and the like, whereas clear bases include sodium stearate/glycerin mixtures.

Moistening Bases

This base is used to produce solid, hard sticks that must be moistened to become "activated." When the stick is moistened, a concentrated solution of the drug forms at the tip of the stick. When applied, the drug will exert its effect topically. A styptic pencil containing alum or aluminum sulfate is an example of this type of stick. It is possible that some drugs that are not stable in other forms would be stable in a dry, hard crystalline stick.

Preparation

Certain characteristics are required of a good stick. It should spread easily without excessive greasiness. It should be uniform, stable, and free from mottling. Conversely, it should not sweat, crumble, or crack.

To prepare a stick, one should have familiarity with waxes. Some waxes such as carnauba have high melting points; others such as beeswax, paraffin, and cocoa butter have lower melting points. There are also the waxy fatty acids such as spermaceti and stearic acid and the waxy alcohols such as cetyl and stearyl alcohol. Table 14-1 lists the melting and congealing points of various waxes, oils, and PEGs. It is soon obvious that no single waxy substance serves the purpose alone. The high-melting-point waxes must be blended with the low-melting-point waxes to produce a combination that will soften at body temperature. Adding lubricants will minimize the coherence of the waxes and make the product easier to spread. By balancing these ingredients, one eventually develops a stick that has the desired physical properties for its application. The formulator's goal is to prepare a combination of waxes that will soften at body temperature and will still contain lubricants and other ingredients that promote the absorption and emollient effects.

The consistency of the stick is determined by the melting point of the waxes. To change the consistency, one must adjust the melting point by changing the percentage of the wax with the highest melting point.

Table 14-1. Melting and Congealing Points/Ranges of Waxes, Oils, and PEGs

Item	Melting Point/ Range (°C)	Congealing Point/ Range (°C)
Waxes		
Carnauba wax	81–86	
Cetostearyl alcohol	48–55	
Cetyl alcohol	45–50	
Cetyl esters wax	43–47	
Cholesterol	147–150	
Cocoa butter	30–35	
Emulsifying wax	48–52	
Glyceryl monostearate	≥ 55	
Hard fat	27–44	
Microcrystalline wax	54–102	
Paraffin		47–65
Polyoxyl 40 stearate		37–47
Propylene glycol monostearate		≥ 45
Purified stearic acid		66–69
Stearic acid		≥ 54
Stearyl alcohol	55–60	
White wax	62–65	
Yellow wax	62–65	
Oils		
Castor oil		−10 to −18
Corn oil	−18 to −10	
Cottonseed oil		0 to −5
Hydrogenated castor oil	85–88	
Hydrogenated vegetable oil	61–66	
Oleic acid		≤ 10
Peanut oil		−5
Polyoxyl 40 hydrogenated castor oil	20–30	
Soybean oil		−10 to −16
Polyethylene glycols		
PEG 300		4 to 8
PEG 1500	44–48	
PEG 3350	54–58	
PEG 6000	58–63	

One should mold a batch all at once, taking care that the mixture does not grow cold and require reheating. All trimmings and scraps, together with any sticks rejected because of mold marks or pin holes, should be kept separate from the regular batch. This material can be remelted and will produce sticks that are as good as the others.

The formulator should keep in mind a number of hints when preparing a product. Vitamins E and A can be added to a preparation for enhancing emollient and skin care effects. Zinc oxide or para-aminobenzoic acid acts as a sunblock. Perfume sticks can be prepared by adding an appropriate perfume oil.

When medication sticks are prepared, a constant-temperature dry bath filled with sand or salt at about 35°C to 40°C provides the proper temperature for softening and melting fatty acid and cocoa butter bases; 55°C to 65°C provides the proper temperature for softening and melting PEG bases in a minimum of time.

Physicochemical Considerations

The ingredients used to formulate sticks have unique properties. A listing of the individual ingredients and their advantages and disadvantages follows.

Oils

Vegetable oils, such as olive oil and sesame oil, have a tendency to rancidity.

Mineral oils resist rancidity, but their ability to dissolve certain ingredients is limited. They also tend to make the product smear and run off. They can be used in small proportions to enhance gloss.

Castor oil is a unique vegetable oil that has a high viscosity. High viscosity helps to delay the settling of ingredients from the molten stick mass; it also lessens the tendency of the applied stick to smear and run off.

Butyl stearate has been widely used in the preparation of sticks. A pure grade has no disagreeable odor and does not turn rancid.

Fatty esters of lower alcohols are generally similar in properties to butyl stearate.

Cocoa butter is widely used because it melts on application at about body temperature. However, it tends to "bloom" or come to the surface in an irregular fashion, which could produce unsightly craters or excrescences, a characteristic that can be overcome by the use of commercially available fatty acid bases (Fattibase).

Petrolatum is quite stable, produces good gloss, and is thus useful in preparing sticks.

Lanolin and absorption bases enhance the incorporation of water-containing ingredients and are useful in preparing sticks.

Lecithin improves smoothness, emollience, and ease of application.

Waxes

Carnauba wax is one of the harder waxes, so a small percentage raises the melting point and the strength.

Candelilla wax has a lower melting point than carnauba and must be used in larger proportions to obtain equal effects.

Beeswax is the traditional stiffening agent for sticks and is still used extensively. If used as the only wax, it produces a rather dull stick that does not apply easily. Hard waxes yield a better gloss.

Paraffins are too weak and brittle to be of much value in sticks, although small amounts can improve gloss. Immiscibility with castor oil can limit their use in some applications. Hydrogenated castor oil is a brittle white wax that yields a high gloss but little strength.

Synthetic waxes of many types are available. Each must be judged on its own merits.

Water-Soluble Bases

PEGs and their ethers are available in great variety. They are quite water soluble and are easy to remove from the skin.

Propylene glycol monoesters have relatively good solvent power and are found in some sticks. Sodium stearate-propylene glycol combinations are widely used for deodorant sticks and are good for the application of topical drugs. This type of base melts at body temperature, is colorless, and rubs in nicely.

A pleasant fragrance is one factor in determining consumer acceptance of some sticks. When selecting flavoring oils, one must ensure that those to be applied near or on the lips are free from irritating effects (burning) and disagreeable tastes.

Quality Control

Quality control procedures that can be used in preparing medication sticks include weight variation, melting point, and physical observation. Also, it is advisable to prepare extra medication sticks and place them in storage over the expected use or life of the prescription. If adverse changes are observed in the dosage form in storage, the patient can be contacted and the remaining sticks recalled. See the Standard Operating Procedure (SOP) "Performing Quality Assessment of Medication Sticks."

Packaging/Storage/Labeling

Sticks should be packaged in 5-g, 25-g, or other appropriate tube sizes (Figure 14-1), depending on the application. The sticks should be kept out of the reach of children and out of heat and direct sunlight. It is best to store at either 5°C or 25°C, depending on the composition of the stick. Appropriate labeling of these products includes "For External Use Only," "Do Not Take Internally," "Keep Out of Reach of Children," and "Protect from Heat."

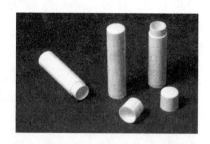

Figure 14-1. Applicator tube.

Stability

Medication sticks are generally considered dry and thus provide a stable dosage form as long as they are protected from moisture and heat. According to Chapter <795>, "Pharmacy Compounding,"[1] sticks prepared with the use of a manufactured product have a beyond-use date of 25% of the time remaining on the product's expiration date or 6 months, whichever is earlier. If the product is prepared from USP/NF ingredients, a beyond-use date of 6 months is appropriate, unless evidence is available to support other dating. Because many of these products do not contain water, the active drug should remain stable. However, using heat in the preparation could result in drug degradation. The formulator should estimate a reasonable beyond-use date.

Patient Counseling

When counseling a patient about medications sticks, the pharmacist must take into account the active drug and the method of application. In general, the patient should be told to apply the stick only to the involved area and not to surrounding skin. In addition, the patient should apply the medication liberally over the area but only as needed. The surface of the stick should be cleaned with a clean tissue after each use, and, to avoid transmitting infection, the product should not be shared with others.

Sample Formulations

Three categories of bases and ingredient-specific formulations for medication sticks are discussed in the following section: soft opaque, soft clear, and hard. Sample formulations are presented for illustrative purposes only. These sticks can be used in many ways, depending on the active ingredients incorporated into the formulation.

Soft Opaque Sticks

Several formulations for bases can be used to prepare soft opaque sticks. Nine such base formulations, followed by sample formulations for preparations containing active drugs, are presented in this section.

Sample Bases

 Stick Formulation No. 1 (A general purpose, water-repellent base)

Beeswax	34 g
Cocoa butter	8 g
Lanolin	6 g
Petrolatum	18 g
Paraffin wax	10 g
Talc (optional)	16 g
Perfume (optional)	1 g
Active drug	qs

1. Weigh or measure the ingredients.
2. Triturate the active drug with the petrolatum mass until smooth.
3. Melt the beeswax, cocoa butter, paraffin, and lanolin and add the petrolatum base; stir thoroughly and slowly sift in the active drug and talc (optional) while mixing.
4. Add perfume, stir, and pour into molds or containers.

Stick Formulation No. 2 (A softer, general purpose, water-repellent base)

Talc (optional)	19 g
Petrolatum	20 g
Paraffin wax	30 g
Cocoa butter	15 g
Beeswax	10 g
Perfume (optional)	1 g
Active drug	qs

1. Weigh or measure the ingredients.
2. Mix the active drug and talc with the petrolatum and triturate until smooth.
3. Melt the waxes and the cocoa butter with the petrolatum mixture; mix thoroughly, and then add the perfume and pour into molds.

Stick Formulation No. 3 (Stiff stick that will take up some water)

White beeswax	31 g
Paraffin	5 g
Cocoa butter (Fattibase)	7 g
Aquabase	34.5 g
Castor oil, tasteless	4 g
Perfume	0.9 g
Preservative	0.1 g
Butyl stearate	5 g

1. Weigh or measure the ingredients.
2. Mix the butyl stearate and the castor oil.
3. Melt the Aquabase using mild heat.
4. Add the butyl stearate–castor oil mixture to the Aquabase and mix thoroughly.
5. Melt the beeswax, paraffin, and cocoa butter and mix with the mixture prepared in step 4.
6. Mix thoroughly and add the perfume and preservative. Heat until the temperature of the mass reaches 45°C; keep the temperature of the batch at this point while filling the molds.

Stick Formulation No. 4 (Hard, firm stick)

White petrolatum	70.75 g
Cetyl alcohol	3 g
Lanolin	10.5 g
White beeswax	5.25 g
Cetyl esters wax	10.5 g

1. Weigh or measure the ingredients.
2. Melt the cetyl esters wax, white beeswax, and cetyl alcohol together and mix well.
3. Melt the lanolin and white petrolatum together and mix well.
4. Mix the melt from step 2 to the melt in step 3 by stirring.
5. Cool to about 45°C and fill molds.

 Stick Formulation No. 5 (Water-repellent stick)

Carnauba wax	10 g
White beeswax	15 g
Lanolin	5 g
Cetyl alcohol	5 g
Castor oil	65 g

1. Weigh or measure the ingredients.
2. Melt the carnauba wax, white beeswax, and cetyl alcohol together.
3. Add the lanolin and castor oil and mix well.
4. Cool to about 45°C and fill molds.

Stick Formulation No. 6 (Smooth stick that will absorb some water)

White wax	36 g
Beeswax, yellow	18 g
Cocoa butter	19 g
Absorption base (Aquabase)	5.5 g
Mineral oil	9.5 g
Oleyl alcohol	3 g
Absorption Base[a]:	
Petrolatum	94 g
Cholesterol	3 g
Cetyl alcohol	3 g

1. Weigh or measure the ingredients.
2. Melt the white wax and yellow wax together.
3. Melt the absorption base and cocoa butter together.
4. Add the melt from step 2 to the melt from step 3.
5. Add the mineral oil and oleyl alcohol and mix well.
6. Cool to about 45°C and pour into molds.
7. For the absorption base, melt the cetyl alcohol and cholesterol together; add the petrolatum, mix well, and cool.

[a]*Alternative absorption base.*

Stick Formulation No. 7 (Lip balm base)

White wax NF	5 g
White petrolatum USP	95 g

1. Weigh or measure the ingredients.
2. Melt the white wax in a beaker using low heat.
3. Add the white petrolatum and mix thoroughly with a stirring rod until uniform.
4. Cool until thick and pour into an ointment jar for storage at room temperature until used.

Stick Formulation No. 8 (Lip balm base)

White wax NF	30 g
Cetyl esters wax NF	30 g
Mineral oil USP	40 g

1. Weigh or measure the ingredients.
2. Melt the white wax and cetyl esters wax in a beaker.
3. Stir in the mineral oil.
4. Cool until thickened.
5. Pour into an ointment jar for storage until used.

 Stick Formulation No. 9 (Lip balm base)

Glyceryl monostearate NF	20 g
Span 80	2 g
Oil-in-water emulsion base	78 g (Dermabase)

1. Weigh or measure the ingredients.
2. Melt the glyceryl monostearate at 55°C–70°C in a beaker.
3. Add the Span 80 and mix thoroughly.
4. Heat the emulsion base to about 60°C and pour into the other melted mixture.
5. Stir rapidly.
6. Cool and pour into an ointment jar until used.

Ingredient-Specific Soft Opaque Sticks

 Camphor Ice-Type Product (For insect stings)

Powdered camphor	20 g
Light beeswax	18 g
White petrolatum	15 g
Cetyl esters wax	47 g

1. Weigh or measure the ingredients.
2. Melt the cetyl esters wax, beeswax, and petrolatum.
3. Mix the ingredients. When the temperature drops to about 50°C, add the camphor and mix well.
4. Fill the molds and cool.

℞ Acyclovir Lip Balm[a], Plain

	Formula 1	Formula 2
Acyclovir (200 mg capsules)	#6	#6
Span 80	0.5 g	
Glyceryl monostearate	5 g	
Water-in-oil emulsion base (Dermabase)	19.5 g	
Polyethylene glycol base (Polybase)		25 g

[a]*These formulas can be modified by incorporating lidocaine, PABA, or other ingredients as needed.*

Formula 1

1. Weigh or measure the ingredients.
2. Heat the glyceryl monostearate to about 55°C to 70°C and add the Span 80, followed by the acyclovir powder, which has been previously removed from the capsules and comminuted to obtain a fine, uniform powder.
3. Heat the water-in-oil emulsion base; add the melted glyceryl monostearate mixture to the base; stir and remove from heat.
4. Stir rapidly, cool, and pour into tubes or molds.

Formula 2

1. Weigh or measure the ingredients.
2. Heat the PEG base to about 55°C.
3. Empty the acyclovir capsules into a mortar and reduce the particle size to a fine powder.
4. Add these powders to the melted base and mix thoroughly.
5. Cool to just above the melting point of the product, until it starts to thicken.
6. While stirring, pour into the lip balm molds or tubes.

℞ Lidocaine 30% Lip Balm[a]

Lidocaine	1.5 g
Polyethylene glycol 4000	1 g
Polyethylene glycol 400	2.5 g

1. Weigh or measure the ingredients.
2. Melt the PEG bases together at about 55°C.
3. Add the powder to the melted base and mix until evenly dispersed.
4. Cool to just above the melting point of the product, until it starts to thicken.
5. While stirring, pour into the lip balm molds or tubes.

[a]*Alternative formulation: Replace PEG bases with 3.5 g of Polybase.*

℞ Camphor–Phenol–Menthol (CPM) Lip Balm

Camphor	1%
Phenol	0.5%
Menthol	1%
Lip balm base	qs

1. Weigh or measure the ingredients.
2. Mix the camphor, phenol, and menthol until a eutectic liquid forms.
3. Melt the lip balm base in a beaker using gentle heat.
4. Remove from heat and add the eutectic mixture to the base while it is still fluid and mix thoroughly with a stirring rod.
5. Pour into lip balm molds or tubes. Cool and package.

℞ Analgesic Medication Stick

Methyl salicylate	35 g
Menthol	15 g
Sodium stearate	13 g
Purified water	12 mL
Propylene glycol	25 g

1. Weigh or measure the ingredients.
2. Gently heat and melt the sodium stearate.
3. Mix the purified water with the propylene glycol and add to the melted sodium stearate.
4. Mix thoroughly, remove from heat, and allow the base to cool slightly.
5. Dissolve the menthol in the methyl salicylate; add this solution to the base and mix thoroughly.
6. As the product begins to thicken, continue to mix and pour into either 5-g or 20-g stick containers.
7. Allow to harden at room temperature.

℞ Clear Stick Base

Sodium stearate	7 g
Alcohol	65 g
Propylene glycol	25 g
Cyclomethicone	3 g

1. Weigh or measure the ingredients.
2. Melt the sodium stearate.
3. Mix the alcohol, propylene glycol, and cyclomethicone and add to the melted sodium stearate.
4. Mix well, cool slightly, and pour into stick molds.

Hard Sticks

Hard sticks, or styptic pencils, are used to stop the flow of blood from cuts. There are two types of styptic pencils: those with a hard crystalline structure and those with a wax base.

℞ Styptic Pencil (Hard with Aluminum Sulfate)

Ammonium chloride	7 g
Aluminum sulfate	27 g
Ferric sulfate	40 g
Copper sulfate	26 g

1. Mix the ingredients together; heat in a porcelain-lined vessel until they fuse.
2. While the mass is molten, pour into molds.

℞ Styptic Pencil (Crayon type)

Titanium dioxide	3.7 g
Alum	18 g
Aluminum chloride	15 g
Oxyquinoline sulfate	2.3 g
Cocoa butter (Fattibase)	22 g
Cetyl esters wax	19 g
Petrolatum	13 g
Lanolin	7 g

1. Weigh or measure the ingredients.
2. Triturate the alum, titanium dioxide, and aluminum chloride.
3. Add enough petrolatum to make a viscous paste.
4. Mix the rest of the petrolatum with the oxyquinoline sulfate.
5. Melt the cocoa butter, cetyl esters wax, and lanolin; stir in the alum, petrolatum mixture, and then the oxyquinoline mixture.
6. Pour into molds.

℞ Moisturizing/Cold Sore Stick

Vitamin E oil	1.1 g
Lysine	1.1 g
Silica gel	120 mg
Polyethylene glycol 4500	7 g
Polyethylene glycol 300	14 mL

1. Accurately weigh/measure each of the ingredients.
2. Melt the bases together at about 55°C.
3. Mix the vitamin E oil, lysine, and silica gel together and add to the melted bases.
4. Turn off heat and mix until uniform.
5. Pour into tubes and cool.
6. Package and label.

Standard Operating Procedure (SOP)

Performing Quality Assessment of Medication Sticks

Purpose of SOP

The purpose of this procedure is to provide a method of documenting uniformity between batches and to conduct quality assessment tests and observations of medication sticks.

Materials

The following items are used in one or more of the assessment tests:

- Balance
- Graduates
- Beaker
- Weight

Procedure

The appropriate tests should be conducted and the results/observations recorded on the worksheet "Quality Assessment Form for Medication Sticks" (Figure 14-2).

Weight.

- Accurately weigh the product on a balance.

Specific Gravity. To calculate the specific gravity, one must know the weight and volume of the product.

- Record the weight of the individual dosage form or a tube/package of the dosage forms (tared weight).

The steps in determining the volume of water displaced include the following:

1. Place 5 mL of water in a 10-mL graduate.
2. Add the dosage form and read the water level.

3. Subtract 5 mL from the water level measurement in step 2 to determine the volume of water occupied by the dosage form.
4. If the dosage form floats, place a weight attached to a paper clip in the graduate before adding the water to the 5-mL mark. Then, wrap one end of the paper clip around the dosage form to hold it below the water surface and place it in the graduate. Proceed as in step 3.

Calculations.   Once the weight and volume of the product are known, the specific gravity is calculated by dividing the weight (grams) by the volume (milliliters):

$$SG = w \text{ (g)}/v \text{ (mL)}$$

Active Drug Assay Results. As appropriate, representative samples of the product should be assayed for active drug content by a contract analytical laboratory. Stability can be assessed by storing the product at room, refrigerated, and/or frozen temperatures and having the assay repeated on the stored samples.

Color of Product. It may be advisable to use a color chart for determining the actual color of the product.

Clarity. Clarity is evaluated by visual inspection. On the worksheet (Figure 14-2), 1 is the clearest and 5 is the least clear on the scale provided.

Texture-Surface.

▸ Observe the product to determine smoothness of the surface.

Appearance.

▸ Determine whether the product appears dry or oily/moist.

Feel.

▸ Touch the product to determine whether it is sticky (tacky) or hard (plastic) or bounces back (elastic).

Melting Test. This test is performed for fatty acid, cocoa butter, and oil-based products as follows:

1. Heat a 200-mL beaker of water to 37°C on a magnetic stirring unit that is set at about 50 rpm.
2. Add a dosage unit to the water. (Note: It may be necessary to add a weight to these dosage units to pull them below the water surface.)
3. After 30 minutes, record your observations as Yes, No, or the appropriate number with 1 being the most melted on the scale provided.

Dissolution Test. This test is performed for polyethylene glycol, gelatin, and water-soluble products as follows:

1. Perform steps 1 and 2 of the melting test.
2. After 30 minutes, record your observations as Yes, No, or the appropriate number with 1 being the most dissolved on the scale provided.

Physical Observation.

▸ Describe the appearance and organoleptic qualities of the product.

Physical Stability.

- Prepare a few additional dosage forms, package, and label "For Physical Stability Observations." Weekly, observe the product for signs of discoloration, dryness, cracking, mottling, mold growth, and so forth. Record a descriptive observation on the form (Figure 14-2) at each observation interval. Sufficient lines are provided for observations for 8 weeks or approximately 60 days.

Reference

1. Expert Review Panel on Pharmacy Compounding Practices. Pharmacy compounding. *United States Pharmacopeia 25/National Formulary 20.* Rockville, Md: United States Pharmacopeial Convention; 2000.

Quality Assessment Form for Medication Sticks

Product _____ Date _____

Lot/Rx number_____ Dosage form: Medication sticks _____

Characteristic	Theoretical	Actual	Normal Range
Weight/volume	_____	_____	_____
Specific gravity	_____	_____	_____
Active drug assay results	_____	_____	_____
Initial assay	_____	_____	_____
After storage No. 1	_____	_____	_____
After storage No. 2	_____	_____	_____
Color of product	_____	_____	_____
Clarity	Clear	1 2 3 4 5	Opaque
Texture—Surface	Smooth	1 2 3 4 5	Rough
Appears dry	Yes	1 2 3 4 5	No
Appearance	Dry	1 2 3 4 5	Oily/moist
Feels tacky	Yes	1 2 3 4 5	No
Feels plastic	Yes	1 2 3 4 5	No
Feels elastic	Yes	1 2 3 4 5	No
Melting test	Yes	1 2 3 4 5	No
Dissolution test	Yes	1 2 3 4 5	No

Sample set aside for physical stability observation: Yes   No

If yes, results: Date   Observation

_____   _____
_____   _____
_____   _____
_____   _____
_____   _____
_____   _____
_____   _____
_____   _____
_____   _____
_____   _____
_____   _____

Figure 14-2. Sample worksheet for quality assessment of medication sticks.

Chapter 15

Solutions

Pharmacists are often called on to compound solution products for many routes of administration, including oral, topical, rectal, vaginal, ophthalmic, and otic. The most common solution dosage form is the oral liquid, which includes solutions, syrups, elixirs, and the like. The preparation techniques for most of these liquid dosage forms are similar.

Definitions/Types

Solutions are liquid preparations containing one or more drug substances that are molecularly dispersed in a suitable solvent or a mixture of mutually miscible solvents. Oral liquids are intended for oral administration and contain one or more substances with or without flavoring, sweetening, or coloring agents dissolved in water or cosolvent—water mixtures. They can be either formulated for direct oral administration to the patient or dispensed in a concentrated form that requires dilution before dispensing or administration.

Topical solutions are generally aqueous but may contain cosolvent systems such as various alcohols or other organic solvents with or without added active ingredients. Oftentimes, the term *lotion* is used to designate solutions or suspensions that are applied topically.

Syrups are concentrated aqueous preparations of a sugar or sugar-substitute with or without flavoring agents and medicinal substances. Syrups can serve as pleasant-tasting vehicles for active drugs.

Elixirs are clear, sweetened, hydroalcoholic solutions that are usually flavored and are suitable for drugs that are insoluble in water alone but soluble in water—alcohol mixtures. Less sweet and less viscous than syrups, elixirs are generally less effective in masking taste. Elixirs can contain different solvents as cosolvent systems, for example, water, alcohol, glycerin, sorbitol, propylene glycol, and polyethylene glycol 300.

Aromatic waters can be used for both internal and external purposes. They are clear, saturated aqueous solutions of volatile oils or other aromatic or volatile substances. For compounding purposes, they are generally prepared with volatile oils and water.

Historical Use

Solutions are one of the oldest dosage forms. Myrrh, laudanum, and other tinctures are mentioned in literature dating back to biblical times. The composition and preparation of earlier solutions (e.g., fluid extracts, tinctures, spirits, and potions) were simpler than that of contemporary preparations. Solutions prepared today can be buffered, preserved, flavored, sweetened, adjusted for pH and osmolality range, and protected against oxidation.

Applications

An oral liquid may be the most appropriate dosage form for a patient for a number of reasons. The most common reasons why a pharmacist may compound an oral liquid dosage form include the following:

- Many drug products are not commercially available as oral liquids.
- Infant, pediatric, and some psychiatric patients, as well as patients of advanced age, cannot swallow solid dosage forms.
- Some products are therapeutically better in liquid form.
- The bulk of some preparations makes oral liquids more feasible.
- Some patients, such as patients in a nursing home or those who are incarcerated, are administered oral liquids to prevent them from placing tablets or capsules under the tongue and not swallowing them at the time of administration.
- Patients on enteral feeding methods require a liquid dosage form.
- Oral liquid dosage forms are diverse and have varying dosage strengths.
- Drugs are often more bioavailable from oral liquids than from solids.

Solubilization

The preparation of many dosage forms requires the preparation of a solution even though the final product may not be a solution. The proper selection of a solvent depends on the physicochemical characteristics of the solute and the solvent as well as the purpose of the solution in the formula.

The actual solubility of a substance represents the sum of the various factors involved in the transport of a solute particle from the solid phase to the solution phase. The driving force for dissolution is the interaction of the solvent molecules with the solute molecules or solute ions. The actual process of dissolution involves (1) the breaking of interionic or intermolecular bonds in the solute, (2) the separation of the molecules of the solvent to provide space in the solvent for the solute, and (3) the interaction between the solvent and the solute molecule or ion. A number of forces of attraction are involved in the dissolution process, including van der Waals, dipole–dipole, and ionic forces.

A good general rule to remember is the one learned in chemistry class: "Like dissolves like." Generally, polar solutes will dissolve in polar solvents; nonpolar solutes will dissolve in nonpolar solvents. The difficulty one encounters is that many solutes are of intermediate polarity.

If appropriate, official solvents should be used in pharmaceutical compounding. Currently, there are a number of official solvents listed in the *United States Pharmacopeia 25/National Formulary 20 (USP 25/NF 20)* that will be briefly discussed. Generally, all solvents should be preserved in tight containers, and those that are flammable should be stored away from excessive heat and/or sources of sparks or flame. The oils should be stored to avoid exposure to excessive heat.

Composition

The composition of solutions can range from quite simple to very complex. The choice of active ingredient, intended use, patient characteristics, and, potentially, the environment in which the product will be stored can affect its composition.

Oral liquids generally contain the active drug with or without cosolvent systems, flavorings, sweeteners, colorings, preservatives, buffering agents, antioxidants, or other ingredients. A drug is generally more susceptible to degradation in an aqueous solution. Adding buffers to adjust the pH, preservatives, and antioxidants can prevent degradation from occurring. Flavorings and sweeteners can make a drug with a disagreeable taste or odor more palatable, thereby increasing patient acceptance of the product and ease of administration. For physiologic reasons, other additives are used to bring the solution within a suitable osmolality range.

pH

pH is important in drug product formulation, especially because it involves drug solubility, activity, absorption, stability, sorption, and patient comfort. pH is related to certain physical characteristics, such as the viscosity of some polymers used as gel-forming agents and in suspensions. Tables 15-1 and 15-2 list acidifying agents and alkalizing agents that are used to adjust pH.

pH adjustment is critical in maintaining drugs in solution. A slight increase or decrease in pH can cause some drugs to precipitate from a solution. Conversely, a slight adjustment of pH can aid in solubilizing some drugs. Drug activity can be related to pH, depending on whether the ionized or the nonionized form is desired. Drug stability, in many cases, directly depends on the pH of the environment (dosage form). pH:degradation profiles are of great value in selecting the proper pH for optimum stability of a product. Sorption of a drug can occur to various excipients, packaging components, and administration sets/components. The sorption can be pH related, depending on which species, ionized or nonionized, is sorbed to the material. Patient comfort and, ultimately, compliance can depend on the proper pH of the product. In some cases, a compromise must be reached between the drug requirements and the patient preferences. This compromise can often be handled by adjusting the pH for optimum drug stability and by using a low buffer capacity, so, when it is administered, the patient's physiologic buffers will quickly move the pH to the physiologic range.

Vehicles

Vehicles used in oral solutions include primarily water, ethanol, glycerin, syrups, and various blends of these ingredients. A greater variety of vehicles is available for topical solutions. Most of the vehicles used for oral solutions, as well as acetone, isopropanol, propylene glycol, the polyethylene glycols, collodion, many oils, and numerous polymers, can be used in topical preparations. Another vehicle, dimethyl sulfoxide (DMSO), has limited use in topical solutions. Although oral solutions are usually ready to administer, they sometimes have to be diluted or prepared before administering to the patient. This preparation is especially true of products that are not very stable. A list of official solvents is shown in Table 15-3; some selected oleaginous vehicles are listed in Table 15-4.

Table 15-1. Physicochemical Characteristics of Acidifying Agents

Acidifying Agent	Physical Form	% Strength	Solubility		Specific Gravity	Solution pH (%)[a]	Container Specifications
			Water	Alcohol			
Acetic acid NF	Liquid	36.5	Misc	Misc	1.04		T
Acetic acid, glacial USP	Liquid	100	Misc	Misc	1.05		T
Citric acid USP	Solid	100	VS	FS	—	2.2 (1)	T
Fumaric acid NF	Solid	100	SlS	Sol	—	2.45 (saturated)	W
Hydrochloric acid NF	Liquid	37.5	Misc	Misc	1.18	0.1 (10)	T
Hydrochloric acid, diluted NF	Liquid	10	Misc	Misc	1.06	0.1	T
Lactic acid USP	Liquid	88	Misc	Misc	1.21		T
Malic acid NF	Solid	100	VS	FS	—	2.35 (1)	W
Nitric acid NF	Liquid	70	Misc	Misc	1.41		T
Phosphoric acid NF	Liquid	87	Misc	Misc	1.71		T
Phosphoric acid, diluted NF	Liquid	10	Misc	Misc	1.06		T
Propionic acid NF	Liquid	100	Misc	Misc	0.99		T
Sodium phosphate monobasic USP	Solid	100	FS	PrIn	—	4.3 (5)	W
Sulfuric acid NF	Liquid	98	Misc	Misc	1.84		T
Tartaric acid NF	Solid	100	VS	FS	—	2.2 (1.5)	W

[a] Aqueous solutions.

Table 15-2. Physicochemical Characteristics of Alkalizing Agents

Alkalizing Agent	Physical Form	% Strength	Solubility		Specific Gravity	Solution pH (%)[a]	Container Specifications
			Water	Alcohol			
Ammonia solution, strong NF	Liquid	29	Misc	Misc	0.90	—	T
Ammonium carbonate NF	Solid	100	FS	—	—		T, LR
Diethanolamine NF	Liquid	100	Misc	Misc	1.088	11 (0.1 N)	T, LR
Monoethanolamine	Liquid	100	Misc	Misc	1.012	12.1 (0.1 N)	T, LR
Potassium hydroxide NF	Solid	100	FS	FS	—		T
Sodium bicarbonate USP	Solid	100	Sol	IS	—	8.3 (0.1 M)	W
Sodium borate NF	Solid	100	Sol	IS	—		T
Sodium carbonate NF	Solid	100	FS	—	—		W
Sodium hydroxide NF	Solid	100	FS	FS	—		T
Sodium phosphate dibasic USP	Solid	100	FS	SIS	—	9.1 (1)	T
Trolamine NF	Liquid	100	Misc	Misc	1.12	10.5 (0.1 N)	T, LR

[a]Aqueous solutions.

Table 15-3. Physicochemical Characteristics of Official Solvents

Solvent	Miscibility			General Use		Specific Gravity	Boil Point	Freeze Point	Flammable
	Water	Alcohol	Oil	External	Internal				
Acetone	Misc	Misc	—	Yes	—	0.789	56	—	Yes
Alcohol	Misc	Misc	—	Yes	Yes	—	78	—	Yes
Alcohol, diluted	Misc	Misc	—	Yes	Yes	0.936	—	—	—
Amylene hydrate	Misc	Misc	—	—	—	0.805	100	—	—
Benzyl benzoate	Immisc	Misc	—	Yes	Yes	1.118	—	18	—
Butyl alcohol	Misc	Misc	—	—	—	—	—	—	—
Corn oil	Immisc	SlS	Misc	Yes	Yes	0.918	—	—	—
Cottonseed oil	Immisc	SlS	Misc	Yes	Yes	0.918	—	—	Yes
Diethylene glycol monoethyl ether	Misc	Misc	PartMisc	Yes	—	0.991	198	—	Yes
Ethyl acetate	Misc	Misc	Misc	Yes	—	0.896	—	—	Yes
Glycerin	Misc	Misc	Immisc	Yes	Yes	1.249	—	—	No
Hexylene glycol	Misc	Misc	—	—	—	0.919	—	—	—
Isopropyl alcohol	Misc	Misc	—	Yes	—	0.785	—	—	Yes
Methyl alcohol	Misc	Misc	—	Yes	—	—	65	—	Yes
Methylene chloride	—	Misc	Misc	Yes	—	1.320	40	—	Yes
Methyl isobutyl ketone	SlS	Misc	—	Yes	—	—	—	—	Yes
Mineral oil	Immisc	Immisc	Misc	Yes	Yes	0.870	—	—	No
Peanut oil	Immisc	VSS	Misc	Yes	Yes	0.916	—	—	No
Polyethylene glycol									
300	Misc	Misc	—	Yes	Yes	1.12	—	−11	No
400	Misc	Misc	—	Yes	Yes	1.12	—	6	No
600	Misc	Misc	—	Yes	Yes	1.12	—	20	No
Propylene glycol	Misc	Misc	Immisc	Yes	Yes	1.036	—	—	No
Sesame oil	—	SlS	—	Yes	Yes	0.918	—	—	No
Water	Misc	Misc	Immisc	Yes	Yes	1.00	100	0	No

Table 15-4. Physicochemical Characteristics of Oleaginous Vehicles

Vehicle	Specific Gravity	Refractive Index	Acid Value[a]	Iodine Value[b]	Saponification Value[c]	Container Specifications
Alkyl (C_{12}–C_{15}) benzoate	0.915–0.935	1.483–1.487	≤0.5	—	169–182	T, LR
Almond oil	0.910–0.915	—	—	95–105	190–200	T
Corn oil	0.914–0.921	—	—	102–130	187–193	T, LR
Cottonseed oil	0.915–0.921	—	—	109–120	—	T, LR
Ethyl oleate	0.866–0.874	1.443–1.450	≤0.5	75–85	177–188	T, LR
Isopropyl myristate	0.846–0.854	1.432–1.436	≤1.0	≤1	202–212	T, LR
Isopropyl palmitate	0.850–0.855	1.435–1.438	≤1.0	≤1	183–193	T, LR
Mineral oil	0.845–0.905	—	—	—	—	T, LR
Mineral oil, light	0.818–0.880	—	—	—	—	T, LR
Octyldodecanol	—	—	≤5.0	≤8	≤5	T
Olive oil	0.910–0.915	—	—	79–88	190–195	T
Peanut oil	0.912–0.920	1.462–1.464	—	84–100	185–195	T, LR
Safflower oil	—	—	—	135–150	—	T, LR
Sesame oil	0.916–0.921	—	—	103–116	188–195	T, LR
Soybean oil	0.916–0.922	1.465–1.475	—	120–141	180–200	T, LR
Squalane	0.807–0.810	1.451–1.452	≤0.2	≤4	≤2	T

[a]Acid value is the number of milligrams of potassium hydroxide required to neutralize the free acids in 1 g of the substance. It is a measure of the acidity of the oil.

[b]Iodine value is the number of grams of iodine absorbed, under the prescribed conditions, by 100 g of the substance. It is a measure of the unsaturation of the oil.

[c]Saponification value is the number of milligrams of potassium hydroxide required to neutralize the free acids and saponify the esters contained in 1 g of the substance.

Water is the primary solvent, and *USP 25* lists several different waters, which are clear, colorless, odorless liquids but differ in their preparation, requirements, packaging, and intended use.

Purified water (H_2O, MW 18.02) is water obtained by a suitable process.

Sterile purified water is purified water that is sterilized and suitably packaged. It contains no antimicrobial agent. (Note: It is not to be used for preparations intended for parenteral administration.)

Water for injection is water purified by distillation or by reverse osmosis. Water for injection is intended for use in preparing parenteral solutions.

Sterile water for injection is prepared from water for injection that is sterilized and suitably packaged. It contains no antimicrobial agent or other added substance.

Bacteriostatic water for injection is prepared from water for injection that is sterilized and suitably packaged, containing one or more suitable antimicrobial agents. (Note: Bacteriostatic water for injection must be used with due regard for the compatibility of the antimicrobial agent or agents it contains with the particular medicinal substance that is to be dissolved or diluted.)

Sterile water for irrigation is prepared from water for injection that is sterilized and suitably packaged. It contains no antimicrobial agent or other added substance.

Sterile water for inhalation is prepared from water for injection that is sterilized and suitably packaged. It contains no antimicrobial agents, except where used in humidifiers or other similar devices and where liable to contamination over a period of time, or to other added substances. (Note: Sterile water for inhalation should not be used for parenteral administration or for other sterile compendial dosage forms.)

Preparation

A variety of techniques can be used to prepare an oral liquid dosage form. The most common method is to make a simple solution by dissolving a drug in a solvent. Most materials will dissolve simply by stirring, but others can require heat or a high degree of agitation. Methylcellulose is an example of a material that is initially dispersed in about one third to one half of the total volume of hot water, with the remainder added as ice water or ice. To wet the methylcellulose, one should sprinkle the powder lightly on the surface of the hot water so that it can hydrate. If the powder is added too rapidly, clumps form, making it difficult for inside particles to become wet because they are covered by the outer shell of the hydrated clump. Sometimes an intermediate liquid, such as alcohol or glycerin, can be used before water is added. This intermediate liquid displaces air entrapped in the powder and replaces it with a water-miscible liquid. Then, when water is added, it will wet the powder more easily.

Surfactants aid in solubilizing an ingredient. The surfactant can be either dispersed in the vehicle before the drug is added or mixed with the drug and then added to the vehicle.

A common technique for preparing aromatic waters is to use a solution with a dispersant. The volatile oil is mixed with small pieces of filter paper, talc, or some other appropriate dispersion medium before the water is added. The mixture is agitated and allowed to set for a period of time, with periodic agitation. The aromatic water is then collected by filtration. The purpose of the dispersion medium is to increase the surface area of the oil that is exposed to the water to increase the rate at which the solution is saturated with the oil. When working with aromatic waters, it is important to remember that the addition of a salt will probably "salt out" the volatile oils. (See the box "Hints for Compounding Solutions" for other preparation techniques.)

Hints for Compounding Solutions

- A product should be stirred gently; shaking can entrap air, which causes foaming.
- The use of magnetic stirrers, blenders, and electric mixers can save time and produce uniform products.
- The dissolution step can be speeded up by immersing the beaker in an ultrasonic bath.
- A stirring rod should not be used when adding "sufficient volume" of a solvent to the graduate in which the product is being prepared.
- Either a stirring rod laid across the top of a beaker or an alcohol spray (ethanol for internal solutions) can aid in breaking up a foam; a silicone defoaming agent can also be used.
- Filtration of a liquid helps to produce a clear product. During this process, one should watch the surface of the filter to determine whether the active drug is being inadvertently removed from the preparation.
- One should always know the pH and alcohol concentration of the products being prepared.
- The effectiveness of a preservative can be related to pH. For example, the parabens are generally used within a pH range of 4 to 8, chlorobutanol needs a pH of less than 5, and sodium benzoate is more effective at a pH of about 4 or less.
- Salts should be dissolved in a small quantity of water before a viscous vehicle is added.
- When combining two liquids, one should stir the mixture constantly to lessen the occurrence of incompatibilities resulting from concentration effects.
- High-viscosity liquids should be added to low-viscosity liquids. The solution should be stirred constantly when these types of liquids are mixed.
- To obtain small quantities of active drugs or excipients, (e.g., flavoring oils) using the dilution or aliquot method, a solvent, not just a liquid, should be used.
- Hydrocolloids should be allowed to hydrate slowly before use.
- Considerations involved in selecting a vehicle include the drug concentration, solubility, pKa, taste, and stability. Other vehicle considerations include pH, flavor, sweetener, color, preservative, viscosity, compatibility and, if indicated, suspending and emulsifying agents.
- When preparing elixirs, it is advisable to dissolve the alcohol-soluble constituents in the alcohol and the water-soluble constituents in the water. The aqueous solution should then be added to the alcohol solution by stirring, to maintain as high an alcohol concentration as possible.
- Talc can be used to remove excess flavoring oils. This removal is accomplished by adding 1 to 2 g of talc per 100 mL of solution and then filtering. During the filtration process, the first portions are returned to the filter until a clear filtrate is obtained.
- Cosolvent systems (e.g., mixtures of water, alcohol, glycerin, and propylene glycol) can aid in clarifying solutions that are hazy or cloudy because of poor solubility in water.

Physicochemical Considerations

To prepare a successful oral liquid product, the pharmacist must confront and overcome several technical difficulties. Unstable drugs are even more unstable in solution; poorly soluble drugs must be solubilized or suspended; and bad-tasting drugs must be masked to produce a palatable product. The formulation of a successful product thus depends on a combination of scientific acuity and pharmaceutical art.

Physicochemical, pharmaceutical, and patient factors must be taken into account during the preparation of an oral liquid dosage form. The physicochemical and stability characteristics of the active drug determine the oral liquid dosage form that can be prepared (i.e., syrups, elixirs, suspensions). Factors to be considered in formulating an oral liquid dosage form include the following:

- Physical and chemical properties of the ingredients.
- Order of mixing and adjuvants.
- Pharmaceutical techniques required.
- Incompatibilities in preparation and storage.
- Stability and potency of the ingredients.
- Proper labeling, including accessory labels.

When preparing an oral liquid, the pharmacist should consider the drug's concentration, solubility, pKa, taste, and stability. Vehicle considerations include pH, flavor, sweetener, color, preservative, viscosity, compatibility, and, if indicated, suspending and emulsifying agents. The drug's concentration and solubility in various solvents will dictate the type of dosage form to prepare. For example, if the drug is water soluble, a syrup can be prepared; however, if it is soluble in water–alcohol–glycerin cosolvent systems, an elixir is appropriate. If the drug is insoluble, a suspension can be formulated, but, if the drug is an oil, an emulsion is the form of choice. The following points should be considered when solubilizing drugs:

- Small particles dissolve faster than large particles.
- Stirring increases the dissolution rate of a drug.
- The more soluble the drug, the faster is its dissolution rate.
- When working with a viscous liquid, the dissolution rate of the drug is decreased.
- An increase in temperature generally leads to an increase in the solubility and dissolution rate of a drug.
- Adding an electrolyte can increase or decrease the solubility of a nonelectrolyte drug.
- An alkaloidal base, or any nitrogenous base of relatively high molecular weight, is generally poorly soluble unless the pH of the medium is decreased (i.e., conversion to a salt occurs).
- The solubility of poorly soluble acidic substances is increased as the pH of the medium is increased (i.e., conversion to a salt occurs).

The pH of the vehicle and pKa of the drug partially determine the drug's overall solubility. Slight adjustments in pH can greatly affect the solubility of the drug and should be controlled when preparing a solution. It may also be necessary to buffer the solution to maintain its solubility characteristics.

Another area affected by pH is chemical stability. Various reference sources can be consulted to determine the required pH for maximum stability for specific drugs.

This information can be used to establish guidelines for selecting the best vehicle. An inexpensive pH meter can help predict and prevent pH-related incompatibilities (Figure 15-1).

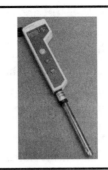

Syrups

Syrups are appropriate for water-soluble drugs. The usual pH requirement for many drugs is slightly to moderately acidic. Thus, flavored syrups can often effectively mask the disagreeable taste of certain drugs.

Figure 15-1. pH meter.

The flavor will remain in the mouth longer because of the syrup's viscosity. Viscosity can cause the active drug to dissolve more slowly in the vehicle during preparation. It is easier to first dissolve the active ingredient in a small quantity of water and then add sufficient quantity to volume with the syrup.

The preservative properties of a syrup depend in part on maintaining a high concentration of sucrose or sugar in the final product. If the sucrose concentration is decreased, it may be necessary to add another preservative (e.g., alcohol) to the product. Table 15-5 lists preservatives that can be used in oral liquids. (See Chapter 5, "Pharmaceutical Compounding Calculations," for an example of how to determine the required quantity of preservatives.)

Some syrup vehicles are listed in Table 15-6. As is evident from this table, most syrups have slightly acidic pH values. Commercially prepared products (e.g., Ora-Sweet, Ora-Sweet SF, and Syrpalta) have pH values of approximately 4.2, 4.2, and 4.5, respectively. The pH of cherry syrup, Coca-Cola syrup, orange syrup, and raspberry syrup are all less than 4. Neutral syrup vehicles include simple syrup (syrup USP) and aromatic eriodictyon syrup. Because the commercially available products contain preservative systems, additional preservatives would not normally be needed unless the vehicle is significantly diluted.

Table 15-5. Common Preservatives for Oral Liquid Products

Preservative	Concentration (%)
Alcohol	15–20
Benzoic acid	0.2
Methylparaben	≤0.2
Potassium sorbate	0.2
Propylparaben	≤0.2
Sodium benzoate	0.2
Sorbic acid	0.2

In some circumstances, fruit juices, especially those that are clear and pulp free such as apple or grape, can be used and "diluted" with syrup to increase sweetness, if necessary. Maple syrup or ice cream sundae toppings such as butterscotch can also be adopted for use, diluted as needed with simple syrup or water. Another interesting approach is the use of soft drink concentrates or lemonade concentrates. These concentrates can be reconstituted with water to a concentrated solution or can be diluted with simple syrup instead of using the water and sucrose formulas

Table 15-6. pH and Alcohol Content of Common Oral Liquid Vehicles

Vehicle	pH	Alcohol Content (%)	Container Specifications
Official USP/NF Vehicles			
Aromatic elixir	5.5–6	21–23	T
Benzaldehyde compound elixir	6	3–5	T, LR
Peppermint water	—	0	T
Sorbitol solution	—	0	T
Suspension structured vehicle	—	0	T, LR
Suspension structured vehicle-SF	—	0	T, LR
Syrup	6.5–7	—	T
Xanthan gum solution	—	0	T, LR
Nonofficial Vehicles			
Acacia syrup	5	—	T
Aromatic eriodictyon syrup	6–8	6–8	T, LR
Cherry syrup	3.5–4	1–2	T, LR
Citric acid syrup	—	<1	T
Cocoa syrup	—	—	T
Glycyrrhiza elixir	—	21–23	T
Glycyrrhiza syrup	6–6.5	5–6	T
Hydriotic acid syrup	—	—	T
Isoalcohol elixir, low	5	8–10	T
Isoalcohol elixir, high	5	73–78	T
Orange flower water	—	0	T
Orange syrup	2.5–3	2–5	T
Raspberry syrup	3	1–2	T, LR
Sarsaparilla compound syrup	5	—	
Tolu syrup	5.5	2–4	T
Wild cherry syrup	4.5	1–2	T
Commercial Branded Vehicles			
Coca-Cola syrup	1.6–1.7	0	
Ora-Sweet	4–4.5	0	T, LR
Ora-Sweet SF	4–4.4	0	T, LR
Syrpalta	4.5	—	T, LR

provided on the commercial package. Still another option is diluting fruit preserves to make syrups. This option is especially noteworthy when using a sugar-free preserve for patients with diabetes. Still other approaches involve diluting a commercial syrup with either simple syrup or a methylcellulose solution; in fact, a 1:1 mixture of simple syrup and methylcellulose solution is commonly used in some areas, flavored to the taste of the patient.

Elixirs

Because elixirs are mixtures of water and alcohol, they dissolve both alcohol-soluble and water-soluble substances, depending on the percentage of each solvent present. Glycerin, which is also present in some elixirs, is comparable in solvent properties to alcohol, but its viscosity causes solutes to dissolve slowly. Propylene glycol is miscible with water and alcohol and is routinely substituted for glycerin.

Elixirs are usually prepared by simple solution; however, care must be taken to keep the alcohol concentration and pH within the range for maximum stability of both the drug and the dosage form. One must consider whether the salt form of the drug (more water soluble) or the free acid or base form (more alcohol soluble) should be used.

The preparation of elixirs involves dissolving the alcohol-soluble components in the alcohol and the water-soluble components in the water. The aqueous phase is generally added to the alcohol solution to maintain the highest alcohol concentration possible. If the situation is reversed, the oils/drug can separate from the solution as soon as the alcohol solution contacts the water. If the product is cloudy, an excess of aromatic oils may have been added. In such cases, talc filtration can be used to produce a clear product. This technique involves adding approximately 1 to 2 g of talc per 100 mL of solution, mixing, and filtering. The portions of the liquid are then refiltered until a clear product is obtained.

Cosolvent systems serve to dissolve not only the active drug but also the flavoring components, as they are often volatile oils. Artificial sweeteners (e.g., saccharin) may be required for sweetening, because sucrose may not be sufficiently soluble in the alcoholic system.

Sample elixir vehicles are listed in Table 15-7. The most common elixir vehicle is aromatic elixir, which has an alcohol content of approximately 22%. Some syrups now contain alcohol, so the distinction between syrups and elixirs is sometimes vague. The two isoalcoholic elixirs (low: 8%–10% alcohol; high: 73%–78% alcohol) can be adjusted to obtain a vehicle of the desired alcohol concentration.

Table 15-7. Elixirs for Use in Common Oral Liquids

Elixir	pH	Alcohol Content (%)
Aromatic elixir	5.5–6.0	21–23
Benzaldehyde compound elixir	6.0	3–5
Isoalcohol elixir (low, high)[a]	5.0	8–10, 73–78

[a]These two elixirs can be mixed in various ratios to obtain the required alcohol concentration.

Quality Control

Quality control procedures include checking the final volume, appearance, odor, clarity, and pH. Small, inexpensive pH meters are available to check the final pH of a product. Products that do not exhibit the expected characteristics should not be dispensed; they may have to be reformulated. See the Standard Operating Procedure (SOP) "Quality Assessment of Oral and Topical Liquids."

Packaging

Solutions can usually be packaged in glass or plastic containers. Oral liquids and some other solutions can be packaged in squeeze bottles for application by spraying (Figure 15-2), in applicator bottles for topical application in small volumes, and in dropper bottles. Many solutions need to be in light-resistant containers.

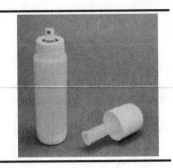

Figure 15-2. Pressure spray bottle.

Storage/Labeling

Oral liquids should generally be stored at room temperature or refrigerated, depending on the characteristics of the active drug. Syrups are often refrigerated to enhance their stability and palatability. If saturated solutions are stored in the refrigerator, precipitation can occur. In many cases, the precipitate will be redissolved when the solution is returned to room temperature. If not, the product can be gently warmed to redissolve the precipitate.

Labels should contain instructions as to type of use (external or internal), proper storage conditions, and beyond-use dates. The statement "Protect from Light" should be on the label. For some solutions, the statement "Shake Well" should also be on the label.

Stability

Physical attributes of liquid dosage forms include clarity, precipitation, mold/bacterial growth, odor, and loss of volume. These attributes can be observed for evidence of instability. Solutions are particularly susceptible to chemical degradation, especially when aqueous vehicles are used. Information on chemical stability can be obtained from the literature or other appropriate sources.

Beyond-use dates for water-containing formulations stored at cold temperatures are no later than 14 days for products prepared from ingredients in solid form. These dates can be extended if valid scientific information on stability supports this extension, as discussed in Chapter 4, "Stability of Compounded Products."

Patient Counseling

Patients should be instructed on how to measure the dose of a liquid product and how to administer it. They should also be informed about shaking the product (if indicated), replacing and tightening the cap, and storing the product properly, including keeping the product out of the reach of children. Patients should be taught how to check the product for physical stability and should be instructed to return it if signs of instability are noted. Instructions on how to dispose of products that have reached their beyond-use date should also be provided.

Sample Formulations

Iontophoretic Solution

℞ Lidocaine Hydrochloride 2% Solution for Iontophoresis

Lidocaine hydrochloride	2 g
Sterile water for injection	100 mL

1. Calculate the quantity of each ingredient required for the prescription.
2. Accurately weigh the lidocaine hydrochloride and measure the sterile water for injection.
3. Dissolve the lidocaine hydrochloride in the sterile water for injection.
4. Package and label.

Oral Solutions

℞ Methylcellulose Oral Liquid Vehicle

Methylcellulose 1% solution		50 mL
Glycerin		3 mL
Preserved flavored syrup	qs	100 mL
Sodium benzoate or		200 mg
potassium sorbate		

1. Calculate the quantity of each ingredient required for the prescription.
2. Accurately weigh or measure each ingredient.
3. Dissolve the sodium benzoate or potassium sorbate in about 1 mL of purified water.
4. Add this solution to the methylcellulose 1% solution.
5. Add the glycerin; then add the preserved flavored syrup to 100 mL and mix well.
6. Package and label.

℞ Flavored Cod Liver Oil

Spearmint oil	0.4 mL
Peppermint oil	0.4 mL
Cod liver oil qs	100 mL

1. Accurately measure the two flavoring oils.
2. Mix the flavoring oils with sufficient cod liver oil to make 100 mL and mix well.
3. Package and label.

Topical Solutions

℞ DMSO 70% Topical Solution (100 g)

Dimethyl sulfoxide   70 g
Alcohol 95% or purified water 30 g

1. Calculate the required quantity of each ingredient for the total amount to be prepared.
2. Accurately weigh/measure each ingredient.
3. In a suitable container, mix the two liquids.
4. Package and label.

℞ Fluconazole 1.5% in Dimethyl Sulfoxide (100 mL)

Fluconazole   1.5 g
Dimethyl sulfoxide   qs   100 mL

1. Accurately weigh the fluconazole powder or obtain from Diflucan tablets.
2. Dissolve the fluconazole powder in DMSO or mix the finely powdered tablets with DMSO.
3. If the tablets were used, filter the product after the fluconazole has gone into solution.
4. Package in a bottle with a glass rod applicator.

Standard Operating Procedure (SOP)

Quality Assessment of Oral and Topical Liquids

Purpose
The purpose of this procedure is to provide a method of documenting quality assessment tests of and to conduct observations on oral and topical solutions, suspensions, and emulsions.

Materials
The following equipment is used in one or more of the assessment tests:

- Balance
- Graduates
- pH meter
- Pycnometer (optional)

Procedure
The appropriate tests should be conducted and the results/observations recorded on the worksheet "Quality Assessment Form for Oral and Topical Liquids" (Figure 15-3).

Weight/Volume.

> ▸ Accurately weigh the product on a balance or measure the quantity in a graduate.

pH.

> ▸ Calibrate the pH meter, and then determine the apparent pH of the product.

Specific Gravity.

> ▸ If a pycnometer is available, make sure it is clean and dry.
> ▸ Weigh the empty pycnometer (W_1); then fill it with the prepared product, being careful not to entrap air bubbles.
> ▸ Weigh the pycnometer a second time (W_2).
> ▸ Subtract the first weight from the second weight to obtain the net weight of the product. Divide this weight (grams) by the volume (milliliters) of the pycnometer to obtain the density/specific gravity of the product:

$$SG = W_1 \, (g) - W_2 \, (g)/V \, (mL)$$

Active Drug Assay Results. As appropriate, have representative samples of the product assayed for active drug content by a contract analytical laboratory. Stability can be assessed by storing the product at room, refrigerated, and/or frozen temperatures and having the assay repeated on the stored samples.

Color of Product. It may be advisable to use a color chart for determining the actual color of the product.

Clarity (solutions). Evaluate clarity by a visual inspection. A light-dark background can be used. On the worksheet (Figure 15-3), 1 is the clearest and 5 is the least clear on the scale provided.

Globule Size Range. Place a drop of the product on a glass plate (microscope slide) and illuminate from the bottom. Estimate the globule size range of the product.

Rheologic Properties/Pourability

Visually determine whether the product pours easily or with difficulty (before and after sitting for a period of time).

Physical Observation

Describe the appearance and organoleptic qualities of the product.

Physical Stability. Prepare an additional quantity of the product, package, and label (for physical stability observations). Weekly, observe the product for signs of discoloration, foreign materials, gas formation, mold growth, and so forth. Record a descriptive observation on the form at each observation interval. Sufficient lines are provided for observations for 8 weeks.

Quality Assessment Form for Oral and Topical Liquids

Product _____   Date_____

Lot/Rx Number_____   Form: Solution   Suspension   Emulsion

Characteristic	Theoretical	Actual	Normal Range
Weight/volume	_____	_____	_____
pH	_____	_____	_____
Specific gravity	_____	_____	_____
Active drug assay results	_____	_____	_____
Initial assay	_____	_____	_____
After storage No. 1	_____	_____	_____
After storage No. 2	_____	_____	_____
Color of product	_____	_____	_____

Clarity (solution)   Clear   1   2   3   4   5   Opaque

Globule size range (emulsion)
    (estimated, mm)   <1 1–2 2–3 >3

Rheologic properties
    (pourability, settling,
    resuspendability)   Good   1   2   3   4   5   Poor

Sample set aside for physical stability observation: Yes   No

    If yes, results   Date   Observation

    _____   _____

    _____   _____

    _____   _____

    _____   _____

    _____   _____

    _____   _____

    _____   _____

    _____   _____

    _____   _____

    _____   _____

    _____   _____

    _____   _____

    _____   _____

Figure 15-3. Sample worksheet for quality assessment of oral and topical liquids.

Chapter 16

Suspensions

Definitions/Types

When components of a formula are not soluble, either a suspension or an emulsion (as described in Chapter 17, "Emulsions") is often indicated. A *suspension* is a two-phased system consisting of a finely divided solid dispersed in a solid, liquid, or gas. Suspensions are appropriate when the drug to be incorporated is not sufficiently soluble in an ordinary solvent or cosolvent system. A good suspension ensures that the drug is uniformly dispersed throughout the vehicle. *Oral suspensions* are liquid preparations in which solid particles of the active drug are generally dispersed in a sweetened, flavored, and, sometimes, viscous vehicle. As their name implies, these preparations are taken orally.

Topical suspensions are liquid preparations containing solid particles dispersed in a suitable liquid vehicle that are intended for application to the skin. These preparations are sometimes called lotions (e.g., calamine lotion).

Historical Use

The first suspensions were possibly simple preparations of vegetable or earth products mixed with water. Mixing the drug with water made it easier to take orally or apply topically. This dosage form was a simple way of converting powdered leaves, bark, clays, and the like to a fluid preparation that not only would be easier to administer but also would increase patient acceptance of the preparation.

Applications

When drugs are not soluble in a solvent, they should be placed in a suitable vehicle for administration. A suitable vehicle to be used in a suspension would have the necessary viscosity to keep the drug particles suspended separately from each other but would be sufficiently fluid to allow the preparation to be poured from the container. Suspensions can be prepared for oral internal use or for topical use; they can even be prepared for ophthalmic, otic, and nasal applications. The suspension dosage form can enhance the stability of a drug that is poorly stable in solution. Using an insoluble form of the drug places more of the drug in the suspended form, not in solution, and thus the drug is not available for solution degradation.

Composition

Suspensions usually contain insoluble particles, a liquid medium, a suspending agent/surfactant/viscosity enhancer, and a preservative. They can also contain a flavoring/perfume agent and a sweetener. The order in which these ingredients are blended is important to the stability of the preparation.

Preparation

To prepare a suspension, the pharmacist must first obtain uniform, small particles of the drug. This is accomplished through particle size reduction, which was discussed in Chapter 9, "Powders and Granules." Once this step is completed, the active insoluble material should be thoroughly wetted before it is mixed with the vehicle. Hydrophilic materials are best wetted with water-miscible liquids (e.g., glycerin), whereas hydrophobic substances can be wetted with nonpolar liquids or with the use of a surfactant. A general guideline is to use the minimal amount of wetting agent required to produce the desired product.

After the drug and wetting agent have been combined to form a thick paste, the vehicle can be added with constant stirring. Methylcellulose preparations are best prepared by dispersing the polymer in about one third to one half of the total volume of hot water, followed by adding the remaining water as ice water or ice. Many polymers can be sprinkled onto rapidly agitating water to improve their dispersion.

Physicochemical Considerations

Sample suspension vehicles are listed in Table 16-1. If a good suspension vehicle is unavailable, one can usually prepare a 0.5% to 5% methylcellulose dispersion. A 0.5% to 1.5% sodium carboxymethylcellulose dispersion can also be prepared. The viscosity required depends on the active drug's tendency to settle, which, in turn, is related to the powder's density and particle size. Table 16-2 provides a list of the concentrations of viscosity-increasing agents that will yield a viscosity of 800 centipoise (cP). After the suspending agent is prepared, it can be mixed 1:1 with a flavored syrup.

Viscosity and Rheology

Viscosity plays an important role in a number of different dosage forms. It is an important factor in maintaining drugs in suspension, enhancing the stability of emulsions, altering the release rate of drugs at sites of application, and making it easier to apply drugs to various parts of the body so they do not run off. Compounding pharmacists routinely use viscosity to enhance stability of numerous preparations. As seen in Table 16-1, there are many different viscosity-increasing agents with different physical properties and, consequently, different applications and uses. Physical properties of importance include solubility in different solvents, pH range of maximum viscosity, and rheologic characterization. (See Appendix V, "Viscosity-Increasing Agents for Aqueous Systems" for information on properties of commonly used suspending/thickening agents.)

Viscosity is an important factor in rheology, the study of flow. *Viscosity* is defined as the force required to move one plane surface past another under specified conditions when the space between is filled by the liquid in question. More conve-

Table 16-1. Suspending Agents and Vehicles for Compounding Suspensions

Suspending Agent	Final Concentration (%)
Acacia NF	2.0–5.0
Carbomer resins NF	0.5–5.0
Carboxymethylcellulose sodium USP	0.5–1.5
Colloidal silicon dioxide NF	1.5–3.5
Methylcellulose USP	0.5–5.0
Tragacanth NF	0.5–2.0

Vehicle	pH	Alcohol Content (%)
Cologel[a]	4	5
Ora-Plus	4–4.5	0
Suspendol-S	5.3–6	0

[a]No longer available.

Table 16-2. Concentration of Viscosity-Increasing Agents Required to Obtain a Viscosity of 800 cP

Viscosity Agent	% Concentration Required
Acacia	35[a]
Bentonite	6.3
Carboxymethylcellulose, low	4.1
Carboxymethylcellulose, medium	1.9
Carboxymethylcellulose, high	0.7
Methylcellulose 100 cP	3.5
Methylcellulose 400 cP	2.4
Methylcellulose 1500 cP	1.7
Tragacanth	2.8
Veegum	6.0

[a]Concentration of acacia required to yield a viscosity of 600 cP.

niently, it can be considered as a relative property with water as the reference material that is assigned a viscosity of 1 cP. If a liquid has a viscosity 10 times that of water, it is assigned a viscosity of 10 cP. Fluids generally fall into Newtonian or nonNewtonian flow categories.

Newtonian flow reflects a liquid whose viscosity does not change with increasing shear rate, as, for example, with water. Regardless of how much shear is applied, its viscosity remains at 1 cP. Other Newtonian liquids include many pure substances, such as glycerin, alcohol, propylene glycol, and the like.

NonNewtonian flow involves substances that fail to follow the Newton equation of flow and include materials such as colloidal solutions, emulsions, liquid suspensions, and ointments. There are three types of nonNewtonian flow: plastic, pseudoplastic, and dilatant. *Plastic flow* is characterized by materials (such as petrolatum) that have a certain yield value and whose viscosity decreases with increasing shear rate. *Pseudoplastic* materials (such as polymer solutions) do not have a yield value, and their viscosity decreases with increasing shear rate; they are also called "shear-thinning" systems. *Dilatant* materials (such as pastes) actually increase in volume when sheared, and the viscosity increases with increasing shear rate; they are also called "shear-thickening" systems and, generally, have a high percentage of solids in their formulations.

Thixotropy is a type of flow that is a reversible gel to sol transition on stressing; it reverts back to a gel on standing. This characteristic is desirable for increasing the physical stability of suspension dosage forms. They thicken on standing and stabilize the suspension and become thinner on shaking, which makes pouring and application easier.

Depending on the desired characteristics of the final formulation, one can select Newtonian or nonNewtonian flow properties and formulate accordingly. For example, a gel of Pluronic F-127 exhibits reverse thermal gelling. It is fluid at colder temperatures and becomes a gel at warmer temperatures. This type of product is good for application to the skin, where it "sets up" and delivers the drug over a longer time period.

Preparation Methods

Most viscosity-increasing agents are best dispersed by pouring the powder slowly and steadily into vigorously stirred water with continued stirring during hydration. A second method is to mix the agent with another water-soluble substance, such as sucrose, before adding to water. A third method is to form a paste of the agent with a water-miscible liquid, such as alcohol or glycerin, before adding to water. Some agents are best dispersed initially in hot water, and then the remaining water is added as cold or ice water. These methods will aid in minimizing the "clumping" that can occur with these polymers and that makes their preparation more difficult.

One characteristic of a good suspension is its resuspendability. The product can be observed over time to determine its settling and caking tendencies. In formulating the suspension, the pharmacist should make sure it is not too thick, because the product may be difficult to pour, especially if it has been refrigerated.

Quality Control

Quality control involves checking certain characteristics of the suspension. These characteristics include weight/volume, extent of settling, ease of dispersibility, appearance, odor, and pourability. The measured and observed characteristics should be documented, and, if possible, the product should be periodically checked for these characteristics.

The amount of settling can be measured by allowing the product to sit for a day and then measuring the height of the settled particles. If necessary, formulation changes can be made to reduce the amount of settling. Measuring the height of the settled particles in different batches of the same product can be used as a general guide in determining the consistency of preparation.

Packaging/Storage/Labeling

Suspensions should be packaged in tight containers that have an opening large enough to easily pour a viscous liquid. Sufficient headspace should be allowed for ease of shaking.

These preparations should be stored at room temperature or refrigerated, depending on the physicochemical characteristics of the active drug and the supporting matrix.

The instruction "Shake Well Before Using" or "Shake Well Before Taking" should always appear on the label of a suspension preparation. In addition, these preparations should be labeled as to whether they are for internal or external use.

Stability

Suspension dosage forms should be observed for the following physical attributes: uniformity, settling, caking, crystal growth, and difficulty in resuspending, as well as mold/bacterial growth, odor, and loss of volume. Suspensions are less susceptible to chemical degradation than are solutions, but, if water is present, they generally have a short beyond-use date.

Beyond-use dates for water-containing suspensions are no later than 14 days after preparation, when stored at cold temperatures, for products prepared from ingredients in solid form. This period is extended if valid scientific information is available to support greater stability, as discussed in Chapter 4, "Stability of Compounded Products."

Patient Counseling

Patients should be instructed to always shake the suspension before taking or applying it. They should also be instructed on how to shake suspensions. These preparations should be either shaken vigorously or mixed using a rolling action. Patients should be counseled on the proper storage of suspensions and the proper method for measuring doses.

Sample Formulations

Rx **Spironolactone Suspension**

Spironolactone		200 mg
Cetylpyridinium chloride, monohydrate		10 mg
Potassium sorbate		150 mg
Xanthan gum		200 mg
Magnesium aluminum silicate		1 g
Citric acid, anhydrous		60 mg
Sucrose		20 g
Purified water	qs	100 mL

1. Calculate the quantity of each ingredient required for the prescription.
2. Accurately weigh or measure each ingredient.
3. Place the spironolactone powder in a mortar and add the cetylpyridinium chloride, which has previously been dissolved in 15 mL of purified water; mix to form a paste.
4. Place 20 mL of purified water in a beaker on a magnetic stirrer and stir; sprinkle the xanthan gum on the stirred water.
5. Add the stirred water mixture to the beaker containing the spironolactone mixture.
6. Dissolve the potassium sorbate in 50 mL of purified water; place this solution on a magnetic stirrer and stir.
7. Sprinkle the magnesium aluminum silicate onto the stirred water prepared in step 6; make sure it is thoroughly dispersed.
8. Add the sucrose and citric acid to the mixture prepared in step 6, using heat if necessary; cool to room temperature.
9. Add to the spironolactone and xanthan gum mixture prepared in step 5.
10. Add sufficient purified water to volume and mix well.
11. Package and label.

℞ Progesterone Oral Suspension

Progesterone, micronized		4 g
Glycerin		5 mL
Methylcellulose 1% solution		50 mL
Flavored syrup	qs	100 mL

1. Calculate the quantity of each ingredient required for the prescription.
2. Accurately weigh or measure each ingredient.
3. Place the progesterone powder in a mortar and wet with the glycerin to obtain a thick, smooth paste.
4. Slowly add the methylcellulose solution to the paste while triturating.
5. Pour the mixture into a graduated cylinder.
6. Add small quantities of flavored syrup to the mortar and mix; then add these portions to the graduated cylinder.
7. After transferring all the material to the graduated cylinder, add sufficient flavored syrup to volume and mix thoroughly.
8. Package and label.

℞ Progesterone Enema

Progesterone, micronized		20 g
Povidone		10 g
Purified water	qs	100 mL

1. Calculate the quantity of each ingredient required for the prescription.
2. Accurately weigh or measure each ingredient.
3. Wet the povidone with about 15 mL of water to form a paste.
4. Using a magnetic stirrer, add about 60 mL of water and stir until a clear solution is obtained.
5. Add the micronized progesterone and mix well.
6. Add the remaining water to volume and mix thoroughly.
7. Package and label.

Xanthan Gum Suspension Vehicle

Xanthan gum		300 mg
Sodium saccharin		100 mg
Aspartame		200 mg
Propylene glycol		5 mL
Syrup or other preserved vehicle	qs	100 mL

1. Calculate the quantity of each ingredient required for the prescription.
2. Accurately weigh or measure each ingredient.
3. Place the xanthan gum, sodium saccharin, and aspartame in a mortar; triturate the ingredients, using a pestle.
4. Add the propylene glycol and make a smooth paste.
5. Add the syrup in small portions and pour into a graduated cylinder, rinsing the mortar into the cylinder until 100 mL of suspension is prepared.
6. Mix well.
7. Package and label.

℞ Wound Care Mixture

Phenol		200 mg
Zinc oxide		12 g
70% Ethanol		
Calcium hydroxide solution	aa qs	100 mL

1. Calculate the quantity of each ingredient required for the prescription.
2. Accurately weigh or measure each ingredient.
3. Prepare 100 mL of the vehicle, using equal parts of 70% ethanol and calcium hydroxide solution (lime water).
4. Dissolve the phenol in about 75 mL of the vehicle prepared in step 3.
5. Sprinkle the zinc oxide powder on the phenol–vehicle mixture.
6. Add additional vehicle to the zinc oxide–phenol mixture to make 100 mL of suspension. (Discard the remainder of the vehicle.)
7. Package and label.

Sugar-Free Suspension Structured Vehicle USP

Xanthan gum		200 mg
Saccharin sodium		200 mg
Potassium sorbate		150 mg
Citric acid		100 mg
Sorbitol		2 g
Mannitol		2 g
Glycerin		2 mL
Purified water	qs	100 mL

1. Calculate the required quantity of each ingredient for the total amount to be prepared.
2. Accurately weigh/measure each ingredient.
3. Place 30 mL of purified water in a beaker on a hot plate/stirrer.
4. Using moderate heat, stir to form a vortex and slowly sprinkle the xanthan gum into the vortex.
5. In a separate beaker, dissolve the saccharin sodium, potassium sorbate, and citric acid in 50 mL of purified water.
6. Using moderate heat, incorporate the sorbitol, mannitol, and glycerin into this mixture.
7. Add to the previously prepared xanthan gum dispersion.
8. Add sufficient purified water to volume and mix well.
9. Package and label.

R̲x **Metronidazole Benzoate 400 mg/5 mL Oral Suspension**

Metronidazole benzoate		8 g
Glycerin		qs
Flavor		qs
Suspension-structured vehicle or		
sugar-free suspension-structured vehicle or		
commercial oral liquid vehicles	qs	100 mL

1. Calculate the required quantity of each ingredient for the total amount to be prepared.
2. Accurately weigh/measure each ingredient.
3. Mix the metronidazole benzoate powder with sufficient glycerin to form a smooth paste.
4. Add the flavor and mix well.
5. Add sufficient suspension vehicle to volume and mix well.
6. Package and label.

Rx   Misoprostol 0.001% and Lidocaine 0.5% Oral Rinse

Misoprostol		1 mg
Lidocaine hydrochloride		500 mg
Methylparaben		200 mg
Glycerin		10 mL
Cherry flavor, anhydrous		10 µL
Syrup		40 mL
Sodium carboxymethylcellulose 0.25% solution.	qs	100 mL

1. Calculate the required quantity of each ingredient for the total amount to be prepared.
2. Accurately weigh/measure each ingredient and obtain and pulverize five 200 µg misoprostol tablets.
3. Dissolve the methylparaben in the glycerin and add the lidocaine hydrochloride, pulverized misoprostol tablets, and cherry flavor.
4. Add the syrup and sufficient sodium carboxymethylcellulose 0.25% solution to volume and mix well.
5. Package and label.

Stomatitis Preparations (100 mL)

	Kaiser	Kraemer	Powell	Reynolds	Stanford	T-N-D-D
Tetracycline 25 mg/mL suspension	50 mL	—	8 mL	50 mL	48 mL	—
Nystatin oral suspension	12 mL	30 mL	4.8 mL	12 mL	12 mL	—
Hydrocortisone powder	46 mg	—	20 mg	46 mg	46 mg	—
Purified water	qs 100 mL	—	—	—	qs 100 mL	—
Dyclonine 1% solution	—	22.5 mL	—	—	—	—
Lemon oil	—	0.25 mL	—	—	—	—
Glycerin	—	qs 100 mL	—	—	—	—
Diphenhydramine 2.5 mg/mL elixir	—	—	qs 100 mL	—	—	—
Chlorpheniramine 0.4 mg/mL syrup	—	—	—	qs 100 mL	—	—
Chlorpheniramine 4 mg tablets	—	—	—	—	#5	—
Tetracycline	—	—	—	—	—	1.25 g
Nystatin	—	—	—	—	—	1,666,667 units
Diphenhydramine HCl	—	—	—	—	—	125 mg
Dexamethasone	—	—	—	—	—	333 µg
Xanthan gum	—	—	—	—	—	200 mg
Aspartame	—	—	—	—	—	200 mg
Saccharin sodium	—	—	—	—	—	100 mg
Flavor	—	—	—	—	—	qs
Simple syrup	—	—	—	—	—	qs 100 mL

1. Calculate the required quantity of each ingredient for the total amount to be prepared.
2. Accurately weigh/measure each ingredient.
3. Select the appropriate method of preparation:

▸ Kaiser: Mix the hydrocortisone powder with a small amount of the tetracycline syrup until smooth. Slowly add the remaining tetracycline syrup, mix in the nystatin suspension, and add sufficient purified water to volume and mix well.

▸ Kraemer: Add the lemon oil to about 100 mL of glycerin followed by the dyclonine solution and nystatin oral suspension. Add sufficient glycerin to volume and mix well.

▸ Powell: Mix the hydrocortisone powder with a small amount of the tetracycline suspension. Add the remainder of the tetracycline suspension followed by the nystatin oral suspension and the diphenhydramine elixir and mix well.

▸ Reynolds: Mix the tetracycline and nystatin suspension. Slowly add the hydrocortisone (previously dissolved in 15 mL of ethanol) with constant stirring. Add sufficient chlorpheniramine syrup to volume and mix well.

▸ Stanford: Thoroughly pulverize the chlorpheniramine tablets and blend in the hydrocortisone powder. Add the tetracycline syrup in portions with thorough mixing followed by the nystatin oral suspension. Add sufficient purified water to volume and mix well.

▸ T-N-D-D: Blend the tetracycline, nystatin, diphenhydramine hydrochloride, dexamethasone, xanthan gum, aspartame, and saccharin powders and mix well. Add 90 mL of simple syrup, in portions, with thorough mixing after each addition. Add the desired flavor and mix well. Add sufficient simple syrup to volume and mix well.

4. Package and label.

R̶x̶ Triple Estrogen 0.25 mg/drop in Oil Suspension

Estriol	0.2 mg/drop
Estrone	0.025 mg/drop
Estradiol	0.025 mg/drop
Saccharin	100 mg
Tangerine oil (flavor)	qs
Sesame oil	qs

1. Accurately determine the number of drops per milliliter depending on the dropper:container being used. Using a dropper, count the number of drops to make a volume of 2 mL. Divide by 2 to get the number of drops per mL.
2. This formula calls for 0.25 mg of the triple-estrogen mixture per drop. To determine the quantity of each of the estrogens needed per mL, multiply the concentration (0.25 mg per drop) times the number of drops per mL. Multiply result times the number of mL to be prepared to get the quantity for the prescription.
3. Accurately weigh/measure each of the ingredients.
4. Mix the estriol, estrone, and estradiol in a suitable oil, such as sesame oil. Add the sweetener and flavor and mix well. Add additional sesame oil to volume and mix well.
5. Package and label.

R̶x̶ Progesterone 100 mg/mL Sublingual Drops

Progesterone, micronized		1 g
Silica gel, micronized		200 mg
Saccharin		100 mg
Flavor (mild)		qs
Almond oil/peanut oil	qs	10 mL

1. Calculate the required quantity of each ingredient for the total amount to be prepared.
2. Accurately weigh/measure each ingredient.
3. Mix the progesterone, silica gel, and saccharin in a mortar.
4. Add a small quantity of the vehicle (oil) to make a paste.
5. Add the flavor and mix well.
6. Add sufficient vehicle to volume and mix well.
7. Package and label.

℞ Minoxidil 5% and Finasteride 0.1% Topical Liquid

Minoxidil		5 g
Finasteride		100 mg
Propylene glycol		20 mL
Ethanol 95%		70 mL
Purified water	qs	100 mL

1. Calculate the required quantity of each ingredient for the total amount to be prepared.
2. Accurately weigh/measure each ingredient; count out the number of finasteride (Proscar).
3. Thoroughly pulverize the finasteride tablets, add to the ethanol, mix well, and filter.
4. To the filtrate, add the propylene glycol and minoxidil.
5. Mix well until all dissolved.
6. Add sufficient purified water to volume and mix well.
7. Package and label.

Chapter 17

Emulsions

Definitions/Types

incapable of mixing

Emulsions are heterogeneous systems consisting of at least one immiscible liquid that is intimately dispersed in another liquid in the form of droplets, or "globules,"whose diameters generally exceed 0.1 μm. Emulsions are also defined as thermodynamically unstable mixtures of two essentially immiscible liquids and an emulsifying agent to hold them together. The process of combining these ingredients is termed *emulsification*.

An emulsion consists of a dispersed phase (internal phase or discontinuous phase), a dispersion medium (external phase or continuous phase), and a third component, known as an emulsifying agent. The diameter of the dispersed-phase globules is generally in the range of about 0.1 to 10 μm, although some can be as small as 0.01 μm or as large as 100 μm.

Emulsions are used as a dosage form whenever two immiscible liquids must be dispensed in the same preparation. Ordinarily, the mixture has both a polar and a nonpolar component, each of which is a liquid. When the dispersed phase is nonpolar (oil) and the dispersion medium is polar (water), the emulsion is known as an oil-in-water (o/w) emulsion. When the dispersed phase is water and the dispersion medium is oil, the emulsion is of the water-in-oil (w/o) type. Generally, emulsions for internal use are of the o/w type, and those for external use can be of either type. Water-in-oil emulsions are insoluble in water, are not water washable, will absorb water, are occlusive, and can be "greasy." Conversely, o/w emulsions are miscible with water, are water washable, will absorb water, are nonocclusive, and are nongreasy.

Creams are opaque, soft solids or thick liquids consisting of medications that are dissolved or suspended in water-removable (i.e., vanishing cream) or emollient bases. They are intended for external application and can be either type of emulsion. The term "cream" is often applied to soft, o/w, cosmetically acceptable types of preparations. Creams are usually applied to moist, weeping lesions because they have a somewhat drying effect in that the lesions' fluids are miscible with the aqueous external phase of creams.

Lotions are fluid emulsions or suspensions designed for external application. They have a lubricating effect and thus are applied to intertriginous areas, that is, areas where the skin rubs together, such as between the fingers, between the thighs, or under the arms.

Historical Use

The term "emulsion" is derived from the word "emulsus." The verb associated with this word, "emulgere," means "to milk out." Emulsion originally referred to the milky liquid extracted from almonds but in time was used to refer to any milky fluid. Although emulsions still have a milky appearance, the term now commonly refers to a dispersion of immiscible liquids.

Applications

Topical creams and lotions are popular forms of emulsions for external use. Internally, emulsions are used to dispense oil and aqueous drugs together, to mask the taste of unpleasant oily drugs, and sometimes to enhance the absorption of selected drugs. Emulsions containing high caloric oil can be administered intravenously to severely debilitated patients.

Composition

Emulsions generally contain three components: a lipid phase, an aqueous phase, and an emulsifier. The compounding pharmacist has the greatest flexibility in the choice of an emulsifier. Common emulsifiers are listed in Table 17-1.

Table 17-1. Emulsifiers and Stabilizers for Use in Emulsions

Carbohydrates	High Molecular Weight Alcohols
Acacia	Cetyl alcohol
Agar	Glyceryl monostearate
Chondrus	Stearyl alcohol
Pectin	**Surfactants**
Tragacanth	Anionic
Proteins	Cationic
Casein	Nonionic
Egg yolk	**Solids**
Gelatin	Aluminum hydroxide
	Bentonite
	Magnesium hydroxide

Preparation

Emulsions do not form spontaneously when liquids are mixed. Rather, they require energy input, such as mechanical agitation, ultrasonic vibration, or heat, to break up the liquids, which thereby increases the surface area of the internal phase.

Emulsions can be prepared by both manual and mechanical methods. These methods can involve the use of a mortar and pestle, a bottle for shaking, beakers, an electric mixer or a mechanical stirrer, a hand homogenizer, and sonifiers. A mortar and pestle can be used with both the English and the Continental methods of emulsification, which are described later. For best results, the mortar should have rough surfaces to help shear the liquid into small globules.

The English Method, also called the wet gum method, relies on the use of mucilages or dissolved gums. The ratio of oil:water:emulsifier often ranges from 2 to 4:2:1 for forming the primary emulsion, as shown in Table 17-2. The mucilage is made by adding a small quantity of water to the hydrocolloid (e.g., acacia) and then triturating the mixture until uniform. Oil is added in small quantities by using rapid trituration. The resulting mixture will be thick and viscous. More water is added slowly, and the emulsion is triturated rapidly until complete.

Table 17-2. Component Ratios for the Preparation of Primary Emulsions

Oil	Acacia	Tragacanth
Fixed oils	4:2:1	40:20:1
Mineral oil	3:2:1	30:20:1
Linseed oil	2:2:1	20:20:1
Volatile oils	2:2:1	20:20:1

The Continental Method, known as the dry gum method, involves rapid mixing of the hydrocolloid with the oil for a short time, after which the water is added all at once with rapid trituration. When a snapping sound is heard, the primary emulsion has formed. More water is then added slowly with rapid trituration until the emulsion is complete. The ratio of oil:water:emulsifier for preparing the primary emulsion is generally about 4:2:1.

The bottle method (shaking) is another approach to preparing emulsions that contain volatile oils and other nonviscous oils. This method eliminates the splashing problem that sometimes occurs when a mortar and pestle are used. The bottle method, which is a variation of the dry gum method, involves mixing the powder (emulsifier) and oil in a bottle and then shaking the bottle with short, rapid movements. The required quantity of water is added all at once, and the mixture is again shaken rapidly to form the primary emulsion (4:2:1 ratio). If more water is required, it is added in small amounts, with the bottle shaken after each addition. The oil and gum should *not* be allowed to remain in contact too long, as the gum can imbibe the oil and partially waterproof the powder.

The beaker method is often used with synthetic emulsifying agents. The prescription ingredients are generally divided into two separate phases: oil and water. Each phase is heated individually to about 60°C to 70°C, if needed. The internal phase is then stirred into the external phase. Finally, the product is removed from the heat and stirred gently and periodically until it has cooled (congealed).

A mechanical stirrer (mixer) with various impellers can be used to prepare an emulsion. The unit's propeller should be placed directly into the system to be emulsified. Mixers are available commercially and can be found in department stores and gourmet kitchen stores (Figure 17-1).

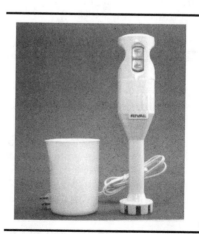

Figure 17-1. Two-speed mixer.

Hand homogenizers function by forcing the mixture of liquids through a small inlet orifice at a high pressure. This shearing action causes the globules to break up.

Incorporating Materials into a W/O Emulsion

Oils and insoluble powders can be incorporated directly into an emulsion by using a pill tile and spatula or a mortar and pestle. A levigating agent may be needed if large amounts of insoluble powders are required for the formulation. In many w/o emulsions, sufficient emulsifying agent is available to emulsify a larger quantity of the aqueous solution of the drug, which can be incorporated by using a pill tile with a spatula or a mortar and pestle or gentle heat from a water bath. When using heat, the pharmacist should make sure that the preparation is not held at a high temperature for too long because some loss of water can occur. This loss of water would change the volume of the product. Adding oily ingredients usually poses no problem. Some crystalline drugs may need to be dissolved in oil before being incorporated, if possible. In this case, it may be necessary to use the base form rather than the salt form of the drug. Adding water to these emulsions is difficult unless an excess quantity of the emulsifier is present.

Incorporating Materials into an O/W Emulsion

A pill tile and spatula or a mortar and pestle are also used to incorporate insoluble powders and aqueous solutions into emulsions. It may be advisable to use a levigating agent, such as glycerin or propylene glycol, when mixing the insoluble powder with the emulsion. Crystalline materials should be dissolved in a small quantity of water before they are added to the emulsion. Water-soluble materials should also be dissolved in a small amount of water before the solution is incorporated into the base. Because there is usually an excess of emulsifying agent, a small quantity of oil can be incorporated directly into the base. However, if larger amounts of oil are required, it may be necessary to add a small quantity of an o/w surfactant to help disperse the oil uniformly in the vehicle. It is generally easy to add water-soluble ingredients.

Using heat to incorporate an ingredient into an o/w vehicle can cause the product to lose water. Thus, it is necessary to work quickly. If water is lost, the volume of the product will change; moreover, if it is a semisolid, it may tend to become stiff and "waxy." (See the box "Hints for Compounding Emulsions" for additional preparation suggestions.)

Hints for Compounding Emulsions

- It is advisable to dissolve the oil-soluble ingredients in the oil phase and the water-soluble ingredients in the aqueous phase.
- Light, rapid trituration is more effective than heavy, slow trituration when using a mortar and pestle.
- Under a given set of conditions, an o/w emulsion can be more easily produced with glass equipment, whereas w/o emulsions can be more easily prepared with water-repellent plastic equipment. This ease of preparation could be related to the "wettability" of the external phase when it comes into contact with the surface of the equipment.
- Water and oil phases should be added slowly under constant agitation.
- If heat is used, the aqueous phase should be a few degrees warmer than the oil phase.

Physicochemical Considerations

The pharmacist must consider a number of factors before compounding an emulsion. These factors include the purpose and route, whether internal or external, of the drug, the concentration of the active drug, the liquid vehicle, the physicochemical stability of the drug, preservatives, buffers, solubilizers, emulsifying agents, viscosity enhancers, colors, and flavors.

Two immiscible liquids in contact with each other will tend to maintain as small an interface as possible. Consequently, mixing these liquids together will be difficult. If the liquids are shaken together, spherical droplets will form because the liquids generally maintain as small a surface area as possible. There will be interfacial tension between the two liquids. With the addition of a surfactant, the liquids will become miscible because the molecules of the agent will tend to be oriented between the two phases, with the polar ends in the polar phase and the nonpolar ends in the nonpolar phase.

An emulsifying agent makes the globules less likely to coalesce, or join together to form larger globules, which eventually causes the two liquids to separate. The stability of an emulsion depends on the properties of the emulsifier and the film it forms where the two phases interface. This film, which should form rapidly during the emulsification process, should be both tough and elastic.

Emulsifying agents aid in forming emulsions through three different approaches: (1) reduction of interfacial tension, as described earlier, (2) formation of a rigid interfacial film, and (3) formation of an electrical double layer. If the concentration of the emulsifier is sufficiently high, a rigid film can form between the immiscible phases. This film can act as a mechanical barrier to the coalescence of the globules. An electrical double layer minimizes coalescence by producing electrical forces that repulse approaching droplets.

Emulsifying agents can be divided into three different categories: (1) surfactants, (2) hydrophilic colloids, and (3) finely divided solid particles. Surfactants are adsorbed at oil:water interfaces to form monomolecular films, resulting in a decrease in interfacial tension, whereas hydrophilic colloids form multimolecular films that surround the dispersed particles. The finely divided solid particles are adsorbed at the interface between the two liquid phases of the globules and create a film of particles around the dispersed globules. As can be seen, the one common feature of each of these agents is that they form a film.

Hydrophile–Lipophile–Balance (HLB) System

The HLB system is used to describe the characteristics of a surfactant. The system consists of an arbitrary scale to which HLB values are experimentally determined and assigned. If the HLB value is low, the number of hydrophilic groups on the surfactant is small, which means it is more lipophilic (oil soluble) than hydrophilic (water soluble). For example, according to Table 17-3, Span 80 has an HLB value of 4.3 and is oil soluble. Conversely, if the HLB value is high, there are a large number of hydrophilic groups on the surfactant, which makes it more hydrophilic (water soluble) than oil soluble. Tween 20, for example, has an HLB value of 16.7 and is water soluble. A number of types of surfactants and their HLB ranges are listed in Table 17-4, and some of their physicochemical characteristics are shown in Table 17-5.

Antifoaming agents include alcohol, ether, castor oil, and some surfactants. These agents dissipate foam by destabilizing the air:liquid interface, which allows the liquid to drain away from the air pocket.

Table 17-3. HLB Values of Emulsifiers

Commercial Name	Chemical Name	HLB Value
Acacia	Acacia	12.0/8
Arlacel 83	Sorbitan sesquioleate	3.7
Bryj 30	Polyoxyethylene lauryl ether	9.7
Glyceryl monostearate	Glyceryl monostearate	3.8
Methocel 15 cP	Methylcellulose	10.5
Myrj 45	Polyoxyethylene monostearate	11.1
Myrj 49	Polyoxyethylene monostearate	15.0
Myrj 52	Polyoxyl 40 stearate	16.9
PEG 400 monoleate	Polyoxyethylene monoleate	11.4
PEG 400 monolaurate	Polyoxyethylene monolaurate	13.1
PEG 400 monostearate	Polyoxyethylene monostearate	11.6
Pharmagel B	Gelatin	9.8
Potassium oleate	Potassium oleate	20.0
Sodium lauryl sulfate	Sodium lauryl sulfate	40
Sodium oleate	Sodium oleate	18
Span 20	Sorbitan monolaurate	8.6
Span 40	Sorbitan monopalmitate	6.7
Span 60	Sorbitan monostearate	4.7
Span 65	Sorbitan tristearate	2.1
Span 80	Sorbitan monooleate	4.3
Span 85	Sorbitan trioleate	1.8
Tragacanth	Tragacanth	13.2
Triethanolamine oleate	Triethanolamine oleate	12
Tween 20	Polyoxyethylene sorbitan monolaurate	16.7
Tween 21	Polyoxyethylene sorbitan monolaurate	13.3
Tween 40	Polyoxyethylene sorbitan monopalmitate	15.6
Tween 60	Polyoxyethylene sorbitan monostearate	14.9
Tween 61	Polyoxyethylene sorbitan monostearate	9.6
Tween 65	Polyoxyethylene sorbitan tristearate	10.5
Tween 80	Polyoxyethylene sorbitan monooleate	15.0
Tween 81	Polyoxyethylene sorbitan monooleate	10.0
Tween 85	Polyoxyethylene sorbitan trioleate	11.0
N/A	Diethylene glycol monolaurate	6.1
N/A	Ethylene glycol distearate	1.5
Pluronic F-68	Poloxamer	17.0
Lauroglycol	Propylene glycol monostearate	3.4
N/A	Sucrose dioleate	7.1

N/A = not applicable.

Emulsifying agents are surfactants that reduce the interfacial tension between oil and water, thereby minimizing the surface energy through the formation of globules. *Wetting agents*, however, aid in attaining intimate contact between solid particles and liquids.

Detergents used in cleaning reduce surface tension and wet a surface as well as any foreign material. When a detergent is used, the foreign material will be emulsified, foaming can occur, and the foreign material will then wash away.

Table 17-4. HLB Ranges of Surfactants

	HLB Range	Surfactants
Low	1–3	Antifoaming agents
	3–6	Emulsifying agents (w/o)
	7–9	Wetting agents
	8–18	Emulsifying agents (o/w)
	13–16	Detergents
High	16–18	Solubilizing agents

Surfactants can act as solubilizing agents by forming micelles. For example, a surfactant with a high HLB would be used to increase the solubility of an oil in an aqueous medium. The lipophilic portion of the surfactant would entrap the oil in the lipophilic (interior) portion of the micelle. The hydrophilic portion of the surfactant surrounding the oil globule would, in turn, be exposed to the aqueous phase.

An HLB value of 10 or higher means that the agent is primarily hydrophilic, whereas an HLB value of less than 10 means it would be lipophilic. For example, Spans have HLB values ranging from 1.8 to 8.6, which is indicative of oil-soluble or oil-dispersible molecules. Consequently, the oil phase will predominate, and a w/o emulsion will be formed. Tweens have HLB values that range from 9.6 to 16.7, which is characteristic of water-soluble or water-dispersible molecules. Therefore, the water phase will predominate, and o/w emulsions will be formed.

Blending of Surfactants

Often a blend of emulsifiers produces a more stable emulsion than does the use of a single emulsifier with a correctly calculated HLB. Because the HLB numbers are additive, the HLB value of a blend can be readily calculated. Table 17-6 lists the required HLB values for some common lipid materials to aid the pharmacist in preparing o/w emulsions.

Surfactants can be blended by direct ratios and proportions. For example, if 20 mL of an agent with an HLB value of 9.65 is required, then two surfactants, one with an HLB value of 8.6 and one with an HLB value of 12.8, can be blended in a 3:1 ratio. The following quantities of each surfactant will be required:

$3/4$	$\times$	8.6	=	6.45	(15 mL)
$1/4$	$\times$	12.8	=	3.20	(5 mL)
Total HLB			=	9.65	(20 mL)

To calculate the HLB required for the emulsifier in the formulation shown below, the following method is used:

		% of Oil Phase	Required HLB		Portion of HLB
Petrolatum	25 g	56 (25 g/45 g) $\times$	8	=	4.5
Cetyl alcohol	20 g	44 (20 g/45 g) $\times$	15	=	6.7
Emulsifier	2 g				
Preservative	0.2 g				
Pure water qs ad	100 g				

Approximate HLB value for emulsifier = 4.5 + 6.7 = 11.2

Table 17-5. Selected Physicochemical Characteristics of Wetting and/or Solubilizing Agents

| Item | Physical State | Solubility | | Container Specifications |
		Water	Alcohol	
Benzalkonium chloride	Gel	VS	VS	T
Benzethonium chloride	Solid	Sol	Sol	T, LR
Cetylpyridinium chloride	Solid	VS	VS	W
Docusate sodium	Solid	SpS	FS	W
Nonoxynol 9	Liquid	Sol	Sol	T
Octoxynol 9	Liquid	Misc	Misc	T
Poloxamer(s)	Solid	FS	FS	T
Polyoxyl 35 castor oil	Liquid	VS	Sol	T
Polyoxyl 40 hydrogenated castor oil	Paste	VS	Sol	T
Polyoxyl 10 oleyl ether	Semisolid/ liquid	Sol	Sol	T
Polyoxyl 20 cetostearyl ether	Solid	Sol	Sol	T
Polyoxyl 40 stearate	Solid	Sol	Sol	T
Polysorbate 20	Liquid	Sol	Sol	T
Polysorbate 40	Liquid	Sol	Sol	T
Polysorbate 60	Liquid/gel	Sol	—	T
Polysorbate 80	Liquid	VS	Sol	T
Sodium lauryl sulfate	Solid	FS	—	W
Sorbitan monolaurate	Liquid	IS	—	T
Sorbitan monooleate	Liquid	IS	—	T
Sorbitan monopalmitate	Solid	IS	[a]	W
Sorbitan monostearate	Solid	[b]	—	W
Tyloxapol	Liquid	Misc	—	T

[a]*Soluble in warm absolute alcohol.*

[b]*Dispersible in warm water.*

Table 17-6. Required HLB Values for Some Common Lipid Materials Used in O/W Emulsions

Lipid Material	Required HLB	
	W/O	O/W
Beeswax	4	9–12
Carbon tetrachloride		16
Carnauba wax	12	
Castor oil	6	14
Cetyl alcohol		15
Cottonseed oil	5	6–10
Kerosene		14
Lanolin, anhydrous	8	10–12
Lauric acid		15–16
Lauryl alcohol		14
Methyl silicone		11
Mineral oil, light/heavy	5	11–12
Oleic acid		17
Olive oil	6	14
Paraffin wax	4	10–11
Petrolatum	5	7–12
Stearic acid	6	15
Stearyl alcohol		14

Preserving an Emulsion

Because emulsions will support microbiological growth, contamination can occur during the preparation stage or during use. To minimize contamination, the work area and equipment should be kept clean, and every attempt should be made to produce an uncontaminated product. However, if the product is going to be stored for any length of time, a preservative may have to be added.

A preservative must be nontoxic, stable, compatible, and inexpensive; in addition, it must have an acceptable taste, odor, and color. It should also be effective against a wide variety of bacteria, fungi, and yeasts.

The preservative should be concentrated in the aqueous phase because bacterial growth will normally occur there. Additionally, because the nonionized form of the preservative is more effective against bacteria than the ionized form, most of the preservative should be in the nonionized state. To be effective, the preservative must be neither bound nor adsorbed to any agent in the emulsion or the container. Preservatives can partition into the oil phase and lose their effectiveness. Examples of preservatives that are often used in emulsions are shown in Table 17-7. The parabens (methylparaben, propylparaben, butylparaben) are considered to be some of the most satisfactory preservatives for emulsions.

Oils and fats can become rancid, which causes the product to have an unpleasant odor, appearance, and taste. Antioxidants can prevent rancidity. The following agents are examples of antioxidants used in emulsions:

‣ Ascorbic acid.
‣ Ascorbyl palmitate.

Table 17-7. Preservatives Used for Emulsions

Preservative	% Concentration
Alcohol	15
Benzoic acid, sodium benzoate (pH ≤ 4)	0.05–0.1
Benzyl alcohol (pH >5)	1–4
Chlorobutanol[a]	0.5
Imidazolidyl urea (Imidurea)	0.05–0.5
Mercurials	0.005
Organic mercurials	
Phenylmercuric nitrate	0.002–0.004
Phenylmercuric acetate	0.002–0.004
Thimerosal	0.005–0.02
Parabens[b]	
Methylparaben	0.05–0.3
Propylparaben	0.02–0.2
Butylparaben	0.02–0.2
Quaternary ammonium compounds	
Benzalkonium chloride	0.002–0.1
Sorbic acid (pH <6)	0.1–0.2

[a]*Chlorobutanol needs a pH <5; it will also sorb to plastic.*

[b]*Generally used in pairs. Low water solubility; poor taste. May degrade at a pH >8. Use at pH 4–8.*

- ‣ Butylated hydroxyanisole.
- ‣ Butylated hydroxytoluene.
- ‣ Gallic acid.
- ‣ 4-Hydroxymethyl-2,6-*di-tert*-butylphenol.
- ‣ Propyl gallate.
- ‣ Sulfites.
- ‣ L-Tocopherol.

Flavoring an Emulsion

When selecting an appropriate flavoring agent, the pharmacist should take into consideration the dispersion medium (external phase) of the emulsion. For example, if a flavoring oil is used and most of the oil partitions into the internal phase as an o/w emulsion, the flavor will be reduced in strength. Oils can be incorporated by using small quantities of surfactants. Usually surfactants with HLB values of 15 to 18 are used, often in conjunction with a surfactant with an HLB value in the range of 8 to 12. As a general rule, it is necessary to have from three to five times as much surfactant as oil (flavoring) to ensure solubilization. For best results, the oil should be mixed with the surfactants before it is added to the aqueous phase. Because this technique can cause the flavor to lose some of its potency, another approach is to use a cosolvent system to incorporate the flavor. The use of ethanol, glycerin, or some appropriate solvent often provides acceptable results.

Determining the Type of Emulsion

The pharmacist should know whether an emulsion is o/w or w/o in case other ingredients must be added. Determining the type of emulsion can be accomplished by some simple tests, including the drop dilution test, dye solubility test, electrical conductivity test, and filter paper test. The drop dilution test is based on the principle that an emulsion is miscible with its external phase. This test is performed by simply dropping a small quantity of the emulsion onto a surface of water. If the drop is miscible with the water, it will spread, indicating that water is the external phase (i.e., an o/w emulsion). The dye solubility test is based on the principle that a dye disperses uniformly throughout an emulsion if it is soluble in the external phase. This test is performed by adding a small quantity of a water-soluble dye (powder or solution) to the emulsion. If the dye diffuses uniformly throughout the emulsion, water is the external phase (i.e., an o/w emulsion). The principle under-lying the electrical conductivity test is that water conducts an electric current and oils do not. Generally, o/w emulsions tend to conduct electricity better than do w/o emulsions, if the required equipment is available. The filter paper test involves putting a drop of emulsion onto a clean piece of filter paper. If the drop spreads rapidly into the filter paper, it is an o/w emulsion, because water (the external phase) tends to spread more rapidly throughout the filter paper than does oil. Table 17-8 lists some commercial emulsion bases and indicates whether they are o/w or w/o emulsions.

Table 17-8. Commercial Emulsion Bases

Product	Type	Emulsifier
Allercreme Skin Lotion	O/W	Triethanolamine stearate
Almay Emulsion Base	O/W	Fatty acid glycol esters
Cetaphil	O/W	Sodium lauryl sulfate
Dermovan	O/W	Fatty acid amides
Eucerin	W/O	Wool wax alcohols
HEB Base	O/W	Sodium lauryl sulfate
Keri Lotion	O/W	Nonionic emulsifiers
Lubriderm	O/W	Triethanolamine stearate
Neobase	O/W	Polyhydric alcohol esters
Neutrogena Lotion	O/W	Triethanolamine lactate
Nivea Cream	W/O	Wool wax alcohols
pHorsix	O/W	Polyoxyethylene emulsifiers
Polysorb Hydrate	W/O	Sorbitan sesquioleate
Velvachol	O/W	Sodium lauryl sulfate

One can prepare a multiple emulsion by adding another external phase to the emulsion. For example, the pharmacist could combine a w/o emulsifier (e.g., sorbitan monooleate) with liquid petrolatum and then add an aqueous phase to form a w/o emulsion. This step would be followed by dispersing an o/w emulsifying agent (e.g., Tween 80) and the original w/o emulsion in an aqueous solution to form a final w/o/w emulsion. An o/w/o emulsion can be prepared in a similar fashion. Possible uses of multiple emulsions include detoxification, drug targeting/localization, prolonged-acting dosage forms, and potential application in cosmetics.

Quality Control

Quality control involves both observing physical attributes and checking calculations. The final volume of the prepared emulsion should be confirmed with the prescription. The physical appearance and smell should be noted and recorded. Observations should include the color of the emulsion and a description of the size of the globules. A microscope can be used to study a portion of the emulsion so that an approximate range of globule sizes can be recorded. The emulsion should be checked for signs of creaming, coalescence, and mold/bacterial growth. Emulsions are subject to chemical degradation, especially when aqueous vehicles are used.

Packaging/Storage/Labeling

It is important to package emulsions in tight containers to minimize the evaporation of water from the product. If the preparation is a liquid, the container should have sufficient headspace to allow shaking of the product. Oral liquids should be packaged in bottles that have an opening large enough to allow easy pouring of the product. Squeeze bottles work fine for topical liquid emulsions, whereas tubes or pump containers work well for viscous creams.

Emulsions should be stored at room temperature or refrigerated. They should be protected from temperature extremes. Their labels should include the instruction "Shake Well."

Stability

Beyond-use dates for water-containing formulations are no later than 14 days, when stored at cold temperatures, for products prepared from ingredients in solid form. These dates can be extended if there is valid scientific information to support stability, as discussed in Chapter 4, "Stability of Compounded Products."

The stability of an emulsion can be enhanced by (1) decreasing the globule size of the internal phase, (2) obtaining an optimum ratio of oil to water, and (3) increasing the viscosity of the system. Because the oil-to-water ratio (concentration of active ingredient:oil) is frequently determined by the referring primary care provider, the compounding pharmacist's efforts to enhance the emulsion's stability are directed at the other two factors.

If the size of the globule is reduced to less than 5 μm, the stability and dispersion of the emulsion will increase. This reduction can be accomplished both with the shearing action of a mortar and pestle and with a homogenizer.

The optimum phase:volume ratio is generally obtained when the internal phase is about 40% to 60% of the total quantity of the product. As the percentage of the internal phase increases, the viscosity of the product will also increase. A linear relationship exists between the viscosity of the emulsion and the viscosity of the continuous or external phase. The viscosity of an emulsion generally increases on aging.

Enhancing the viscosity of the external phase will tend to enhance the stability of the emulsion. To improve the viscosity, the pharmacist can add a substance that is soluble in or miscible with the external phase of the emulsion. In the case of o/w emulsions, hydrocolloids can be used, whereas for w/o emulsions, waxes and viscous oils as well as fatty alcohols and fatty acids are appropriate.

Of major importance to the compounding pharmacist is the physical stability of the emulsion. The emulsion is stable when it retains its original appearance, odor, color, and other physical properties and when no creaming or coalescence occurs.

Creaming

Creaming occurs when the globules flocculate and concentrate in one specific part of the emulsion. This action creates an unsightly product and causes the drug to be distributed unevenly. In o/w emulsions, creaming can be identified when one sees the oil globules gather and rise to the top. This situation occurs because the oil is generally less dense than the water phase. Creaming is easily reversible because the dispersed globules are still surrounded by the protective film. In some cases shaking can redistribute the emulsion.

Three methods that are used to minimize creaming are (1) to enhance the viscosity of the external aqueous phase, (2) to reduce the size of the globules to a very fine state with a homogenizer, and (3) to adjust the densities of both the internal and the external phases so that their densities are the same. Thus, neither phase would tend to rise to the top or settle at the bottom.

Coalescence

Contrary to creaming, coalescence (i.e., breaking) is an irreversible process because the film that surrounds the individual globules is destroyed. Altering the viscosity may help to stabilize globules and to minimize their tendency to coalesce. An optimum viscosity can be determined experimentally.

Another factor is the phase:volume ratio, or the ratio of the internal volume to the total volume of the product. The maximum phase:volume ratio that can be achieved is 74%, assuming that the particles are perfectly spherical. In general, a phase:volume ratio of about 50%, which approximates loose packing of spherical particles (i.e., a porosity of 48% of the total bulk volume of a powder), yields a reasonably stable emulsion.

Phase Inversion

Phase inversion occurs when an emulsion inverts from one form to another, that is, from o/w to w/o or w/o to o/w. Phase inversion, which is the basis for the Continental Method of emulsion preparation described earlier, can result in the formation of a better emulsion. Monovalent cations tend to form o/w emulsions, whereas divalent cations tend to form w/o emulsions. If sodium stearate is used to form an o/w emulsion and then a calcium salt is added to form calcium stearate, the emulsion inverts from an o/w to a w/o type. The Continental Method uses a small proportion of water in the presence of a large proportion of oil. The nucleus of the initial emulsion, or primary emulsion, is of the w/o type; however, when water is added in small quantities, the emulsion inverts to an o/w type.

Patient Counseling

The patient should be instructed on how to shake the emulsion and how to measure the required dose. Instruction should also be provided on the proper recapping and storage of the bottle, as well as on how to determine if the emulsion has become physically unstable.

Sample Formulations

R_X Ivermectin 0.8% Cream Rinse

Ivermectin		480 mg
Polyethylene glycol 300		10 mL
Hair conditioner/cream rinse	qs	60 mL

1. Calculate the quantity of each ingredient required for the prescription.
2. Accurately weigh or measure each ingredient.
3. Add the ivermectin powder to the polyethylene glycol 300 and mix well.
4. Incorporate sufficient commercial cream rinse product to make 60 mL and mix well.
5. Package and label.

(Note: Most hair conditioners/cream rinses are o/w emulsions.)

R_X Dry Skin and Massage Lotion

Safflower oil		30 mL
Glycerin		20 mL
Rose oil (or other oil)		2 mL
Polysorbate 80		2 mL
Benzyl alcohol		1 mL
Purified water	qs	100 mL

1. Calculate the quantity of each ingredient required for the prescription.
2. Accurately measure each ingredient.
3. Mix the safflower oil, rose oil, and polysorbate 80.
4. Mix the glycerin with the benzyl alcohol, and add 45 mL of purified water to form the aqueous phase.
5. Add the oil–polysorbate 80 mixture to the aqueous phase and mix well.
6. Use a hand homogenizer or a high-speed mixer, if available, to enhance the emulsification process.
7. Package and label.

Chapter 18

Ointments, Creams, and Pastes

Topical dosage forms have been used throughout human history; for instance, ointments are mentioned in the Bible on many occasions. These dosage forms, which include salves, ointments, pastes, and compresses, are used to deliver a drug topically to the skin to treat various disorders.

Topically applied pharmaceuticals have three main functions: (1) to protect the injured area from the environment and permit the skin to rejuvenate, (2) to provide skin with hydration or to produce an emollient effect, and (3) to convey a medication to the skin for a specific effect, either topically or systemically. If the dosage form is a semisolid, how much of the drug penetrates the skin is determined by (1) the amount of pressure applied and the vigor with which it is rubbed, (2) the surface area covered, (3) the condition of the skin, (4) the base used, and (5) the use of occlusive dressings.

Definitions/Types

Ointments are semisolid preparations that are intended to be applied externally to the skin or mucous membranes. Ointments soften or melt at body temperature; they should spread easily and should not be gritty.

Creams are opaque, soft solids or thick liquids intended for external application. Creams consist of medications dissolved or suspended in water-soluble or vanishing cream bases and can be either a water-in-oil (w/o) or an oil-in-water (o/w) type of emulsion. The term *cream* is most frequently applied to soft, cosmetically acceptable types of preparations.

Pastes are thick, stiff ointments that ordinarily do not flow at body temperature and thus protectively coat the areas to which they are applied. They usually contain at least 20% solids.

Historical Use

The Greek word *miron* and the Latin word *unguentum* were combined to form the modern word *ointment*. Early ointments were primarily oils that were used as anointing preparations. Changes in early ointment preparations resulted in the development of pastes (preparations with a high content of solids), cerates (preparations with a high content of waxes), and creams (emulsified ointments).

Applications

The decision to use an ointment, a paste, a cream, or a lotion (emulsion) depends not only on considerations of how much skin penetration of the medication is desired but also on the characteristics of the skin to which the product is being applied. For example, ointments (oleaginous bases) are generally used on dry, scaly lesions because their emollient properties will aid in rehydrating the skin. They also stay on the skin longer. Ointments are formulated as topical, rectal, and ophthalmic preparations. Pastes are topical preparations that are typically applied to an area that requires protection. Creams are usually applied to moist, weeping lesions because they have a "drying" effect in that the lesions' fluids are miscible with the aqueous external phase of creams. Creams are formulated as topical, rectal, and vaginal preparations. Because of their lubricating effect, lotions are generally applied to intertriginous areas, that is, areas where the skin rubs together, such as between the fingers, between the thighs, or under the arms. Based on these considerations, the pharmacist should not substitute one of these dosage forms for another without the consent of the prescriber.

Topical ointment bases are classified according to two different methods: (1) the degree of skin penetration and (2) the relationship of water to the composition of the base. These methods are summarized in Tables 18-1 and 18-2.

Table 18-1. Classification of Ointment Bases Based on Skin Penetration

Base Type	Skin Penetration	Example Bases
Epidermic[a]	None or very little	Oleaginous
Endodermic[b]	Into the dermis	Absorption
Diadermic[c]	Yes, into and through the skin	Emulsion, water soluble

[a]*Epidermic refers to the external layer of the skin, or epidermis.*
[b]*Endodermic refers to the internal layer of the skin, or dermis.*
[c]*Diadermic refers to going through the skin.*

Composition

In addition to the active drug, ingredients in topical preparations can include stiffeners, oleaginous components, aqueous components, emulsifying agents, humectants, preservatives, penetration enhancers, and antioxidants. Some of these ingredients will be discussed in greater detail in the "Preparation" and "Physicochemical Considerations" sections.

Stiffeners generally include waxes that have high melting points (e.g., white wax). The waxes blend into oleaginous bases to enhance the viscosity of a preparation.

Humectants, such as glycerin, propylene glycol, or polyethylene glycol (PEG) 300, can be added to a preparation to decrease the evaporation rate of water from the preparation, especially just after its application to the skin.

Antioxidants, such as butylated hydroxy toluene, are sometimes required to delay the rate of rancidification of selected bases.

Penetration (absorption) enhancers are agents that can interact sufficiently with the active drug and the stratum corneum to increase the rate of penetration of a drug through the skin.

Table 18-2. Classification and Characteristics of Ointment Bases

Base Type	Characteristic	Example
Oleaginous	Insoluble in water Not water washable Will not absorb water Emollient Occlusive Greasy	White petrolatum White ointment
Absorption	Insoluble in water Not water washable Anhydrous Can absorb water Emollient Occlusive Greasy	Hydrophilic petrolatum Aquabase Aquaphor
W/O emulsion	Insoluble in water Not water washable Will absorb water Contains water Emollient Occlusive Greasy	Cold cream Lanolin, hydrous Hydrocream Eucerin Nivea
O/W emulsion	Insoluble in water Water washable Will absorb water Contains water Nonocclusive Nongreasy	Hydrophilic ointment Dermabase Velvachol Unibase
Water soluble	Water soluble Water washable Will absorb water Anhydrous or hydrous Nonocclusive Nongreasy	PEG ointment

Preparation

Most of the techniques discussed here are directed toward incorporating ingredients into commercially prepared bases. If a base must be extemporaneously prepared from individual ingredients, the principles discussed in Chapter 17, "Emulsions," will apply, as well as those discussed later.

Manual Methods of Preparation

Manual methods of ointment preparation primarily involve using a pill tile and spatula or a mortar and pestle. Ointment pads and various hard, clean surfaces have also been used. Ointment pads, however, can absorb moisture and tear unless one works quickly. The surface used must be clean and nonshedding and should provide for ease of mixing. The advantage of a pill tile is that it can be used for particle size reduction as well as for mixing the ointment. Pill tiles are easy to clean and should allow no carryover of materials from one preparation to the next. In some situations, mixing in a plastic bag is convenient and less messy.

Mechanical Methods of Preparation

To prepare large quantities of ointments, the pharmacist may want to invest in mixers, which range from handheld propeller types to kitchen mixers with paddles or blades. In fact, if regular supply sources do not have the type of equipment desired, the pharmacist may find it at gourmet kitchen shops, which are excellent sources of unusual equipment. Electronic mortars and pestles (the Unguator) are gaining widespread acceptance and offer the advantage of mixing and dispensing in the same container.

Preparation of Oleaginous Bases

White petrolatum and white ointment are examples of oleaginous bases. Official ointment bases are shown in Table 18-3. An example of an extemporaneously prepared prescription using an oleaginous base is 5% sulfur in white petrolatum.

The preparation of an oleaginous-based ointment is rather simple. After obtaining the desired quantities of the individual ingredients, the pharmacist finely pulverizes the powder on a pill tile with a spatula. When incorporating insoluble

Table 18-3. Selected Physicochemical Characteristics and Packaging for Official Ointment Bases

Vehicle	Melting Point (°C)	Specific Gravity	Container Specifications
Diethylene glycol monoethyl ether	—	0.991	T
Lanolin	38–44	0.932–0.945[a]	W
Ointment, hydrophilic	—	—	T
Ointment, white	—	—	W
Ointment, yellow	—	—	W
Polyethylene glycol ointment	—	—	W
Petrolatum	38–60	0.815–0.880[b]	W
Petrolatum, hydrophilic	—	—	W
Petrolatum, white	38–60	0.815–0.880[b]	W
Rose water ointment	—	—	T, LR
Squalane	—	0.807–0.810	T
Vegetable oil, hydrogenated, type II	20–50	—	T

[a]At 15°C.
[b]At 60°C.

Table 18-4. Levigating Agents for Use in Preparing Ointments

Aqueous Systems and O/W Dispersions

Agent	Specific Gravity
Glycerin	1.25
Propylene glycol	1.04
PEG 400	1.13

Oleaginous Systems and W/O Dispersions

Agent	Specific Gravity
Castor oil	0.96
Cottonseed oil	0.92
Mineral oil, heavy	0.88
Mineral oil, light	0.85
Tween 80	—

powders by using a levigating agent, the pharmacist should follow the technique of geometric dilution to ensure that the active ingredient is thoroughly mixed with the vehicle. For example, a few drops of mineral oil can be used to levigate sulfur before it is mixed with white petrolatum. The sulfur–mineral oil mixture would be mixed with an equal quantity of white petrolatum. Then more white petrolatum equal in quantity to the new mixture would be added; the process is repeated until all of the white petrolatum has been added. A levigating agent can also be used with a small quantity of melted base. Examples of levigating agents are shown in Table 18-4.

Heat should be used when preparing a base containing ingredients with high melting points. Generally, a water bath or direct heat is used. Water baths are used for low-temperature applications, whereas direct heat is used for preparations that require higher temperatures. When using direct heat (a hot plate), the pharmacist must be careful not to scorch the product. Microwaves can be used either to heat the product directly or to heat the water for preparing a water bath. Using a microwave with a carousel will minimize the occurrence of "hot spots," which are areas with high temperatures caused by uneven heating. When heat is used, materials with the highest melting points are placed in a container that has been set on the heat source. The container is heated until the materials melt. The rest of the ingredients are then added according to their decreasing melting points, beginning with the highest and moving downward. The product is thoroughly mixed and then cooled. During the cooling process, the product is stirred occasionally; however, cooling should not be too rapid because the product can become lumpy. When cool, the product is packaged and labeled.

Oleaginous bases are often used to prepare pastes. Heat makes the preparation process easier by allowing a high percentage of powders to be introduced into the base. The product must be stirred thoroughly during the cooling process, however, to prevent the solids from settling.

Stiffening Agents

Many pharmaceutical preparations require the adjustment of viscosity, or "stiffness" to produce the desired characteristics that can make them useful and acceptable by patients. Ointments, creams (emulsions), medication sticks, pastes, suppositories, and other dosage forms can require stiffening agents. Generally, stiffening agents have higher melting points (generally greater than about 50°C but less than about 100°C) and, when blended with materials with lower melting points, will raise the lower melting point materials to within an acceptable range for patient use. Excessive quantities, however, will produce a product that will not melt or soften appropriately and will produce a stiff or grainy product.

The term *stiffening agents* is ordinarily applied to oleaginous ingredients, such as those included in this collection. Their incorporation into dosage forms usually involves the use of heat. Generally, it is advisable to have the different phases of a product heated to approximately the same temperature before combining them to prevent premature solidification, which might occur if, for example, a melt of a wax is poured into a cool aqueous mixture. When combining materials with different melting points, it is often best to first melt the material with the highest melting point and then add the lower melting point materials as the temperature is lowered. This process minimizes the necessity of bringing all materials up to the melting point of the highest ingredient. Stiffening agents for ointments are listed in Table 18-5.

Preparation of Absorption Bases

If a w/o emulsifying agent is added to an oleaginous base, an absorption base is formed. Examples of these bases include hydrophilic petrolatum, Aquabase, and Aquaphor. Example prescriptions include 1% hydrocortisone incorporated into Aquabase and 3% crude coal tar/3% polysorbate 80 in Aquabase.

Ointments using an absorption base can be prepared by using the same techniques as with an oleaginous base, that is, incorporation directly into the base or with the use of heat. Other options, however, depend on the material(s) to be incorporated. Levigation can be used to incorporate a water-insoluble powder. For absorption bases, such as Aquabase or Aquaphor, the choice of the levigating agent depends on where the drug should be, that is, in the external phase or in the internal phase if water is going to be added to the base. In the latter case, water, glycerin, alcohol, or propylene glycol can generally be used and should be taken up into the internal phase of the finished product. Mineral oil can be used if the ingredient should stay in the continuous phase of the product.

Before a water-soluble ingredient is added, it should be dissolved in a small quantity of water. The water can then be incorporated into the base by using either a pill tile and spatula or a mortar and pestle. If large quantities of water or an aqueous solution are to be incorporated, using heat can be the best approach. It may be necessary to add an additional emulsifying agent and a preservative. The preservative would be needed because water will usually support microbial growth. Another alternative would be to assign a short expiration date, such as 2 weeks. The base can be melted by using a water bath, after which the aqueous phase is added by stirring. The final product should be stirred continuously during cooling.

Preparation of W/O Emulsion Bases

Water-in-oil emulsion bases can be prepared by adding water to an absorption base. Commercial preparations are also available. They include Hydrocream, Eucerin, Nivea, and cold cream. An example of an extemporaneous preparation is 2% miconazole in Hydrocream.

Table 18-5. Physical Properties of *United States Pharmacopeia 25/National Formulary 20* Stiffening Agents

Substance	Melting Range (°C)	Flashpoint Range (°C)	Density (g/mL)	Solubility				
				Water	Alcohol	Chloroform	Ether	Fixed Oils
Castor oil, hydrogenated	85–88	316	1.023	IS	—	Sol	—	—
Cetostearyl alcohol	48–55	150	0.820	PrIn	Sol	—	Sol	—
Cetyl alcohol	46–52	—	0.907	PrIn	FS	—	Sol	Misc
Cetyl esters wax	43–47	—	0.830	PrIn	PrIn	Sol	—	Sol
Hard fat	27–44	—	—	PrIn	SlS	—	FS	—
Paraffin	—	—	—	IS	IS	FS	FS	FS
Synthetic paraffin	—	—	—	—	—	SlS	—	—
Stearyl alcohol	55–60	191	0.812	PrIn	Sol	Sol	Sol	Sol
Wax, emulsifying	50–54	>55	0.940	IS	Sol	FS	FS	—
Wax, white	62–65	245–258	0.955	PrIn	SpS	Sol	FS	Sol
Wax, yellow	62–65	245–258	0.955	PrIn	SpS	Sol	FS	Sol

Oils and insoluble powders can be incorporated directly by using a pill tile and spatula or a mortar and pestle. A levigating agent may be needed if large amounts of insoluble powders are required. If Hydrocream or Eucerin is used as the base, the levigating agent should be miscible with the oil phase (i.e., mineral oil).

In many of the w/o emulsion bases, however, sufficient surfactant is available to further emulsify a reasonable quantity of an aqueous solution of a drug, which can be incorporated by using a pill tile with a spatula or a mortar and pestle or gentle heat from a water bath. When using heat, the pharmacist should make sure that the preparation is not held at a high temperature for too long, because a loss of water can occur. This loss results in a thicker ointment/cream.

Preparation of O/W Emulsion Bases

Oil-in-water emulsion bases are usually elegant preparations and are known as the "vanishing cream" types of preparations because they disappear, or vanish, on application. These bases include Dermabase, Velvachol, and hydrophilic ointment USP. Various concentrations of triamcinolone, urea, or retinoic acid have been included in these bases as extemporaneous preparations.

Insoluble powders and aqueous solutions can be incorporated by using a pill tile and spatula or a mortar and pestle. Water-soluble materials can be added by dissolving the powder in a small quantity of water and incorporating the solution into the base. A small quantity of an oil can be directly incorporated into the base, as there is usually excess emulsifying agent. If a larger amount of an oil is required, it may be necessary to add a little o/w surfactant to help the oil disperse uniformly throughout the vehicle.

If an o/w emulsion base, such as Dermabase or Velvachol, is used, the levigating agent should be water, glycerin, propylene glycol, PEG 300 or 400, alcohol, or some liquid that is miscible with water.

If heat is used to incorporate an ingredient into an o/w vehicle, the pharmacist must work quickly because water can be lost rather rapidly from the product. This loss could make the product stiff and waxy, thereby causing it to lose its elegant character.

To prevent an o/w emulsion from drying too rapidly on the skin, the pharmacist can add a humectant such as glycerin, propylene glycol, 70% sorbitol, or PEG 300 or 400 to the formulation in a concentration of around 2% to 5%.

Preparation of Water-Soluble Bases

PEG 400 (600 g) and PEG 3350 (400 g) are examples of water-soluble bases. Incorporating 20% benzocaine into any of these bases yields a nice ointment that can be easily removed by washing. Water-soluble ingredients can be dissolved in a small quantity of water and mixed with the base by using a pill tile and spatula or a mortar and pestle. Insoluble powders can be levigated with a small quantity of PEG 300, glycerin, or propylene glycol and then mixed with the base. To enhance stability, the pharmacist should mix an intermediate solvent such as glycerin or propylene glycol with oils before they are incorporated into a water-soluble base. If large quantities of water or aqueous solutions are to be added, the use of gentle heat or a water bath to prepare the product can be preferable.

The box "Hints for Compounding Ointments, Creams, and Pastes" provides additional suggestions for preparing these dosage forms.

Hints for Compounding Ointments, Creams, and Pastes

Ointments

- Mixtures of two or more ointments can be combined by mixing them in a plastic bag.
- Ointments can be removed from plastic bags and placed directly into tubes by cutting one corner of the plastic bag and squeezing the contents directly into the ointment tube or jar. This step makes cleanup very easy.
- A few drops of mineral oil or other suitable solvent can enhance the workability of drugs that build up electrostatic forces, such as sulfur.
- Volatile solvents should not be used when levigating powders, because the solvent will evaporate and leave crystals of drug behind.
- When oil and aqueous phases are mixed together, it is helpful to heat the aqueous phase a few degrees higher than the oil phase before mixing. The aqueous phase tends to cool faster than the oil phase.
- Ointments should be cooled until just a few degrees above solidification before they are poured into tubes or jars. This step will minimize "layering" of the ointment in the packaging.
- Heat softens ointments and makes filling jars and tubes easier. Heating must be done cautiously to prevent stratification of the ingredients.
- When a base is being prepared, the ingredient with the highest melting point should be melted first, and then the heat should be gradually reduced. The remaining ingredients should be added in the order of the highest to lowest melting point until a uniform mixture is obtained. This process will ensure that the ingredients will be exposed to the lowest possible temperature during the preparation process and thus will enhance the stability of the final product.
- If a water-containing base is used and the drug is water soluble, the drug should be dissolved in a minimum quantity of water before incorporating it into the base.

Creams

- Whether an emulsion is o/w or w/o can be determined by placing a drop of the emulsion on the surface of water. If the drop spreads out, it is of the o/w type because the external phase of the emulsion is miscible or continuous with water. If the emulsion remains in a "ball," it is probably of the w/o type because of immiscibility.
- If no active drugs are present, creams can be softened by heating in a microwave for a short time at a low power setting.
- A humectant, such as glycerin, propylene glycol, sorbitol 70%, or PEG 300 or 400, added to a cream will minimize evaporation. These humectants can be added in a 2% to 5% concentration.
- Use of low heat when preparing creams will minimize evaporation of water.
- Hand homogenizers can aid in preparing emulsions.
- Generally, the smaller the globule size, the more stable will be the emulsion.
- Before volatile oils are added, it is best to cool the preparation. Temperatures of less than 78°C work well with many bases. If alcoholic solutions of flavors are to be added, the preparation should be cooled below the boiling point of alcohol before the addition takes place.
- The quantity of surfactant required to prepare a good emulsion is generally about 0.5% to 5% of the total volume.
- Lotions can often be prepared from creams (o/w emulsions) by diluting the cream with water or an aromatic water such as rose water. To do this task

Hints for Compounding Ointments, Creams, and Pastes (cont.)

successfully, the pharmacist usually must add the water slowly while stirring continuously. This process will also dilute the preservative, however, which could lead to bacterial growth. Therefore, a short beyond-use date should be assigned to this product.

Pastes

- Levigating agents are generally not used when preparing pastes that are characterized by relatively high percentages of solids. The easiest method of preparing pastes involves the fusion technique (heat). Heat improves the workability of pastes.
- Products prepared by using fusion should be cooled before they are placed in tubes or jars. If poured while hot, they tend to separate on cooling. They should be cooled to the temperature at which they are viscous fluids and then poured into containers.
- If a product is too stiff and difficult to apply, the pharmacist should decrease the concentration of the waxy components.

General Considerations

- Insoluble materials need to be in a very fine state of subdivision before incorporation into the base or vehicle.
- Levigating agents must be compatible with the vehicle used. For oleaginous bases, a small quantity of the base (melted or at room temperature) or mineral oil works best. For absorption bases, it depends on where the drug should be (i.e., in the external or internal phase if water is going to be added to the base). Generally, water, glycerin, alcohol, or propylene glycol can be used and should be taken into the internal phase of the finished product. Mineral oil can be used if the ingredient should stay in the continuous phase of the product.

  For emulsion bases, the levigating agent should generally be selected based on the external phase of the emulsion. For example, if an o/w emulsion base is used, the levigating agent should be water, glycerin, propylene glycol, PEG 300, alcohol, or some liquid that is miscible with water.

  If a w/o emulsion base is used, the levigating agent should be miscible with the oil phase (i.e., mineral oil). For PEG ointment and other water-soluble bases, water, glycerin, or propylene glycol can be used.
- When insoluble powders are incorporated by using a levigating agent, the technique of geometric dilution should be followed to ensure thorough mixing of the active ingredient with the vehicle. For example, a few drops of mineral oil can be used to levigate sulfur before mixing with white petrolatum. The sulfur—mineral oil mixture would be mixed with an equal quantity of white petrolatum. Then another quantity of white petrolatum equal to the new mixture would be added, and the process repeated until all the white petrolatum was added.
- When incorporating soluble powders, use solvents that have low vapor pressure (e.g., water, glycerin, and propylene glycol). Volatile solvents should not generally be used, especially in oleaginous bases, because the solvent may evaporate and the drug may, in turn, be crystallized out in the base and cause irritation on application to the skin.
- Before adding volatile ingredients, whether flavors or active drugs, cool the product a little. The melt should still be fluid, but not hot, to allow uniform mixing without evaporative loss of ingredients. Temperatures less than 78°C work well with many bases, but lower temperatures would be required if alcohol and volatile materials were present.

Hints for Compounding Ointments, Creams, and Pastes (cont.)

- When working with aqueous systems, use heat for as short a time and as low a temperature as feasible. This action will minimize the quantity of water lost through evaporation.
- If a product is too stiff and difficult to apply, try decreasing the concentration of the waxy components.
- Generally, drugs can be incorporated into ointments, creams, and pastes easily on a pill tile with a spatula. If large quantities of solids are to be incorporated, it may be advisable to use heat to melt the base before incorporating the drug.
- For maximum stability, keep the product anhydrous, if possible.
- Unless otherwise instructed, when a pharmacist is adding several powders to a topical vehicle, it is best to add the powders one at a time with thorough mixing after each addition. This action ensures maximum stability and uniformity of the final product.

Physicochemical Considerations

Problems involved in ointment preparation include drug degradation, discoloration, the separation of ointment components, and the development of a rancid odor. To check whether problems with incompatibility are possible, the pharmacist should refer to the appropriate information sources. Because potent products are now being used topically, preparing an ineffective product can be expensive and wasteful.

One potential problem involves Plastibase (Squibb). When compounding a product that uses Plastibase, the pharmacist should not apply heat, as Plastibase will not regain its viscosity on cooling. Plastibase is a shock-cooled product consisting of mineral oil gelled with polyethylene.

Absorption Enhancers

Absorption enhancers facilitate the absorption of drugs through the skin. These excipients have attracted more attention in the general scientific literature as the transdermal route of administration has grown more popular. It appears that some of these materials have a direct effect on the permeability of the skin, whereas others augment percutaneous absorption by increasing the thermodynamic activity of the penetrant, thus creating a greater concentration gradient across the skin. Absorption enhancers that have a direct effect can be either common or not-so-common chemicals, including solvents, surfactants, and chemicals such as urea and N,N-diethyl-m-toluamide.

Because of its occlusive nature, water is the most prevalent absorption enhancer, even in "anhydrous" systems. The classic absorption enhancer is dimethyl sulfoxide. Other solvents, such as laurocapram (Azone), have been shown to be quite effective, even in concentrations below 5%, because they are retained in the stratum corneum for a period of time, which prolongs their effect.

Surfactants also function as absorption enhancers, but they can cause irritation, thereby limiting their usefulness. Examples of absorption enhancers used in ointments and creams are shown in Table 18-6.

Table 18-6. Examples of Penetration-Enhancing Agents

Water

Alcohols (methanol, ethanol, propanol, butanol, pentanol, benzyl alcohol, hexanol, octanol, nonanol, decanol, 2-butanol, 2-pentanol)

Fatty alcohols (caprylic, decyl, lauryl, 2-lauryl, myristyl, cetyl, stearyl, oleyl, linoleyl, linolenyl alcohols)

Fatty acids (valeric, heptanoic, pelagonic, caproic, capric, lauric, myristic, stearic, oleic, caprylic, isovaleric, neopentanoic, neoheptanoic, neononanoic, trimethyl hexanoic, neodecanoic, isosteric)

Fatty acid esters (aliphatic: isopropyl n-butyrate, isopropyl n-hexanoate, isopropyl n-decanoate, isopropyl myristate, isopropyl palmitate, octyldodecyl myristate)

Alkyl (ethyl acetate, butyl acetate, methyl acetate, methyl valerate, methyl propionate, diethyl sebacate, ethyl oleate)

Polyols (propylene glycol, polyethylene glycol, ethylene glycol, diethylene glycol, triethylene glycol, dipropylene glycol, glycerol, propanediol, butanediol, pentanediol, hexanetrio)

Alkyl methyl sulfoxides (dimethyl sulfoxide, decylmethyl sulfoxide, tetradecyl methyl sulfoxide)

Pyrrolidones (2-pyrrolidone, N-methyl-2-pyrrolidone, N-(2-hydroxyethyl) pyrrolidone)

Anionic surfactants (docusate sodium, sodium lauryl sulfate, sodium laurate)

Cationic surfactants (quaternary ammonium salts, benzalkonium chloride, cetylpyridinium chloride)

Amphoteric surfactants (lecithins, cephalins, alkylbetamines)

Nonionic surfactants (monoglycerides, diglycerides, and triglycerides; poloxamers; Miglyol; Spans; Tweens)

Bile salts (sodium cholate; sodium salts of taurocholic, glycolic, desoxycholic acids)

Organic acids (salicylic acid, citric acid, succinic acid)

Amides (urea, dimethyl acetamide, diethyltoluamide, dimethyl formamide, dimethyl octamide, dimethyl decamide, diethanolamide, triethanolamide)

Water Repellents

Silicon-containing personal care products were introduced in 1950 with Revlon's "Silicare." The benefits of incorporating silicone into topical preparations continue to expand, and this expansion is partly due to their safety and positive performance characteristics. The silicones are widely used as water-repelling agents, as well as in many topical formulations. They lubricate without feeling oily, reduce "stickiness" or that "tacky" feeling associated with many lotions and creams, provide for water-repelling characteristics, and enhance and stabilize "foams." A list of official water-repelling agents is shown in Table 18-7.

Preservation

Unless water is present in the product, there is generally no need to incorporate a preservative into an ointment. If the product does contain water, however, as in the case of emulsion bases, a preservative would normally be required. Selecting a preservative and determining the concentration required to preserve the product are sometimes difficult. (See Chapter 17, "Emulsions," for additional information on preserving this type of product.)

Table 18-7. Selected Physicochemical Characteristics and Packaging for Official Silicones

Silicone	Nominal Viscosity (centistoke)	Specific Gravity	Refractive Index	Container Specifications
Cyclomethicone NF	—	—	—	T
Dimethicone	20	0.946–0.954	1.3980–1.4020	T
	100	0.962–0.970	1.4005–1.4045	
	200	0.964–0.972	1.4013–1.4053	
	350	0.965–0.973	1.4013–1.4053	
	500	0.967–0.975	1.4013–1.4053	
	1000	0.967–0.975	1.4013–1.4053	
	12,500	—	1.4015–1.4055	
	30,000	0.969–0.977	1.4010–1.4100	
Silicone USP	575	0.967	1.402	T

Quality Control

Quality control involves checking the final product for the following characteristics: final product weight, visual appearance, color, odor, viscosity, pH, homogeneity/phase separation, particle size distribution, and texture. The pharmacist should document the observations as a product record. (See Standard Operating Procedure (SOP) "Quality Assessment of Ointments/Creams/Pastes."

Packaging/Storage/Labeling

Ointments can generally be packaged in tubes and jars. Creams can be packaged in tubes and jars as well as in syringes, applicators, and pump dispensers. Because of their high viscosity, pastes are generally dispensed in jars. It is usually best to minimize the headspace in a container to decrease loss of water and the tendency toward rancidity. Pump dispensers, tubes, syringes, push-button plastic jars, and applicators are generally preferable to standard jars because the latter tend to

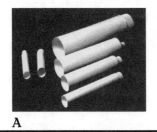 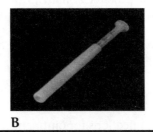 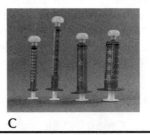

A   B   C

Figure 18-1. Packaging devices for ointments and creams: *A*, collapsible plastic ointment tubes; *B*, calibrated vaginal cream applicator; *C*, syringes with tip caps.

become contaminated easily. Figure 18-1 shows some of the devices commonly used to package these dosage forms.

Ointments should generally be kept at room temperature and away from excessive heat. Labeling of preparations should be appropriate for the mode of administration.

Stability

Ointments are relatively stable, especially if they are in an oleaginous, anhydrous absorption, or anhydrous, water-soluble base. If water is present, as in the emulsion bases, the product is often less stable. Both physical stability (appearance, feel, odor, color) and chemical stability (the active drug and the base ingredients) must be considered. Because the base ingredients are relatively stable, the stability of the active drug is a major determinant of the product's overall stability. In projecting a beyond-use date, one can usually look at commercial products containing the active drug to get a reasonable approximation. It is always best to be conservative when establishing the beyond-use date for an extemporaneously prepared product, especially if water is present, because water supports microbial growth. Generally, only a 2-week supply should be dispensed if the preparation contains water and lacks a preservative.

Ointments are best packaged in tubes or in syringes, if feasible. Such packaging leaves minimal space for air, and the product can be kept clean during administration. Ointment jars, although widely used, expose the preparation to air when opened and to microbial contamination, particularly when ointment is removed with the fingers. One means to lessen contamination is to use an implement similar to a tongue depressor to remove the required quantity of ointment from a jar for application. Pharmacies that prepare large quantities of ointments often use plastic tubes and a tube sealer.

When determining the stability of an ointment, the pharmacist should observe such physical attributes as changes in consistency and separation of a liquid, the formation of granules or grittiness, and drying. For creams, one should take note of emulsion breakage, crystal growth, shrinkage resulting from water loss, and gross microbial contamination. Ointments and emulsions are susceptible to chemical degradation, especially when water is present. Information on chemical stability is generally obtained from the literature or from other appropriate sources. Beyond-use dates for water-containing formulations are no later than 14 days, when stored at cold temperatures, for products prepared from ingredients in solid form. These dates can be extended if valid scientific information is available to support the stability of the product, as discussed in Chapter 4, "Stability of Compounded Products." If a manufactured product is used to prepare nonaqueous liquids or anhydrous preparations, the beyond-use date is 25% of the time remaining on the product's expiration date or 6 months, whichever is earlier. If the product is prepared from USP/NF ingredients, a beyond-use date of 6 months is appropriate, unless evidence is available to support other dating.

Patient Counseling

Counseling for proper applications for ointments, creams, and pastes may differ depending on the dosage form, active ingredients, and desired therapeutic outcomes. Generally, only a thin film of an ointment or a cream is desired. A sufficient quantity is removed from the container and applied and gently rubbed into the area, unless otherwise indicated. Instruct the patient not to wash the area for a few hours to allow the drug to have sufficient time to have an effect. Pastes are often placed on an area but not necessarily rubbed in, because of their viscosity. Pastes are generally used for a protectant effect and should not be removed until indicated. Removal of creams (o/w) is relatively easy by using warm water and, if necessary, soap. Removal of ointments and pastes will require warm water, soap, and some mechanical action. If the area is covered, for example, by clothing, it may be advisable to use a protective pad over the area to prevent the preparation from being removed by the clothing. Usually, it is best to continue using the preparation for a short while after the symptoms or injury has been resolved, depending on the specific situation.

Unless otherwise indicated, ointments, creams, and pastes should be stored at room temperature away from children, heat, and direct sunlight.

Sample Formulations

Bases

 White Ointment

White wax	50 g
White petrolatum	950 g

1. Calculate the quantity of each ingredient required for the prescription.
2. Accurately weigh each ingredient.
3. Put the white wax in a suitable container and melt the wax, using a water bath.
4. Add the white petrolatum and mix until uniform.
5. Cool, package, and label.

 Hydrophilic Petrolatum

Cholesterol	30 g
Stearyl alcohol	30 g
White wax	80 g
White petrolatum	860 g

1. Calculate the quantity of each ingredient required for the prescription.
2. Accurately weigh each ingredient.
3. Place the stearyl alcohol, white wax, and white petrolatum in a suitable container and melt the ingredients, using a water bath.
4. Add the cholesterol and stir until the mixture is blended completely.
5. Remove the mixture from the bath and stir until congealed.
6. Package and label.

Cold Cream

Cetyl esters wax	125 g	7,5
White wax	120 g	7,2
Mineral oil	560 g	33,6
Sodium borate	5 g	0,3
Purified water	190 mL	11,4
		60g

1. Calculate the quantity of each ingredient required for the prescription.
2. Accurately weigh or measure each ingredient.
3. Reduce the cetyl esters wax and the white wax to small pieces; melt the pieces, using a water bath.
4. Add the mineral oil and continue heating the mixture until it reaches 70°C.
5. Dissolve the sodium borate in the purified water, which has been warmed to 70°C. Add the warm mixture gradually to the melted oleaginous mixture.
6. Remove the mixture from the heat; stir rapidly and continuously until the mixture has congealed.
7. Package and label.

Hydrophilic Ointment

Methylparaben		0.25 g
Propylparaben		0.15 g
Sodium lauryl sulfate		10 g
Propylene glycol		120 g
Stearyl alcohol		250 g
White petrolatum		250 g
Purified water	qs	1000 g

1. Calculate the quantity of each ingredient required for the prescription.
2. Accurately weigh or measure each ingredient.
3. Melt the stearyl alcohol and the white petrolatum, using a steam bath. Warm the mixture to about 75°C.
4. Dissolve the other ingredients in the water and warm the mixture to 75°C. Add this mixture to the stearyl alcohol–white petrolatum mixture.
5. Remove the mixture from the heat; stir rapidly and continuously until the mixture has congealed.
6. Package and label.

Polyethylene Glycol Ointment

Polyethylene glycol 3350	400 g
Polyethylene glycol 400	600 g

1. Calculate the quantity of each ingredient required for the prescription.
2. Accurately weigh each ingredient.
3. Heat the polyethylene glycols to 65°C, using a water bath.
4. Mix the ingredients well, remove from heat, and stir until the mixture has congealed.
5. Package and label.

Ingredient-Specific Formulations

R℞ **Anthralin 1% in Lipid Crystals Cream (100 g)**

Anthralin		1 g
Glyceryl laurate		7 g
Glyceryl myristate		21 g
Citric acid		1 g
Sodium hydroxide		140 mg
Purified water	qs	100 g

1. Calculate the quantity of each ingredient required for the prescription.
2. Accurately weigh or measure each ingredient.
3. Heat the glyceryl laurate and glyceryl myristate to about 70°C and incorporate the anthralin powder.
4. Heat the citric acid and sodium hydroxide in 70 mL of purified water to 70°C.
5. Add the oil phase (step 3) to the aqueous phase (step 4) and mix well; continue heating at 70°C for 15 minutes.
6. Cool the mixture to about 40°C.
7. Slowly continue cooling the mixture, with stirring, to room temperature; this is a controlled cooling step.
8. Package and label.

(Note: Use glass or plastic equipment when working with this preparation; avoid contact with metal utensils.)

℞ Bismuth Iodoform Paraffin Paste (BIPP)

Bismuth subnitrate	25 g
Iodoform	50 g
Mineral oil (sterilized)	25 g

1. Calculate the quantity of each ingredient required for the prescription.
2. Accurately weigh or measure each ingredient.
3. If the mineral oil is not already sterile, sterilize it using dry heat.
4. Mix the powders with the mineral oil to form a smooth paste.
5. Package and label.

℞ Estradiol Vaginal Cream

Estradiol	200 mg
Glycerin	qs
Hydrophilic ointment	100 g

1. Calculate the quantity of each ingredient required for the prescription.
2. Accurately weigh or measure each ingredient.
3. Levigate the estradiol powder with a few drops of glycerin.
4. Incorporate the hydrophilic ointment or other suitable o/w vehicles geo-metrically, mixing until uniform.
5. Package and label.

(Note: Commercial o/w vehicles can be used and the quantity of estradiol is variable.)

℞ Progesterone 10% Topical Cream

Progesterone, micronized	10 g
Glycerin	5 mL
Oil-in-water cream vehicle	qs 100 g

1. Calculate the quantity of each ingredient required for the prescription.
2. Accurately weigh or measure each ingredient.
3. Add the glycerin to the micronized progesterone and form a smooth paste.
4. Geometrically, incorporate the cream vehicle and mix until uniform.
5. As an option, run through a roller ointment mill.
6. Package and label.

℞ Protective Hand Cream (100 g)

Dimethicone	4 g
Stearic acid	6 g
Cetyl alcohol	1.5 g
Mineral oil, light	2.2 g
Triethanolamine	1.5 g
Glycerin	1.8 g
Methylparaben	200 mg
Purified water	82.8 g

1. Calculate the quantity of each ingredient required for the prescription.
2. Accurately weigh or measure each ingredient.
3. Mix the dimethicone, stearic acid, cetyl alcohol, and light mineral oil in a container and heat to about 75°C.
4. Mix the triethanolamine, glycerin, water, and methylparaben in a separate container and heat to about 75°C.
5. Add the oil phase (step 3) to the aqueous phase (step 4) and cool, stirring until the mixture congeals and is at room temperature.
6. Package and label.

℞ Testosterone 2% Ointment

Testosterone propionate	2 g
White petrolatum	98 g

1. Calculate the quantity of each ingredient required for the prescription.
2. Accurately weigh or measure each ingredient.
3. Mix the testosterone propionate with a few drops of mineral oil.
4. Add the white petrolatum geometrically and mix until uniform.
5. Package and label.

℞ Testosterone:Menthol Eutectic Ointment (2% Testosterone)

Testosterone:menthol eutectic mixture	4.33 g
Hydrophilic petrolatum/Aquabase/Aquaphor	95.67 g

1. Calculate the quantity of each ingredient required for the prescription.
2. Accurately weigh each ingredient.
3. Mix the testosterone:menthol eutectic mixture with a small quantity of the base.
4. Geometrically, incorporate the remaining drug into the base and thoroughly mix.
5. Package and label.

The testosterone:menthol eutectic mixture can be prepared as follows:

Testosterone	31.6 g
Menthol	68.4 g
Methyl alcohol	qs

1. Use sufficient methyl alcohol to dissolve both the testosterone and menthol.
2. Allow the alcohol to evaporate while occasionally stirring the mixture. It can take a day or two to evaporate to dryness.
3. After the mixture dries, pulverize it thoroughly and store it in a tight, light-resistant container.

Standard Operating Procedure (SOP)

Quality Assessment of Ointments/Creams/Pastes

Purpose of SOP

The purpose of this procedure is to provide a method of documenting physical quality assessment tests and observations about ointments, creams, and pastes.

Materials

The following items are used in one or more of the quality assessment tests:

- Balance.
- pH meter.
- Pycnometers (optional).
- Graduated cylinders or calibrated syringes.

Procedure

The appropriate tests should be conducted, and the results/observations recorded on the worksheet "Quality Assessment Form for Ointments/Creams/Pastes" (Figure 18-2).

Tests and Observations

Weight/Volume. The product should be accurately weighed on a balance, or the quantity should be measured in a graduated cylinder.

pH. The pH meter should be calibrated; then the pH of the product should be determined.

Specific Gravity.

1. If a pycnometer is available, make sure it is clean and dry.
2. Weigh the empty pycnometer.
3. Fill it with the prepared product, being careful not to entrap air bubbles.
4. Weigh it a second time.
5. Subtract the first weight from the second weight to obtain the net weight of the product.
6. Divide this weight (grams) by the volume (milliliters) of the pycnometer to obtain the density/specific gravity of the product:

$$SG = W \text{ (g)}/V \text{ (mL)}$$

Active Drug Assay Results. As appropriate, representative samples of the product should be assayed for active drug content by a contract analytical laboratory. Stability can be assessed by storage of the product at room, refrigerated, and/or frozen temperatures and having the assay repeated on the stored samples.

Color of Product. It may be advisable to use a color chart to determine the actual color of the product.

Clarity. Clarity is evaluated by visual inspection. (See Figure 18-2 for scale.)

Surface Texture.

1. Observe the product in a container.
2. Note the smoothness of the surface. (See Figure 18-2 for scale.)

Spatula Spread.

1. Spread a small portion of the product out on a pill tile or other flat surface.
2. Note the smoothness of the product. (See Figure 18-2 for scale.)

Globule Size Range.

1. Place a drop of the product on a glass plate (microscope slide) and illuminate from the bottom.
2. Estimate the globule size range of the product.

Appearance. Does the product appear dry or "wet" and oozing with liquid?

Feel. To the touch, is the product sticky (tacky), hard (plastic); does it bounce back (elastic)?

Rheologic Properties.

1. Place a small quantity of the product on a glass plate.
2. Lift one edge of the glass plate up to a 45° angle.
3. Observe whether the product flows easily or remains stationary.

Physical Observation. The appearance and organoleptic qualities of the product should be described.

Physical Stability.

1. Prepare a few additional dosage forms; package and label "For Physical Stability Observations."
2. Weekly, observe the product for signs of discoloration, dryness, cracking, mottling, mold growth, and so forth.
3. Record a descriptive observation on the worksheet (Figure 18-2) at each observation interval. Sufficient lines are provided for 8 weeks or approximately 60 days.

Quality Assessment Form for Ointments/Creams/Pastes

Product _____ Date _____

Lot/Rx Number_____ Form: Ointment Cream Paste Other

Characteristic	Theoretical	Actual	Normal Range
Weight/volume	_____	_____	_____
pH	_____	_____	_____
Specific gravity	_____	_____	_____
Active drug assay results	_____	_____	_____
Initial assay	_____	_____	_____
After storage No. 1	_____	_____	_____
After storage No. 2	_____	_____	_____
Color of product	_____		
Clarity	Clear	1 2 3 4 5	Opaque
Surface texture	Smooth	1 2 3 4 5	Rough
Spatula spread	Smooth	1 2 3 4 5	Rough
Globule size range (estimated, mm)		<1 1–2 2–3 >3	
Appears dry	Yes	1 2 3 4 5	No
Appears weeping	Yes	1 2 3 4 5	No
Feels tacky	Yes	1 2 3 4 5	No
Feels plastic	Yes	1 2 3 4 5	No
Feels elastic	Yes	1 2 3 4 5	No
Rheologic properties (ease of flow)	Easy	1 2 3 4 5	Resistant

Sample set aside for physical stability observation: Yes No

If yes, results: Date Observation

_____ _____

_____ _____

_____ _____

_____ _____

_____ _____

_____ _____

_____ _____

_____ _____

_____ _____

Figure 18-2. Sample worksheet for assessment of ointments/creams/pastes.

Chapter 19

Gels

One of the most versatile delivery systems that can be compounded is the pharmaceutical gel. Gels are an excellent drug delivery system for various routes of administration and are compatible with many different drug substances. Gels containing penetration enhancers are especially popular for administering anti-inflammatory and antinauseant medications. They are relatively easy to prepare and are quite efficacious.

Definitions/Types

According to the *United States Pharmacopeia 25/National Formulary 20 (USP25/NF 20)*, *gels* or *jellies* are semisolid systems consisting of suspensions made up of either small inorganic particles or large organic molecules interpenetrated by a liquid. If the gel mass consists of a network of small discrete particles, the gel is classified as a two-phase system. In a two-phase system, if the particle size of the dispersed phase is large, the product is referred to as a *magma*. Conversely, single-phase gels consist of large organic molecules or macromolecules uniformly distributed throughout a liquid in such a manner that no apparent boundaries exist between the dispersed macromolecules and the liquid. Single-phase gels can be made from synthetic macromolecules or from natural gums (mucilages). The continuous phase is usually aqueous but can also be alcoholic or oleaginous.

Gels are semirigid systems in which the movement of the dispersing medium is restricted by an interlacing three-dimensional network of particles or solvated macromolecules of the dispersed phase. A high degree of physical or chemical cross-linking can be involved. The increased viscosity caused by the interlacing and consequential internal friction is responsible for the semisolid state. A gel can consist of twisted, matted strands often wound together by stronger types of van der Waals forces to form crystalline and amorphous regions throughout the system (e.g., tragacanth and carboxymethylcellulose [CMC]).

Some gel systems are as clear as water in appearance; others are turbid because their ingredients may not be completely molecularly dispersed or they may form aggregates, which disperse light. The concentration of the gelling agents is typically less than 10%, usually in the 0.5% to 2.0% range, with some exceptions.

To appeal to the consumer, gels should have clarity and sparkle. Most gels act as absorption bases and are water washable, water soluble, water absorbing, and greaseless. Gels should maintain their viscosity and character over a wide range of temperatures.

Classification Systems

Gels are categorized according to two classification systems. One system divides gels into inorganic and organic; the other distinguishes them by the classifications hydrogels and organogels. Table 19-1 provides examples of both classification systems.

Table 19-1. General Classification and Description of Gels

Class	Description	Examples
Inorganic	Usually two-phase system	Aluminum hydroxide gel, bentonite magma
Organic	Usually single-phase system	Carbomer, tragacanth
Hydrogels (jellies)	Inorganic	Bentonite, veegum, silica, alumina
	Natural and synthetic gums	Pectin, tragacanth, sodium alginate
	Organic	Methylcellulose, sodium carboxymethylcellulose, Pluronic F-127
Organogels	Hydrocarbon type	Petrolatum, mineral oil/polyethylene gel, Plastibase/Jelene
	Animal/vegetable fats	Lard, cocoa butter
	Soap base greases	Aluminum stearate with heavy mineral oil gel
	Hydrophilic organogels	Carbowax bases (PEG ointment)

Inorganic gels are usually two-phase systems, whereas *organic gels* are generally single-phase systems. Bentonite has been used as an ointment base in about 10% to 25% concentrations. *Hydrogels* contain ingredients that are either dispersible as colloids or soluble in water; they include organic hydrogels, natural and synthetic gums, and inorganic hydrogels. In high concentrations, hydrophilic colloids form semisolid gels, also referred to as *jellies*. Sodium alginate has been used to produce gels that serve as ointment bases. In concentrations greater than 2.5% and in the presence of soluble calcium salts, a firm gel, stable between pH 5 and 10, is formed. Methylcellulose, hydroxyethylcellulose, and CMC sodium are among the commercially available cellulose products that can be used in ointments. They are available in several viscosity types: usually high, medium, and low.

Organogels include the hydrocarbons, animal/vegetable fats, soap base greases, and hydrophilic organogels. Included in the hydrocarbon type is Jelene, or Plastibase, a combination of mineral oils and heavy hydrocarbon waxes with a molecular weight of about 1300. Petrolatum is a semisolid gel consisting of a liquid component together with a "protosubstance" and a crystalline waxy fraction. The crystalline fraction provides rigidity to the structure, whereas the protosubstance or "gel former" stabilizes the system and thickens the gel. The hydrophilic organogels, or polar organogels, are soluble to about 75% in water and are completely washable. They look and feel like petrolatum and are nonionic and stable.

Jellies are a class of gels in which the structural coherent matrix contains a high proportion of liquid, usually water. They are commonly formed by adding a thickening agent such as tragacanth or CMC to an aqueous solution of a drug substance. The resultant product is usually clear and of a uniform, semisolid consistency. Jellies are subject to bacterial contamination and growth; thus, most are preserved with antimicrobials. Jellies should be stored tightly closed because water can evaporate, drying out the product.

Some substances, such as acacia, are termed *natural colloids* because they are self-dispersing in a dispersing medium. Other materials that require special treatment for prompt dispersion are called *artificial colloids*. The special treatment can involve fine pulverization to colloidal size with a colloid mill or a micropulverizer.

An interesting product, a *xerogel*, can be formed when the liquid is removed from a gel, leaving only the framework. Examples include gelatin sheets, tragacanth ribbons, and acacia tears.

Applications

Gels can be used to administer medications orally, topically, intranasally, vaginally, and rectally. They can serve as ointment bases. Examples are Plastibase and mineral oil gels made with aluminum monostearate.

Nasal absorption of drugs from gels has been extensively investigated. Some reports of drugs administered by nasal methylcellulose gels, such as propranolol, show that the drug is better absorbed through the nose than through oral administration. In the future, many more drugs may be administered through nasal gels.

Composition

Examples of gelling agents are acacia, alginic acid, bentonite, carbomer, CMC sodium, cetostearyl alcohol, colloidal silicon dioxide, ethylcellulose, gelatin, guar gum, hydroxyethylcellulose, hydroxypropyl cellulose, hydroxypropyl methylcellulose, magnesium aluminum silicate, maltodextrin, methylcellulose, polyvinyl alcohol (PVA), povidone, propylene carbonate, propylene glycol alginate, sodium alginate, sodium starch glycolate, starch, tragacanth, and xanthan gum.

Preparation

The characteristics of the gelling agents will determine the techniques used in their preparation. Because carbomer gels are used extensively in gel preparations, specific techniques for preparing aqueous dispersions of these resins are presented first, followed by a general discussion of techniques for preparing other gelling agents.

Preparation of Aqueous Dispersions of Carbomer Resins

Carbomer resins are primarily used in aqueous systems, although other liquids can be used as well. In water, a single particle of carbomer will wet rapidly, but, like many other powders, carbomer polymers tend to form clumps of particles when dispersed haphazardly in polar solvents. As the surfaces of these clumps solvate, a layer is formed that prevents rapid wetting of the interior of the clumps. When this situation occurs, the slow diffusion of solvent through this solvated layer determines the mixing or hydration time. To achieve the fastest dispersion of the carbomer, one should take advantage of the small particle size of the carbomer powder by slowly adding it into the vortex of the liquid, which is being stirred rapidly. Almost any device, like a simple sieve, that can sprinkle the powder on the rapidly stirred liquid is useful. A metallic screen will help not only by reducing the particle size but also by diffusing static charge buildup. Generally, the higher the agitation rate of the liquid, the better, but extremely high shear mixers should not be used, as they can break down the polymers and reduce gel viscosity. Propeller or turbine-type mixers running about 800 to 1200 rpm work well. Variable-speed mixers are especially desirable to reduce vortexing when the mixture begins to thicken, and they will incorporate less air into the gel. The propeller should be located close to the bottom of the mixing vessel to minimize incorporating air into the product. The small particle–size powder should be slowly sprinkled over the rapidly agitated water to prevent clumping. Once the powder is incorporated, continued stirring for 10 to 15 minutes at reduced speed is recommended to avoid entrapment of excess air.

A neutralizer is added to thicken the gel after the carbomer is dispersed. Sodium hydroxide or potassium hydroxide can be used in carbomer dispersions containing less than 20% alcohol. Triethanolamine will neutralize carbomer resins containing up to 50% ethanol. Other neutralizing agents include sodium carbonate, ammonia, and borax.

Air bubbles incorporated into the gel should be removed before the neutralizing agent is added. Otherwise, the air will remain entrapped in the product. Air bubbles can be removed by using an ultrasonic unit or by allowing the product to stand. It may be necessary to acidify the gel, remove the air, and neutralize it again. For this procedure, hydrochloric and phosphoric acids should be used in an amount equal to 0.5% of the weight of the carbomer present, *not* the total weight of the product. These acids will not produce the significant salt levels on neutralization that might occur with other acids (e.g., citric or lactic acids).

Cleaning up equipment after preparing carbomer products is facilitated by the use of warm water containing salt, a commercial detergent, and sufficient sodium hydroxide or ammonium hydroxide to a pH of 11 or higher. If the material has dried, the equipment can be soaked in water before this cleaning solution is used. Carbomer resin powders do not support growth of bacteria, mold, or fungi while in powder form. When present in aqueous systems, however, mold and some bacteria can grow. Table 19-2 lists commonly used preservatives and their compatibility with carbomer resins. When added to an aqueous system, 0.1% methylparaben or propylparaben are acceptable preservatives and do not affect the resin's efficiency. Carbomer resins are anionic and can decrease the efficiency of some of the cationic agents.

Table 19-2. Compatibility of Selected Preservatives with Carbomer Gels

Preservative	Concentration	Appearance	Compatible
Benzalkonium chloride	0.01%	Clear	Yes
	0.1%	Cloudy	No
Sodium benzoate	0.01%	Clear	Yes
	0.1%	Cloudy	No
Methylparaben	0.18%	Clear	Yes
Propylparaben	0.02%	Clear	Yes
Thiomersal	0.01%	Clear	Yes
	0.1%	Clear	Yes

Preparation of Other Gelling Agents

Bentonite

Bentonite is added to nonagitated water by sprinkling small portions on the surface of hot water. Each portion is allowed to hydrate and settle in the container. The mixture is allowed to stand for 24 hours, with occasional stirring. The mixture is thoroughly agitated the next day. Glycerin or a similar liquid can be used to prewet the bentonite before mixing with water.

Gelatin Gels

Gelatin gels are prepared by dispersing the gelatin in hot water, and then cooling. An alternative method is to moisten the gelatin with about 3 to 5 parts of an organic liquid that will not swell the polymer, such as ethyl alcohol or propylene glycol; then add the hot water and cool.

Tragacanth

Tragacanth gum tends to form lumps when added to water; therefore, aqueous dispersions are prepared by adding the powder to vigorously stirred water. As noted earlier, ethanol, glycerin, or propylene glycol can be used to prewet the powder. Other powders can be mixed with the tragacanth while dry and then added to the water.

Alginic Acid

Alginic acid can be dispersed in water that is vigorously stirred for approximately 30 minutes. Premixing with another powder or with a water-miscible liquid aids in the dispersion process.

Carboxymethylcellulose Sodium

CMC sodium is soluble in water at all temperatures. The sodium salt of CMC can be dispersed with high shear in cold water before the particles can hydrate and swell to sticky gel grains agglomerating into lumps. Once the powder is well dispersed, the solution is heated with moderate shear to about 60°C for fastest dissolution.

Colloidal Silicon Dioxide

Colloidal silicon dioxide (fumed silica) will form a gel when combined with L-dodecanol and n-dodecane. These gels are prepared by adding the silica to the vehicle and sonicating for about 1 minute to obtain a uniform dispersion. The product is then sealed and stored overnight at about 40°C to complete gelation. This gel is more hydrophobic in nature than the others.

Methylcellulose

Methylcellulose is a long-chain, substituted cellulose that can be used to form gels in concentrations up to about 5%. Because methylcellulose hydrates slowly in hot water, the powder is dispersed with high shear in about one third of the required amount of water at 80°C to 90°C. Once the powder is finely dispersed, the rest of the water is added, with moderate stirring to cause prompt dissolution. Cold water or ice should be used at this point. Anhydrous alcohol or propylene glycol can be used to help prewet the powders. Maximum clarity, fullest hydration, and highest viscosity will be obtained if the gel is cooled to 0°C to 10°C for about an hour. A preservative should be added. A 2% solution of methylcellulose 4000 has a gel point of about 50°C.

Polyvinyl Alcohol

PVA is used at concentrations of about 2.5% in preparing various jellies that dry rapidly when applied to the skin. Borax is a good agent that will gel PVA solutions. For best results, PVA should be dispersed in cold water, followed by hot water. It is less soluble in cold water.

General Preparation Techniques

The active drug can be added before or after the gel is formed. If the active drug does not interfere with the gelling process, it is best to add it before gelling because the drug will be more easily and uniformly dispersed. If the active drug does interfere with gelling, it should be added after gelling occurs, although more effort is required and air can be incorporated into the product.

One easy method of preparation is to place the gel and the active drug in a plastic bag, which is then kneaded to thoroughly mix the drug. After the product is mixed, scissors can be used to snip off one corner of the bag, and then the product can be squeezed into the dispensing container. This approach is similar to the method used for decorating cakes.

When powdered polymers are added to water during gel preparation, they can form temporary gels that slow the dissolution process. As water diffuses into these loose clumps of powder, their exteriors frequently turn into clumps of solvated particles encasing dry powder. The clumps of gel dissolve quite slowly because of their high viscosity and the low diffusion coefficient of the macromolecules. Use of glycerin or another liquid as a wetting/dispersing agent minimizes this occurrence.

Aqueous polymer solutions, especially of cellulose derivatives, are stored for approximately 48 hours after dissolution to promote full hydration, maximum viscosity, and clarity. If salts are to be added, one should add them at this point rather than dissolving them in water before adding the polymer; otherwise, the solutions may not reach their full viscosity and clarity.

The box "Hints for Compounding Gels" provides additional suggestions for preparing this dosage form.

Physicochemical Considerations

Gels and jellies exhibit a number of different characteristics, including imbibition, swelling, syneresis, and thixotropy.

Imbibition is the taking up of a certain amount of liquid by a gel without a measurable increase in volume. *Swelling*, however, is the taking up of a liquid by a gel with an increase in volume. Only those liquids that solvate a gel can cause swelling. The swelling of protein gels is influenced by pH and the presence of electrolytes.

Syneresis is the contraction of a gel caused by the interaction between particles of the dispersed phase. This interaction becomes so great that, on standing, the dispersing medium is squeezed out in droplets, causing the gel to shrink. Syneresis is a form of instability in aqueous and nonaqueous gels. The solvent phase is thought to separate because of the elastic contraction of the polymeric molecules; as swelling increases during gel formation, the macromolecules become stretched and the elastic forces expand. At equilibrium, the restoring force of the macromolecules is balanced by the swelling forces, determined by the osmotic pressure. If the osmotic pressure decreases, such as on cooling, water can be squeezed out of the gel. The syneresis of an acidic gel from *Plantago albicans* seed gum can be decreased by

---

Hints for Compounding Gels

- When gels are prepared, premixing some gelling agents with other powders often aids the dispersion process.
- Adding alcohol to some gels decreases their viscosity and clarity.
- When mixers of any type are used for preparing a gel, the propeller should be kept at the bottom of the container, and formation of a vortex should be dissolved to minimize incorporating air into the product.
- In the preparation of gels, all agents should be dissolved in the solvent/vehicle before adding the gelling agent.
- Any entrapped air in carbomer dispersions should be removed before adding the thickening agent. Air bubbles can be removed by allowing the product to stand for 24 hours or by placing it in an ultrasonic bath. A silicone antifoam agent can be helpful.
- pH is important in determining the final viscosity of carbomer gels.
- Gelatin gels can be prepared by dispersing the gelatin in hot water and then cooling. The procedure can be simplified by (1) mixing gelatin powder with an organic liquid in which it will not swell, such as ethyl alcohol or propylene glycol; (2) adding the hot water; and (3) cooling the gel.
- Tragacanth gels can be prepared by adding the powder to vigorously stirred water. Ethanol, glycerin, or propylene glycol can be used to prewet the powder. Other powders can be mixed with the tragacanth while dry, before adding to the water.
- Generally, natural gums should hydrate about 24 hours to form the best homogenous gel and/or magma.

---

adding electrolytes, glucose, and sucrose and by increasing the gum concentration. pH has a significant effect on the separation of water. At low pH, marked syneresis occurs, possibly because of suppression of ionization of the carboxylic acid groups, loss of hydrating water, and the formation of intramolecular hydrogen bonds. These conditions would reduce the attraction of the solvent for the macromolecule.

Thixotropy is a reversible gel-sol formation with no change in volume or temperature. It is considered a type of non-Newtonian flow.

These characteristics play a role in how some agents form a gel or, once formed, remain as this dosage form. The following discussions of mechanisms of gel formation and the specific physicochemical properties of common gelling agents illustrate this role.

Mechanisms of Gel Formation

As a hot, colloidal dispersion of gelatin cools, the gelatin macromolecules lose kinetic energy. With reduced kinetic energy, or thermal agitation, the gelatin macromolecules are associated through dipole–dipole interaction into elongated or threadlike aggregates. The size of these association chains increases to the extent that the dispersing medium is held in the interstices among the interlacing network of gelatin macromolecules, and the viscosity increases to that of a semisolid. Gums, such as agar, Irish moss, algin, pectin, and tragacanth, form gels by the same mechanism as gelatin.

Polymer solutions tend to cast gels because the solute consists of long, flexible chains of molecular thickness that can become entangled, attract each other by secondary valence forces, and even crystallize. Cross-linking of dissolved polymer molecules also causes these solutions to gel. The reactions produce permanent gels, held together by primary valence forces. Secondary valence forces are responsible for reversible gel formation. For example, gelatin will form a gel when its temperature is lowered to about 30°C, the gel point, but aqueous methylcellulose solutions will gel when heated above about 50°C because the polymer is less soluble in hot water and precipitates. Lower temperatures, higher concentrations, and higher molecular weights promote gelation and produce stronger gels. The reversible gelation of gelatin will occur at about 25°C for 10% solutions, 30°C for 20% solutions, and about 32°C for 30% solutions. Gelation is rarely observed for gelatin above 34°C, and, regardless of concentration, gelatin solutions do not gel at 37°C. The gelation temperature or gel point of gelatin is highest at the isoelectric point. Some water-soluble polymers have the property of thermal gelation; that is, they gel on heating, whereas natural gums gel on cooling. The thermal gelation is reversed on cooling.

Inorganic salts will compete with the water present in a gel and cause gelation to occur at lower concentrations. This process is usually reversible, and the gels will re-form when water is added. Alcohol can cause precipitation or gelation because alcohol is a nonsolvent or precipitant, lowering the dielectric constant of the medium and tending to dehydrate the hydrophilic solute. Alcohol lowers the concentrations at which electrolytes salt out hydrophilic colloids. Phase separation by adding alcohol can cause coacervation.

Properties of Common Gelling Agents

Alginic Acid

Alginic acid is obtained from seaweed that is found throughout the world, and the prepared product is a tasteless, practically odorless, white to yellowish-white, fibrous powder. It is used in concentrations between 1% and 5% as a thickening agent in gels. It swells in water to about 200 to 300 times its own weight without dissolving. Cross-linking with increased viscosity occurs when adding a calcium salt, such as calcium citrate.

Bentonite

Bentonite, a naturally occurring hydrated aluminum silicate, can be used to prepare gels. Aqueous bentonite suspensions retain their viscosity above pH 6 but are precipitated by acids. Alkaline materials, such as magnesium oxide, increase gel formation. Alcohol in significant amounts can precipitate bentonite, and, because bentonite is anionic, the antimicrobial efficacy of cationic preservatives can be reduced. Bentonite exhibits thixotropy: It can form a semirigid gel that reverts to a sol when agitated. The sol will re-form to a gel on standing.

Carbomer

Carbomer (Carbopol) resins were first described in the professional literature in 1955 and are currently used in a variety of pharmaceutical dosage systems, including controlled-release tablets, oral suspensions, and topical gels. The *USP 25/NF 20, British Pharmacopoeia*, United States Adopted Names Council, and Cosmetic, Toiletries and Fragrance Association have adopted the generic name *carbomer* for the Carbopol family of resins. Carbomer resins are allyl pentaerythritol–cross-linked, acrylic acid-based polymers, which have a high molecular weight and are modified with C10 to C30 alkyl acrylates. They are fluffy, white, dry powders with large bulk densities, 2% maximum moisture, and pKa of 6.0 ±0.5. The pH of 0.5% and 1.0% aqueous dispersions are 2.7 to 3.5 and 2.5 to 3, respectively. There are many carbomer resins, with viscosity ranges from 0 to 80,000 cP. pH is important in determining the viscosity of carbomer gels. The resins commonly used in a compounding pharmacy are listed in Table 19-3.

Carbomers 910, 934, 934P, 940, and 1342 are official in the *USP 25/NF 20.* Carbomer 910 is effective at low concentrations when low viscosity is desired and is frequently used for producing stable suspensions. It is the least ion sensitive of these resins.

Table 19-3. Typical Properties of Selected Carbomer Pharmaceutical Resins

Product	Viscosity (cP)[a]	Properties and Uses
Carbomer 907	0–3000	Very water soluble. Good lubricity at low viscosity. A "linear" polymer that is not cross-linked.
Carbomer 910 NF	3000–7000	Effective in low concentrations. Good ion tolerance.
Carbomer 934 NF	30,500–39,400	Good stability at high viscosity. Good for thick formulations, such as medium to high viscosity gels, emulsions, and suspensions. Good for zero order release of products, such as oral and mucoadhesive applications. Excellent for transdermals and topicals.
Carbomer 2984	45,000–80,000	
Carbomer 5984	25,000–45,000	
Carbomer 934P NF	29,400–39,400	
Carbomer 974P NF	29,400–39,400	
Carbomer 940 NF	40,000–60,000	Excellent thickening efficiency at high viscosities and very good clarity. Produces sparkling clear water or hydroalcoholic topical gels.
Carbomer 980 NF	40,000–60,000	
Carbomer ETD 2001	45,000–65,000	
Carbomer 941 NF	4000–11,000	Produces sparkling clear gels with low viscosity. Good stabilizer for emulsions. Effective in moderately ionic systems. More efficient than 934 and 940 at low to moderate concentrations.
Carbomer 981 NF	4000–11,000	
Carbomer ETD 2050	3000–15,000	

[a]*Typical viscosities of a 0.5% solution, pH 7.5, except for carbomer 907, which is a 4.0% solution.*

Carbomer 934 is highly effective in thick formulations such as viscous gels. The two alternative resins, numbers 2984 and 5984, are polymerized in ethyl acetate/cyclohexane in place of benzene. Carbomer 934P is similar to 934 but is intended for oral and mucosal contact applications and is the most widely used carbomer in the pharmaceutical industry. In addition to thickening, suspending, and emulsifying in both oral and topical formulations, the 934 polymer is also used to provide sustained-release properties in the stomach and the intestinal tract for commercial products. Carbomer 940, or 980, its cosolvent alternative, is the most efficient of all the carbomer resins and has good nondrip properties. Carbomer 1342 and its cosolvent analogue, 1382, provide pseudoplastic rheology, which is quite effective in preparing pourable suspensions and stable emulsions and makes them especially good for preparations containing dissolved salts. Carbomer 974P NF differs from carbomer 934P NF in that ethyl acetate rather than benzene is used in its preparation. Carbomers 980 NF and ETD 2001 differ from carbomer 940 NF in that cosolvents are used in place of benzene for their preparation. Such is also the case with carbomers 981 NF and ETD 2050 versus carbomer 941 NF.

Adding alcohol to prepared carbomer gels can decrease their viscosity and clarity. To overcome the loss of viscosity, an increase in the concentration of carbomer may be required; the amount will vary depending on the pH of the product. A preparation at pH 5.5 that goes from 0% to 50% alcohol requires an increase of 0.5% carbomer; similarly, an increase of 0.35% carbomer is required at pH 8.2 when going from 20% to 40% alcohol. Also, gel viscosity depends on the presence of electrolytes and the pH. Generally, a maximum of 3% electrolytes can be added before a rubbery mass forms. Overneutralization will result in decreased viscosity, which cannot be reversed by adding acid. Maximum viscosity and clarity occur at pH 7, but acceptable viscosity and clarity begin at pH 4.5 to 5 and extend to a pH of 11.

Cross-linked carbomer resins can swell in water up to 1000 times their original volume to form gels, when exposed to a pH environment above 4 to 6. Because the pKa of these polymers is about 6, the carboxylate groups on the molecules ionize, resulting in repulsion between the negative particles of the polymer backbone, which contributes to the swelling of the polymer. Determining the molecular weight of the carbomers is difficult. Although the average molecular weights of the polymerized resins are in the order of about 500,000, the actual molecular weight of the cross-linked resin is in the billions.

Other Gelling Agents

CMC in concentrations of 4% to 6% of the medium viscosity grades can be used to produce gels; glycerin can be added to prevent drying. Precipitation can occur at pH values of less than 2; it is most stable at pH levels between 2 and 10, with maximum stability at pH values of 7 to 9. It is incompatible with ethanol.

CMC sodium dispersions are sensitive to pH changes because of the carboxylate group. The viscosity of the product is decreased markedly below pH 5 or above pH 10.

Colloidal silicon dioxide can be used to prepare transparent gels when used with other ingredients of similar refractive index. Colloidal silicon dioxide adsorbs large quantities of water without liquefying. The viscosity is largely independent of temperature. Changes in pH can affect the viscosity: It is most effective at pH values up to about 7.5. At a pH greater than 10.7, the viscosity-increasing properties are reduced, and, at these higher levels, the silicon dioxide dissolves to form silicates with no viscosity-increasing properties.

Magnesium aluminum silicate, Veegum, in concentrations of about 10%, forms firm, thixotropic gels. The material is inert and has few incompatibilities but is best used above pH 3.5. It can bind to some drugs and limit their availability.

Methylcellulose mixtures that contain high concentrations of electrolytes will experience viscosity problems. The electrolytes will salt out the macromolecules and increase their viscosity, ultimately precipitating the polymer.

Plastibase/Jelene is a mixture of 5% low molecular weight polyethylene and 95% mineral oil. The polymer is soluble in mineral oil above 90°C, close to its melting point. When cooled below 90°C, the polymer precipitates and causes gelation. A network of entangled and adhering insoluble polyethylene chains immobilizes the mineral oil. This network probably extends into small crystalline regions. This gel can be heated to about 60°C without a substantial loss of consistency.

Poloxamer, or Pluronic, gels are made from selected forms of polyoxyethylene-polyoxypropylene copolymers in concentrations ranging from 15% to 50%. Poloxamers generally are white, waxy, free-flowing granules that are practically odorless and tasteless. Aqueous solutions of poloxamers are stable in the presence of acids, alkalies, and metal ions. However, they do support mold growth and should be preserved. Commonly used poloxamers include the 124 (L-44 grade), 188 (F-68 grade), 237 (F-87 grade), 338 (F-108 grade), and 407 (F-127 grade) types, which are freely soluble in water. The "F" designation refers to the flake form of the product. The trade name "Pluronic" is used in the United States by BASF Corporation for pharmaceutical- and industrial-grade poloxamers. Pluronic F-127 has low toxicity and good solubilizing capacity and optical properties; thus, it is a good medium for topical drug delivery systems.

Povidone, in the higher molecular weight forms, can be used to prepare gels in concentrations up to about 10%. It has the advantage of being compatible in solution with a wide range of inorganic salts, natural and synthetic resins, and other chemicals. It can also increase the solubility of a number of poorly soluble drugs.

Propylene glycol alginate is used as a gelling agent in concentrations of 1% to 5%, depending on the specific application. The preparations are most stable at a pH of 3 to 6 and should contain a preservative.

Sodium alginate can be used to produce gels in concentrations up to 10%. Aqueous preparations are most stable between pH values of 4 and 10; below pH 3, alginic acid is precipitated. Sodium alginate gels for external use should be preserved, for example, with 0.1% chloroxylenol or the parabens. If the preparation is acidic, benzoic acid can be used. High concentrations will result in increased viscosity up to a point at which the sodium alginate is salted out; this point occurs at about 4% with sodium chloride.

Tragacanth gum has been used to prepare gels that are most stable at pH 4 to 8. These gels must be preserved with either 0.1% benzoic acid or sodium benzoate or a combination of 0.17% methylparaben and 0.03% propylparaben. These gels can be sterilized by autoclaving.

Liqua-Gel (Paddock) is a liquid lubricating gel that is water soluble and non-greasy. It can be used to dissolve or suspend a variety of topically applied dermatologic agents. Liqua-Gel contains purified water, propylene glycol, glycerin, hydroxypropyl methylcellulose, and potassium sorbate. Sodium phosphate and boric acid are used to buffer the gel to a pH of about 5. Diazolidinyl urea and methylparaben and propylparaben are included as preservatives. Liqua-Gel is a clear, colorless, viscous gel with a faint characteristic odor and has a viscosity of about 80,000 cP at 25°C.

Quality Control

The pharmacist should follow standard quality control procedures. These procedures involve checking the appearance, uniformity, weight/volume, viscosity, clarity, pH, and smell of the gels. This information can be documented by using the Standard Operating Procedure (SOP) "Quality Assessment of Gels."

Packaging/Storage/Labeling

Gels generally should be stored in tight containers at refrigerated or room temperatures. This dosage form is commonly dispensed in tubes, jars, squeeze bottles, or pump dispensers (Figure 19-1). Some gels can be dispensed in applicators or syringes. The labels of the containers should include the instruction to keep tightly closed.

Carbomer resins are quite hygroscopic and should be stored in tight containers, away from moisture and extreme temperatures. Moisture does not affect the efficiency of the resins, but high levels make them more difficult to disperse and weigh accurately. Autoclaving appears to have no effect on the viscosity or pH of the prepared gels. Aqueous dispersions of carbomer that have not been neutralized can be stored as stock solutions at concentrations up to 5%.

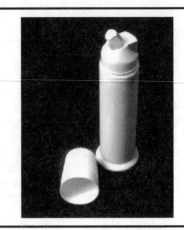

Figure 19-1. Pump dispenser for creams and gels.

Glass, plastic, or resin-lined containers are recommended for storage of carbomer products. Aluminum tubes should be used only when a product has a pH of less than about 6.5. With other metallic materials, a pH of about 7.7 or greater is preferred.

Stability

Gels should be observed for such physical characteristics as shrinkage, separation of liquid from the gel, discoloration, and microbial contamination. Many gels will not promote bacterial/mold growth, nor will they prevent it. Consequently, they should be autoclaved or should contain preservatives. Table 19-2 lists a number of preservatives and concentrations that have been used in preparing gels. Gelling agents in the dry state are usually not a problem.

Beyond-use dates for water-containing formulations are no later than 14 days, when stored at cold temperatures, for products prepared from ingredients in solid form. These dates can be extended if valid scientific information is available to support the stability of the formulation, as discussed in Chapter 4, "Stability of Compounded Products."

Patient Counseling

Patients should be counseled about the proper application of the gel. They should be instructed on how to handle and store the package, as well as the need to keep it tightly closed.

Sample Formulations

Rx Amitriptyline Hydrochloride and Baclofen in Pluronic Lecithin Organogel (100 mL)

Amitriptyline hydrochloride		2 g
Baclofen		2 g
Ethoxy diglycol		5–10 mL
Lecithin:isopropyl palmitate solution		22 mL
Pluronic F-127 gel 20%	qs	100 mL

1. Calculate the quantity of each ingredient required for the prescription.
2. Accurately weigh or measure each ingredient.
3. Combine the amitriptyline hydrochloride and baclofen powders.
4. Add sufficient ethoxy diglycol to form a smooth paste.
5. Add the lecithin:isopropyl palmitate solution and mix well.
6. Add sufficient Pluronic F-127 gel to volume and mix well.
7. Package and label.

Bentonite Magma

Bentonite		50 g
Purified water	qs	1000 mL

1. Calculate the quantity of each ingredient required for the prescription.
2. Accurately weigh the bentonite powder.
3. Sprinkle the bentonite on 800 mL of hot purified water and allow to hydrate for 24 hours, stirring occasionally.
4. Increase the amount of purified water to make 1000 mL. If a mechanical blender is used, place approximately one half of the water in the blender. Add the bentonite while the blender is in operation. Add more purified water to make the volume of 1000 mL, and operate the blender for 10 minutes.
5. Package and label.

R̸ Buspirone Hydrochloride 2.5 mg/0.1 mL in Pluronic Lecithin Organogel

Buspirone hydrochloride	250 mg
Soy lecithin granules	4 g
Isopropyl palmitate	4 g
Potassium sorbate	20 mg
Citric acid	20 mg
Pluronic 20% gel	qs 10 mL

1. Calculate the quantity of each ingredient required for the prescription.
2. Accurately weigh or measure each ingredient.
3. Dissolve the buspirone hydrochloride, citric acid, and potassium sorbate in the Pluronic 20% gel. (Note: The gel will be thinner and easier to work with if kept cold.)
4. Add the soy lecithin granules to the isopropyl palmitate and allow to sit in the refrigerator overnight. (It is advisable to prepare this mixture in advance.)
5. Mix the Pluronic gel solution with the lecithin:isopropyl palmitate in step 4, preferably using high shear, until uniform.
6. Package and label.

R̸ Capsaicin, Ketamine Hydrochloride, and Ketoprofen in Pluronic Lecithin Organogel (100 mL)

Capsaicin		75 mg
Ketamine hydrochloride		2 g
Ketoprofen		10 g
Ethoxy diglycol		10 mL
Lecithin:isopropyl palmitate		22 mL
Pluronic F-127 30% gel	qs	100 mL

1. Calculate the quantity of each ingredient required for the prescription.
2. Accurately weigh or measure each ingredient.
3. Combine the capsaicin, ketamine hydrochloride, and ketoprofen powders.
4. Add sufficient ethoxy diglycol to form a smooth paste.
5. Add the lecithin:isopropyl palmitate solution and mix well.
6. Add sufficient Pluronic F-127 gel to volume and mix well.
7. Package and label.

Clear Aqueous Gel with Dimethicone

Purified water	59.8%
Carbomer 934	0.5%
Triethanolamine	1.2
Glycerin	34.2
Propylene glycol	2.0
Dimethicone copolyol	2.3
Sodium hydroxide	1%

1. Calculate the quantity of each ingredient required for the prescription.
2. Accurately weigh or measure each ingredient.
3. Disperse the carbomer 934 in 20 mL of water.
4. Adjust the pH of the dispersion to 7 by adding sufficient 1% sodium hydroxide solution (about 12 mL is required); then add enough purified water to bring the volume to 40 mL.
5. Add the other ingredients and mix well. Dimethicone copolyol is included to reduce the stickiness associated with glycerin.

R︎ Estradiol Topical Gel

Estradiol	50 mg
70% Isopropyl alcohol	71 mL
Carbomer 940	500 mg
Triethanolamine	670 mg
Purified water	28 mL

1. Calculate the quantity of each ingredient required for the prescription.
2. Accurately weigh or measure each ingredient.
3. Dissolve the estradiol in the 70% isopropyl alcohol.
4. Slowly add the carbomer 940 to this mixture, stirring constantly. A blender or high-speed mixer can be used.
5. Add the triethanolamine to the purified water.
6. Add the triethanolamine solution to the alcohol solution by slowly stirring. Mix thoroughly until the gel is formed. (Note: Slow stirring minimizes the introduction of air into the product.)
7. Package and label.

℞ Estradiol Vaginal Gel

Estradiol	200 mg
Polysorbate 80	1 g
Methylcellulose 2% gel	99 g

1. Calculate the quantity of each ingredient required for the prescription.
2. Accurately weigh or measure each ingredient.
3. Levigate the estradiol with the polysorbate 80.
4. Geometrically add the methylcellulose 2% gel and mix thoroughly.
5. Package and label.

℞ Lidocaine HCl 4%–Epinephrine HCl 0.05%–Tetracaine HCl 0.5% Topical Gel

Lidocaine HCl	4 g
Epinephrine HCl	50 mg
Tetracaine HCl	500 mg
Ascorbic acid	1.7 g
Hydroxyethylcellulose (5000 cP)	1.75 g
Preserved water	qs 100 mL

1. Calculate the quantity of each ingredient required for the prescription.
2. Accurately weigh or measure each ingredient.
3. Dissolve the lidocaine HCl, epinephrine HCl, tetracaine HCl, and ascorbic acid in about 95 mL of preserved water.
4. Slowly, using a magnetic stirrer to form a vortex, sprinkle the hydroxyethylcellulose onto the surface of the moving water, allowing the particles to be wetted before adding additional powder. This action will help prevent clumping and speed up the gelling process.
5. Add sufficient preserved water to volume and mix well.
6. Package and label.

℞ **Lidocaine Hydrochloride 2%, Misoprostol 0.003%, and Phenytoin 2.5% Topical Gel for Decubitus Ulcers**

Lidocaine hydrochloride		2 g
Misoprostol, 200 µg tablets		#15
Phenytoin		2.5 g
Hydroxyethylcellulose		2 g
Methylparaben		200 mg
Glycerin		10 mL
Purified water	qs	100 mL

1. Calculate the quantity of each ingredient required for the prescription.
2. Accurately weigh or measure each ingredient; obtain the 15 tablets of misoprostol.
3. Pulverize the tablets to a fine powder and blend in the remaining powders.
4. Add the glycerin and make a smooth paste.
5. Slowly incorporate sufficient purified water to volume with mixing.
6. Package and label.

 Liquid–Solid Emulsion Gel

Gelatin solution:

Gelatin, 200 bloom		8 g
Phosphate buffer (pH 7)	qs	40 mL

Gel product:

Gelatin solution	40 mL
Long-chain alcohol	10 g

(Note: Liquid–solid emulsion gels can be prepared from gelatin and a selection of an alcohol from a homologous series [e.g., octanol, nonanol, decanol, undecanol, or dodecanol].)

1. Calculate the quantity of each ingredient required for the prescription.
2. Accurately weigh or measure each ingredient.
3. Formulate the aqueous gelatin base such as 20% (weight/weight) 200 bloom gelatin in phosphate buffer (pH 7). Mature the gelatin–water mixture for about 1 hour at room temperature and then melt at 60°C.
4. Leave the molten gel at 60°C for another 2 hours to allow air bubbles to escape.
5. Add 10 g of the long-chain alcohol, which has been preheated to 60°C, to 40 g of the heated molten aqueous gel, and stir at high speed for about 2 minutes.
6. Add the drug to the appropriate phase.
7. Pour the molten mixture onto a plate or between two plates to set or "cast."
8. Cut out circular or other shaped portions of the gel and apply to the skin to release the enclosed drug.

Lubricating Jelly Formula

Methylcellulose 4000 cP		0.8%
Carbomer 934		0.24%
Propylene glycol		16.7%
Methylparaben		0.015%
Sodium hydroxide	qs	pH 7
Purified water	qs ad	100%

1. Calculate the quantity of each ingredient required for the prescription.
2. Accurately weigh or measure each ingredient.
3. Disperse the methylcellulose in 40 mL of hot water (80°C–90°C).
4. Chill overnight in a refrigerator.
5. Disperse the carbomer 934 in 20 mL of purified water.
6. Adjust the pH of the dispersion to 7 by adding sufficient 1% sodium hydroxide solution (about 12 mL is required); and then add enough purified water to bring the volume to 40 mL.
7. Dissolve the methylparaben in the propylene glycol.
8. Carefully mix the methylcellulose, carbomer 934, and propylene glycol fractions to avoid incorporating air.
9. Package and label.

 Methylcellulose Gels

Methylcellulose 1500 cP		1%–5%
Purified water	qs	100%

1. Calculate the quantity of each ingredient required for the prescription.
2. Accurately weigh or measure each ingredient.
3. Add the methylcellulose to about 50 mL of boiling purified water and disperse well.
4. Add the remaining purified water, ice cold, to bring the volume of the gel to 100 mL.
5. Stir until uniform and thickened.
6. Package and label.

℞ Niacinamide 4% Acne Gel

Niacinamide	4 g
Carbopol 940	600 mg
Propylene glycol	20 mL
Ethoxy diglycol	2 mL
Trolamine	3–4 drops
Preserved water	73 mL

1. Calculate the quantity of each ingredient required for the prescription.
2. Accurately weigh or measure each ingredient.
3. Dissolve the niacinamide in the ethoxy diglycol and the preserved water.
4. Mix the Carbopol 940 with the propylene glycol.
5. Incorporate the solution from step 3 into step 4 and mix well.
6. Add the trolamine slowly with thorough mixing until the desired viscosity is obtained.
7. Package and label.

℞ Piroxicam 0.5% in an Alcoholic Gel

Hydroxypropylcellulose	1.75 g
70% Isopropyl alcohol	98.25 mL
Propylene glycol	4.1 mL
Polysorbate 80	1.7 mL
Piroxicam 20 mg capsules	25 capsules

(Note: Piroxicam powder can be used if available.)

1. Calculate the quantity of each ingredient required for the prescription.
2. Accurately weigh or measure each ingredient.
3. Make the hydroxypropylcellulose gel by mixing the hydroxypropylcellulose in the alcohol until a clear gel results.
4. Make a paste with the piroxicam powder (from capsules), the propylene glycol, and the polysorbate 80.
5. Using geometric dilution, add enough hydroxypropylcellulose gel to the paste to make 100 g of the preparation.
6. Package and label.

(Note: It is important to use an alcoholic water mixture, such as 70% isopropyl alcohol, or a gel may not form.)

Poloxamer (Pluronic) Gel Base

Poloxamer F-127 NF		20–50 g
Potassium sorbate NF		0.2 g
Purified water/buffer	qs	100 mL

1. Calculate the quantity of each ingredient required for the prescription.
2. Accurately weigh or measure each ingredient.
3. Add the powders and water to a bottle and shake well.
4. Store in a refrigerator so that the gel will form.
5. Package and label.

 Pluronic Lecithin Organogel (PLO) Gel

Lecithin and isopropyl palmitate liquid	20 mL
(Note: See preparation instructions below.)	
Pluronic 20% gel	80 mL

1. Calculate the quantity of each ingredient required for the prescription.
2. Accurately weigh or measure each ingredient.
3. Mix the two viscous liquids together well. A number of mixing techniques can be used, including plastic bags, pushing the ingredients back and forth between two syringes fitted with a syringe adapter, or simply mixing in a mortar with a pestle. Minimize the incorporation of air.

The lecithin and isopropyl palmitate liquid is prepared as follows:

Soy lecithin, granular	10 g
Isopropyl palmitate NF	10 g
Sorbic acid	0.2 g

1. Calculate the quantity of each ingredient required for the prescription.
2. Accurately weigh or measure each ingredient.
3. Add the soy lecithin granules and the sorbic acid powder to the isopropyl palmitate liquid and allow to set overnight.
4. Mix by rolling or gentle agitation. Do not shake. Since the density of the isopropyl palmitate is about 0.855, a volume of 11.7 mL can be measured.

R̞ **Scopolamine Hydrobromide 0.25 mg/0.1 mL Pluronic Lecithin Organogel (100 mL)**

Scopolamine hydrobromide		250 mg
Soy lecithin/isopropyl palmitate solution		25 mL
Buffer solution (pH 5)		2.5 mL
Poloxamer F-127 gel, 20% dispersion	qs	100 mL

1. Calculate the quantity of each ingredient required for the prescription.
2. Accurately weigh or measure each ingredient.
3. Dissolve the scopolamine hydrobromide in the pH 5 buffer solution.
4. Add the soy lecithin/isopropyl palmitate solution to the ingredients in step 3 and mix well.
5. Add sufficient 20% poloxamer F-127 gel to make 100 mL and mix thoroughly.
6. Package and label.

 Starch Glycerite

Starch	100 g
Benzoic acid	2 g
Purified water	200 g
Glycerin	700 g

1. Calculate the quantity of each ingredient required for the prescription.
2. Accurately weigh or measure each ingredient.
3. Rub the starch and benzoic acid in the water to form a smooth mixture.
4. Add the glycerin and mix.
5. Heat the mixture to 140°C, applying constant, gentle agitation until a translucent mass forms. The heat ruptures the starch grains and permits the water to reach and hydrate the linear and branched starch molecules that trap the dispersion medium in the interstices to form a gel.
6. Package and label.

R_X Vancomycin Gel (Vancomycin Paste, Vanc Paste)

Vancomycin	500 mg
Aspartame	200 mg
Flavor	qs
Sodium benzoate	200 mg
Methylcellulose 2% gel	100 mL

1. Calculate the quantity of each ingredient required for the prescription.
2. Accurately weigh or measure each ingredient.
3. In a mortar, add a small quantity of the methylcellulose 2% gel to the vancomycin, aspartame, and sodium benzoate powders and mix well.
4. Add the flavoring agent and mix well.
5. Add additional methylcellulose 2% gel to almost reach 100 mL.
6. Transfer to a previously calibrated container and add methylcellulose 2% gel to volume.
7. Mix well.
8. Package and label.

Standard Operating Procedure (SOP)

Quality Assessment of Gels

Purpose of SOP
The purpose of this procedure is to provide a method of documenting quality assessment tests and observations on gels.

Materials
The following items are used in one or more of the quality assessment tests:

- Balance.
- pH meter.
- Pycnometers (optional).
- Graduated cylinders or calibrated syringes.

Procedure
The appropriate tests should be conducted, and the results/observations recorded on the worksheet "Quality Assessment Form for Gels" (Figure 19-2).

Tests and Observations
Weight/Volume. The product should be weighed on a balance, or the quantity should be measured in a graduated cylinder.

pH. The pH meter should be calibrated; then the pH of the product determined.

Specific Gravity.

1. If a pycnometer is available, make sure it is clean and dry.
2. Weigh the empty pycnometer.

3. Fill it with the prepared product being careful not to entrap air bubbles.
4. Weigh it a second time.
5. Subtract the first weight from the second weight to obtain the net weight of the product.
6. Divide this weight (grams) by the volume (milliliters) of the pycnometer to obtain the density/specific gravity of the product:

$$SG = W \, (g)/V \, (mL)$$

Active Drug Assay Results. As appropriate, representative samples of the product should be assayed for active drug content by a contract analytical laboratory. Stability can be assessed by storage of the product at room, refrigerated, and/or frozen temperatures and having the assay repeated on the stored samples.

Color of Product. It may be advisable to use a color chart to determine the actual color of the product.

Clarity. Clarity is evaluated by visual inspection.

Surface Texture.

1. Observe the product in a container.
2. Note the smoothness of the surface. (See Figure 19-2 for scale.)

Spatula Spread.

1. Spread a small portion of the product out on a pill tile or other flat surface.
2. Note the smoothness of the product. (See Figure 19-2 for scale.)

Appearance. Does the product appear dry or "wet" and oozing with liquid?

Feel. To the touch, is the product sticky (tacky), hard (plastic); does it bounce back (elastic)?

Rheologic Properties.

1. Place a small quantity of the product on a glass plate.
2. Lift one edge of the glass plate up to a 45° angle.
3. Does the product flow easily or remain stationary?

Physical Observation. The appearance and organoleptic qualities of the product should be described.

Physical Stability.

1. Prepare a few additional dosage forms; package and label "For Physical Stability Observations."
2. Weekly, observe the product for signs of discoloration, dryness, cracking, mottling, mold growth, and so forth.
3. Record a descriptive observation on the worksheet (Figure 19-2) at each observation interval. Sufficient lines are provided for 8 weeks or approximately 60 days.

Quality Assessment Form for Gels

Product _____   Date _____

Lot/Rx Number _____   Form: Gel

Characteristic	Theoretical	Actual	Normal Range
Weight/volume	_____	_____	_____
pH	_____	_____	_____
Specific gravity	_____	_____	_____
Active drug assay results	_____	_____	_____
Initial assay	_____	_____	_____
After storage No. 1	_____	_____	_____
After storage No. 2	_____	_____	_____
Color of product		_____	
Clarity	Clear	1 2 3 4 5	Opaque
Surface texture	Smooth	1 2 3 4 5	Rough
Spatula spread	Smooth	1 2 3 4 5	Rough
Appears dry	Yes	1 2 3 4 5	No
Appears weeping	Yes	1 2 3 4 5	No
Feels tacky	Yes	1 2 3 4 5	No
Feels plastic	Yes	1 2 3 4 5	No
Feels elastic	Yes	1 2 3 4 5	No
Rheologic properties (ease of flow)	Easy	1 2 3 4 5	Resistant

Sample set aside for physical stability observation: Yes   No

If yes, results: Date   Observation

_____   _____
_____   _____
_____   _____
_____   _____
_____   _____
_____   _____
_____   _____
_____   _____
_____   _____

Figure 19-2. Sample worksheet for quality assessment of gels.

Chapter 20

Ophthalmic, Otic, and Nasal Preparations

Compounded products are grouped in this chapter by route of administration rather than by dosage forms. For that reason, the chapter is divided into three major sections: ophthalmic, otic, and nasal preparations.

Ophthalmic Preparations

Definitions/Types

Ophthalmic solutions are sterile, free from foreign particles, and prepared especially for instillation into the eye. *Ophthalmic suspensions* are sterile liquid preparations that contain solid particles in a vehicle suitable for instillation into the eye. *Ophthalmic ointments* are sterile preparations designed for application to the eye. They have an ointment base and may or may not include an active drug.

Historical Use

One of the early treatments of eye conditions with a liquid involved the use of the juice of a liver. This preparation was one of the earlier ones stemming from observations that applying substances topically to the eye was effective. In this case, the vitamin A content of the juice was effective in treating the condition. Throughout history, various plant extracts have been prepared and used for eye conditions. Today's vehicles for ophthalmic liquids include primarily sterile, buffered aqueous systems that contain preservatives.

"Eye salves" were prepared during the period of the early Roman Empire by "medici ocularii," or men who specialized in preparing such salves. One such product was described on a piece of green steatite as containing "crocus of Lucius Vallatinus for affectations of the eyes." Evidence exists that ophthalmic ointments were used throughout the Roman Empire including such outlying areas as Scotland. Ointments developed later used oils and fats as their vehicles. More recently, the petrolatums were used as vehicles for these ophthalmic preparations.

Applications

Ophthalmic preparations are used to treat allergies, bacterial and viral infections, glaucoma, and numerous other eye conditions. The eye is constantly exposed to the atmosphere, dust, pollutants, allergens, bacteria, and foreign bodies. When the eye's natural defensive mechanisms are compromised or overcome, an ophthalmic product, in a solution, suspension, or ointment form, may be indicated. Solutions are used most often to deliver a drug to the eye. Although solutions have a relatively short duration of action, they spread easily over the globe and cover well. Suspensions have a slightly longer duration of action because the particles will usually settle in the lower conjunctival sac and release the drug as the particles dissolve. Ointments have an even longer duration of action. The ointment spreads over the eye and into the conjunctival sac. The active drug is released slowly as the vehicle is slowly removed from the eye.

Composition

In addition to the active drugs, ophthalmic preparations contain a number of excipients, including vehicles, buffers, preservatives, tonicity-adjusting agents, antioxidants, and viscosity enhancers. Ingredients used in the formulation process must be nonirritating to and compatible with the eyes.

Preparation

All preparation must be done in a clean air environment by a qualified aseptic compounding pharmacist. The pharmacist must ensure that all the ingredients are of the highest grade that can be reasonably obtained. The box "Preparation of Ophthalmic Products" lists the steps involved in preparing ophthalmic solutions, suspensions, and ointments. The reader is also referred to the *ASHP Technical Assistance Bulletin on Pharmacy-Prepared Ophthalmic Products* (American Society of Health-Systems Pharmacists, 1993).

Ophthalmic ointments must be prepared so that they do not irritate the eye, do permit diffusion of the drug, and do retain the activity of the drug for a reasonable period of time when stored properly. White petrolatum is the base primarily used for ophthalmic ointments. Aqueous solutions of the drug can be incorporated by using an absorption base, as long as it does not irritate the eye. One example is anhydrous lanolin mixed with white petrolatum. The pharmacist must be aware that surfactants used to make absorption bases can cause eye irritation. Powders incorporated in the preparation must be micronized and sterilized to ensure that the final product is not gritty and thus is nonirritating.

The size of the particles in an ophthalmic suspension must be small enough that they do not irritate and/or scratch the cornea. The micronized form of the drug is required. Ophthalmic suspensions must be free from agglomeration or caking.

Physicochemical Considerations

In preparing ophthalmic solutions, one must consider the general physicochemical parameters: clarity, tonicity, pH/buffers, and sterility. The addition of excipients such as preservatives, antioxidants, and viscosity enhancers, as well as potential incompatibilities between these excipients and active drugs, should be considered.

Preparation of Ophthalmic Products

Solutions

1. Accurately weigh or measure each ingredient.
2. Dissolve the ingredients in about three fourths of the quantity of sterile water for injection and mix well.
3. Add sufficient sterile water for injection to volume and mix well.
4. Take a sample of the solution and determine the pH, clarity, and other quality control factors.
5. Filter through a sterile 0.2-µm filter into a sterile ophthalmic container.
6. Package and label.
7. If a large number of solutions are to be prepared, select a random sample to be assayed and checked for sterility.

Suspensions (Method 1)

1. Accurately weigh or measure each ingredient.
2. Dissolve the ingredients in about three fourths of the quantity of sterile water for injection and mix well.
3. Add sufficient sterile water for injection to volume and mix well.
4. Take a sample of the solution and determine the pH and other quality control factors.
5. Package in a suitable container for autoclaving.
6. Autoclave, cool, and label.
7. If a large number of suspensions are to be prepared, select a random sample to be assayed and checked for sterility.

Suspensions (Method 2)

1. Accurately weigh or measure each ingredient.
2. Sterilize each ingredient by a suitable method.
3. Using aseptic technique, dissolve the ingredients in about three fourths of the quantity of sterile water for injection and mix well.
4. Add sufficient sterile water for injection to volume and mix well.
5. Take a sample of the suspension and determine the pH and other quality control factors.
6. Package and label.
7. If a large number of solutions are to be prepared, select a random sample to be assayed and checked for sterility.

Ointments

1. Accurately weigh or measure each ingredient.
2. Sterilize each ingredient by a suitable method.
3. Using aseptic technique, mix the ingredients with the sterile vehicle.
4. Take a sample of the ointment and determine the quality control factors.
5. Package and label.
6. If a large number of ointments are to be prepared, select a random sample to be assayed and checked for sterility.

Clarity

Ophthalmic solutions must be free from foreign particles. Filtration is generally used to remove these particles and to achieve clarity of the solution. Polysorbate 20 and Polysorbate 80, in a maximum concentration of 1%, can be used to achieve clarity.

Tonicity

Lacrimal fluid has an isotonicity value equivalent to that of a 0.9% sodium chloride solution. However, the eye can tolerate a value as low as 0.6% and as high as 1.8% sodium chloride equivalency. Some ophthalmic solutions will be hypertonic by virtue of the high concentration required of the drug substance. Others will be hypotonic and will require adjustment to attain the proper tonicity range; sodium chloride, boric acid, and dextrose are commonly used for this purpose. The ideal tonicity is 300 mOsm/L; however, a range of 200 to 600 mOsm/L is acceptable. Hypotonicity is a property that can be addressed by the compounding pharmacist; hypertonicity can be addressed only if it is possible to decrease the concentration of some of the components of the formulation.

Pharmacists can use the sodium chloride equivalent method to calculate the quantity of solute that must be added to adjust a hypotonic solution of a drug to be isotonic. A sodium chloride equivalent is defined as the amount of sodium chloride that is osmotically equivalent to 1 g of the drug. For example, the sodium chloride equivalent of ephedrine sulfate is 0.23 (i.e., 1 g of ephedrine sulfate is equivalent to 0.23 g of sodium chloride). See Chapter 5, "Pharmaceutical Compounding Calculations," for example calculations. Table 20-1 lists agents used to adjust tonicity.

pH and Buffering

Ophthalmic solutions are ordinarily buffered at the pH of maximum stability for the drug(s) they contain. The buffers are included to minimize any change in pH that can occur during the storage life of the drug; this change can result from carbon dioxide absorbed from the air or from hydroxyl ions absorbed from a glass container. Changes in pH can affect the solubility and the stability of drugs; consequently, it is important to minimize such fluctuations. The buffer system should be designed so that it maintains the pH throughout the expected shelf life of the product. The buffer capacity should be low enough that, when the ophthalmic solution is dropped into the eye, the buffer system of the tears will rapidly bring the pH of the solution back to that of the tears. Thus, the pharmacist should use a concentration of buffer salt that is effective but as low as possible. Generally, a buffer capacity of less than 0.05 is desired; pH in the range of 4 to 8 is considered optimum.

Sterility

Ophthalmic solutions must be sterile. Sterility is best achieved through sterile filtration, which involves using a sterile membrane filter with a pore size of 0.45 μm or 0.2 μm and filtering into a sterile container. Other methods of sterilizing ingredients or components of ophthalmics include dry heat, steam under pressure (autoclaving; Figure 20-1), and gas sterilization with ethylene oxide.

Preservatives

Because most ophthalmic solutions and suspensions are prepared in multiuse containers, they must be preserved. The preservative used must be compatible with the active drug as well as with all the other excipients in the product. Common preservatives for ophthalmic products are shown in Table 20-2.

Antioxidants

Antioxidants may be required for selected active drug ingredients. Table 20-3 lists a number of antioxidants that can be used in ophthalmic preparations.

Table 20-1. Physicochemical Characteristics of Tonicity Agents

	Solubility (mL)[a]			Sodium Chloride Equivalent (E-1%)	Iso-osmotic Concentration (%)	Volume Needed (mL)[b]	Packaging Containers
Item	Water	Ethanol	Glycerin				
Dextrose	1	100	—	0.16	5.51	6	W
Glycerin	Misc	Misc	Misc	—	2.6	11.7	T
Mannitol	5.5	—	—	—	—	—	W
Potassium chloride	2.8	—	—	0.76	1.19	25.3	W
Sodium chloride	2.8	—	10	1.0	0.9	—	W

[a]Volume of water added to 300 mg of the specific item to produce an isotonic solution.
[b]Volume required to dissolve 1 g of the drug.

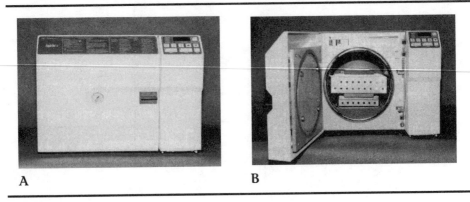

Figure 20-1. Microprocessor-controlled sterilizer/autoclave: *A*, exterior view; *B*, interior view.

Viscosity Enhancers

If an ophthalmic solution is viscous, the product will remain in the eye longer and thereby allow more time for drug absorption and effect. Viscosity enhancers are used to increase the viscosity. The most common is methylcellulose, generally in a concentration of about 0.25% if the 4000 cP grade is used. If methylcellulose is autoclaved, it will come out of solution; however, it can be redispersed after cooling, especially if placed in a refrigerator. Solution viscosity ranging from 25 to 50 cP is common with hydroxypropyl methylcellulose, methylcellulose, or polyvinyl alcohol. With all of these enhancers, however, it is important that the clarity of the solution be maintained. Additives that increase viscosity are shown in Table 20-4.

Tonicity

For comfort during administration, many dosage forms must be "isotonic" with body fluids. This is especially true of parenterals, ophthalmics, and nasal solutions. Pain and irritation at the site of administration can occur if the formulation is either hypertonic or hypotonic.

The tonicity of solutions is a colligative property that depends primarily on the number of dissolved particles in solution (i.e., $KCl \rightarrow K^+ + Cl^-$, two particles. Colligative properties include changes in vapor pressure, boiling point, freezing point, and osmotic pressure; here, we are interested in the latter. *Osmotic pressure* is the pressure that must be applied to a more concentrated solution just to prevent the flow of pure solvent into the solution separated by a semipermeable membrane.

Biologic systems are compatible with solutions having similar osmotic pressures (i.e., an equivalent number of dissolved species). For example, red blood cells, blood plasma, and 0.9% sodium chloride solution contain approximately the same number of solute particles per unit volume and are termed *iso-osmotic* and *isotonic*. If solutions do not contain the same number of dissolved species (i.e., they contain more [hypertonic] or less [hypotonic]), then it may be necessary to alter the composition of the solution to bring them into an acceptable range. An osmol (Osm) is related to a mole (gram molecular weight) of the molecules or ions in solution. One mole of glucose (180 g) dissolved in 1000 g of water has an osmolality of 1 Osm, or 1000 mOsm per kg of water. One mole of sodium chloride (23 + 35.5 = 58.5 g) dissolved in 1000 g of water has an osmolality of almost 2 Osm or 2000 mOsm because sodium chloride dissociates into almost two particles per molecule. In other words, a 1 molal solution of sodium chloride is equivalent to a 2 molal solution of dextrose.

Table 20-2. Preservatives Commonly Used in Ophthalmic, Otic, and Nasal Products

Preservative Name	Usual Conc. (%)	Conc. Range (%)	Max. Conc.[a] (%)	Incompatibilities
Chlorobutanol			0.5	
Quaternary ammonium compounds	0.01	0.004–0.02		Soaps, anionic materials, salicylates, nitrates
Benzalkonium chloride			0.013	
Benzethonium chloride			0.01	
Organic mercurials		0.001–0.01		Certain halides with phenylmercuric acetate
Phenylmercuric acetate			0.004	
Phenylmercuric nitrate			0.004	
Thimerosal			0.01	
Parahydroxybenzoates			0.1	Adsorption by macromolecules

[a]The FDA Advisory Review Panel on OTC Ophthalmic Drug Products (1979) lists these concentrations for preparations that have direct contact with the eye tissues and not for ocular devices such as contact lens products.

Table 20-3. Antioxidants Used for Ophthalmic and Nasal Preparations

Antioxidant	Usual Maximum Concentration (%)
Ethylenediaminetetraacetic acid	0.1
Sodium bisulfite	0.1
Sodium metabisulfite	0.1
Thiourea	0.1

Table 20-4. Viscosity Enhancers for Ophthalmic Preparations

Agent	Usual Maximum Concentration (%)
Hydroxyethylcellulose	0.8
Hydroxypropyl methylcellulose	1.0
Methylcellulose	2.0
Polyvinyl alcohol	1.4
Polyvinylpyrrolidone	1.7

Normal serum osmolality values are in the vicinity of 285 mOsm/kg (often expressed as 285 mOsm/L). Ranges can include values from about 275 to 300 mOsm/L). Pharmaceuticals should be close to this value to minimize discomfort on application to the eyes or nose, or when injected.

Incompatibilities

Because zinc salts can form insoluble hydroxides at a pH above 6.4, a vehicle of boric acid solution can be used. Boric acid solution has a lower pH (about pH 5) and a slight buffering action.

Nitrates or salicylates are incompatible with solutions of benzalkonium chloride. Therefore, benzalkonium chloride should be replaced with 0.002% phenylmercuric nitrate.

Sodium chloride cannot be used to adjust the tonicity of silver nitrate solutions because silver chloride would precipitate. Instead, sodium nitrate should be used to adjust the tonicity, and phenylmercuric nitrate can be used as the preservative in this situation.

Quality Control

The compounding pharmacist should follow standard quality control procedures. These procedures include checking sterility, clarity, appearance, pH, and volume/weight. Sterility can be checked by plating a sample of the product on an agar plate and checking for microbial growth. If this procedure is not feasible, product samples can be sent to a laboratory for testing.

Packaging/Storage/Labeling

Ophthalmic solutions should be packaged in sterile dropper bottles. Individual doses can also be placed in sterile syringes, without needles. Generally, these preparations should be stored at either room or refrigerated temperatures. They should not be frozen. Ophthalmic preparations should be labeled "For the Eye," "Do Not Touch the Eye or Eyelid," "Store as Indicated," and "Dispose after [appropriate date]."

Stability

Beyond-use dates for water-containing formulations are no later than 14 days, when stored at cold temperatures, for products prepared from ingredients in solid form. If nonaqueous liquids are prepared with a manufactured product, the beyond-use recommendation is no later than 25% of the time remaining on the product's expiration date or 6 months, whichever is earlier. For all others, the recommended beyond-use date is the intended duration of therapy or 30 days, whichever is earlier. These beyond-use recommendations can be extended if valid scientific information is available to support the stability of the product, as discussed in Chapter 4, "Stability of Compounded Products."

Patient Counseling

Patients should be instructed on how to administer drops or ointments to the eye. Specifically, they should be cautioned not to allow the tip of the dropper or ointment tube to touch any part of the eye. They should be instructed to allow the drug to fall freely into the eye and not to allow the drug to touch the eye and then be drawn back into the bottle. More information is given in the box "Hints for Administration of Ophthalmic Preparations, p. 327."

Sample Formulations

Vehicles

The steps listed for solutions in the box "Preparation of Ophthalmic Products" on page 327 should be followed to prepare these vehicles.

 Isotonic Sodium Chloride Solution

Sodium chloride USP		0.9 g
Benzalkonium chloride		1:10,000
Sterile water for injection	qs	100 mL

Three buffer solutions have been suggested for certain drugs when they are prepared as ophthalmic solutions. These drugs have been divided into three classes and are listed with the recommended buffer solution for that class.

The following drugs in Class IA can be placed in Buffer Solution IA, which has a pH of about 5:

- Cocaine.
- Dibucaine.
- Neostigmine.
- Phenacaine.
- Piperocaine.
- Procaine.
- Tetracaine.
- Zinc.

 Buffer Solution IA

Boric acid USP		1.9 g
Benzalkonium chloride		1:10,000
Sterile water for injection	qs	100 mL

Some drugs can be incompatible with Buffer Solution IA because of an incompatibility with benzalkonium chloride. Buffer Solution IB contains a different preservative, phenylmercuric nitrate. Sodium sulfite has been added to prevent discoloration/oxidation of some of the drugs in this category. Drugs that are incompatible in Buffer Solution IA but can be prepared by using Buffer Solution IB include the following Class IB drugs:

- Physostigmine.
- Phenylephrine.
- Epinephrine.

Buffer Solution IB

Boric acid USP	1.9 g
Sodium sulfite, anhydrous	0.1 g
Phenylmercuric nitrate	1:50,000
Sterile water for injection qs	100 mL

Drugs in Class II that can be prepared in Buffer Solution II include the following:

- ▸ Atropine.
- ▸ Ephedrine.
- ▸ Homatropine.
- ▸ Pilocarpine.

Buffer Solution II

Sodium acid phosphate, anhydrous	0.560 g
Disodium phosphate, anhydrous	0.284 g
Sodium chloride USP	0.5 g
Disodium edetate	0.1 g
Benzalkonium chloride	1:10,000
Sterile water for injection qs	100 mL

Ingredient-Specific Preparations

℞ Artificial Tears Solution

Polyvinyl alcohol	1.5%
Povidone	0.5%
Chlorobutanol	0.5%
0.9% Sodium chloride solution	qs

1. Calculate the quantity of each ingredient required for the prescription.

2. Accurately weigh or measure each ingredient.

3. Dissolve all ingredients in the sterile 0.9% sodium chloride solution.

4. Filter through a 0.2-μm filter into a sterile ophthalmic container.

5. Package and label.

℞ Cocaine Hydrochloride Ophthalmic Solution

Cocaine hydrochloride		5 g
Ethylenediaminetetraacetic acid		10 mg
Benzalkonium chloride		10 mg
Sterile 0.9% sodium chloride solution	qs	100 mL

1. Calculate the quantity of each ingredient required for the prescription.
2. Accurately weigh or measure each ingredient.
3. Dissolve the cocaine hydrochloride, ethylenediaminetetraacetic acid, and benzalkonium chloride in sufficient sterile 0.9% sodium chloride solution to make 100 mL.
4. Filter through a sterile 0.2-µm filter into a sterile container.
5. Package and label.

℞ Cyclosporine Ophthalmic Solution

Cyclosporine	2%
Corn oil or olive oil	qs

1. Calculate the quantity of each ingredient required for the prescription.
2. Accurately weigh or measure each ingredient.
3. Use alcohol to clean the container to be used for mixing the oral cyclosporine 10% solution and oil.
4. Clean a commercial container of cyclosporine 10% solution with alcohol; open the container and place it in a laminar flow hood for about 24 hours to allow the alcohol to evaporate.
5. Mix four volumes of corn oil or olive oil with one volume of the 10% cyclosporine oral solution; mix thoroughly in the previously cleaned container.
6. Filter through a 0.2-µm filter into a sterile, dry ophthalmic container.
7. Package and label.

℞ Ophthalmic Decongestant Solution

Phenylephrine hydrochloride	0.125%
Polyvinyl alcohol	1.4%
Disodium edetate	0.05%
Sodium acetate	0.1%
Monobasic sodium phosphate	0.1%
Dibasic sodium phosphate	0.05%
Sodium thiosulfate	0.1%
Sterile water for injection qs	100%

1. Calculate the quantity of each ingredient required for the prescription.
2. Accurately weigh or measure each ingredient.
3. Dissolve all the ingredients in sterile water for injection.
4. Filter through a sterile 0.2-µm filter into a sterile container.
5. Package and label.

℞ Ophthalmic Lubricant

White petrolatum	55%
Mineral oil	41.5%
Lanolin alcohol	2%
0.9% Sodium chloride injection	1.5%

1. Calculate the quantity of each ingredient required for the prescription.
2. Accurately weigh or measure each ingredient.
3. Mix the white petrolatum, mineral oil, and lanolin alcohol together, using a water bath.
4. Sterilize the mixture with dry heat.
5. Using aseptic technique, cool the sterile mixture in a laminar flow hood; then incorporate the sterile 0.9% sodium chloride injection and mix.
6. Package in sterile containers.

℞ Tobramycin Fortified Ophthalmic Solution

Tobramycin ophthalmic solution	5 mL
Tobramycin injection, 80 mg/2mL	1 mL

1. Calculate the quantity of each ingredient required for the prescription.
2. Prepare the product using aseptic technique.
3. Accurately measure each ingredient.
4. Mix well, package, and label.

℞ Acetylcysteine 10% Ophthalmic Solution

Acetylcysteine	10%	2 g (10 mL of a 20% solution)
Disodium edetate	0.025%	5 mg
Chlorobutanol	0.5%	100 mg
Artificial tears solution	qs	20 mL

(Note: Prepare in a clean air environment.)

1. Calculate the quantity of each ingredient required for the prescription.
2. Accurately weigh or measure each ingredient.
3. Place the chlorobutanol in a clean, previously sterilized beaker.
4. Add 9 mL of artificial tears solution.
5. Cover and stir (with a magnetic mixer with stir bar) until dissolved.
6. Add the disodium edetate to the solution.
7. Add 10 mL of 20% acetylcysteine oral inhalation solution.
8. Filter the solution through a 0.2-μm filter into a sterile ophthalmic container.
9. Package and label.

℞ Tropicamide–Hydroxyamphetamine Hydrobromide Ophthalmic Solution

Tropicamide		0.25%	250 mg
Hydroxyamphetamine hydrobromide		1%	1 g
Benzalkonium chloride		0.005%	5 mg
Disodium edetate		0.5%	500 mg
Sodium chloride		—	490 mg
Sodium hydroxide or hydrochloric acid to adjust pH to 4.2–5.8			
Sterile water for injection	qs	100%	100 mL

1. Calculate the quantity of each ingredient required for the prescription.
2. Accurately weigh or measure each ingredient.
3. Dissolve the solid ingredients in approximately 50 mL of sterile water for injection.
4. Add the benzalkonium chloride dilution to the solution and mix well.
5. Add sufficient water to make about 90 mL and mix well.
6. Adjust the pH to between 4.2 and 5.8, using the sodium hydroxide or hydrochloric acid.
7. Add sufficient sterile water for injection to make 100 mL.
8. Filter through a 0.2-μm filter into sterile containers.
9. Package and label.

R℞ Tropicamide–Hydroxyamphetamine Hydrobromide Ophthalmic Solution (cont.)

The benzalkonium chloride for this prescription can be prepared as follows:

1. Accurately measure 1 mL of 50% benzalkonium chloride solution.
2. Place in a 100-mL graduated cylinder.
3. Add sufficient sterile water for injection to make 100 mL and mix well.
4. Remove 1 mL of the solution, which contains 5 mg of benzalkonium chloride, and add it to the solution containing the active drug.

R℞ Cefazolin Ophthalmic Solution USP

Cefazolin sodium		350 mg
Thimerosal		2 mg
0.9% Sodium chloride injection	qs	100 mL

(Note: This preparation should be prepared in an aseptic working environment, using aseptic technique, by a validated aseptic compounding pharmacist.)

1. Calculate the quantity of each ingredient required for the prescription.
2. Accurately weigh or measure each ingredient.
3. Dissolve the cefazolin sodium and thimerosal in about 90 mL of the 0.9% sodium chloride injection.
4. Add sufficient 0.9% sodium chloride injection to volume and mix well.
5. Sterilize by filtering through a sterile 0.2-μm filter into sterile ophthalmic containers.
6. Package and label.

R℞ Interferon 10×10^6 μ/mL Ophthalmic Solution

Interferon alfa-2a		100×10^6 μ
Ammonium acetate		7.7 mg
Benzyl alcohol		100 mg
Human albumin		10 mg
Sterile water for injection	qs	10 mL

1. Calculate the quantity of each ingredient required for the prescription.
2. Accurately weigh or measure each ingredient; Roferon-A can be used to provide the interferon alfa. It may be necessary to adjust the final volume depending on the source of the interferon.
3. Dissolve the ammonium acetate, benzyl alcohol, and albumin in about 8 mL of the sterile water for injection.
4. Add the interferon alfa and mix well.
5. Add sufficient sterile water for injection and mix well.
6. Sterilize by filtering through a sterile 0.2-μm filter into a sterile ophthalmic container.
7. Package and label.

℞ Lissamine Green 0.5% Ophthalmic Solution

Lissamine green	500 mg
Sterile water for injection	25 mL
0.9% Sodium chloride injection	qs 100 mL

1. Calculate the quantity of each ingredient required for the prescription.
2. Accurately weigh or measure the appropriate amounts of each ingredient.
3. Dissolve the lissamine green in the sterile water for injection.
4. Add sufficient sterile 0.9% sodium chloride injection to volume and mix well.
5. Sterilize by filtering through a sterile 0.2-μm filter into sterile containers.
6. Package and label.

℞ Tobramycin Sulfate 0.3% and Diclofenac Sodium 0.1% Ophthalmic Solution (100 mL)

Tobramycin sulfate	300 mg
Diclofenac sodium	100 mg
Sodium chloride	806 mg
Sterile water for injection	qs 100 mL

(Note: This preparation should be prepared in a laminar flow hood, using aseptic technique, by a validated aseptic compounding pharmacist.)

1. Determine the total quantity to be prepared and the volume that is required for each component.
2. Accurately weigh or measure each of the ingredients. The tobramycin sulfate can be obtained from 7.5 mL of the tobramycin sulfate 40 mg/mL injection.
3. Dissolve the powders in sufficient sterile water for injection to make about 90 mL of solution.
4. Add the tobramycin sulfate injection, followed by sufficient sterile water for injection to 100 mL and mix well. Adjust the pH to 7 to 8 if necessary.
5. Sterilize by filtering through a sterile 0.2-μm filter into sterile containers.
6. Package and label.

Otic Preparations

Definitions/Types

Otic preparations can be in liquid, ointment, or powder dosage forms. Both *otic solutions* and *suspensions*, the liquid dosage forms, are prepared for instillation into the ear. Solutions are liquid preparations in which all ingredients are dissolved, whereas suspensions are liquid preparations containing insoluble materials. Solutions are also used for irrigating the ear. *Otic ointments* are semisolid preparations that are applied to the exterior of the ear. *Insufflations* are preparations made of finely divided powder that are administered to the ear canal. Insufflating a powder into the ear canal is not too common because the ear lacks fluids and a powder-wax buildup can occur.

Historical Use

Throughout history, medications have been administered to the ear for a local effect. Early otic preparations were applied by soaking materials, such as cloth, wood, or plants, in various oils or extracts from plants or animals and then placing the impregnated materials in the ear. A more recent method of applying otic preparations involves placing a liquid in the ear and inserting a cotton plug to keep the medication from draining out of the ear. This method is still used today, along with the use of ear irrigants, which clean debris from the ear. This debris is the cause of many otic infections.

Applications

Otic irrigating solutions, which can consist of surfactants, weak sodium bicarbonate, boric acid (0.5%–1%), or aluminum acetate solutions, can be warmed to about 37°C before instillation into the ear. These irrigating solutions can be used to remove earwax, purulent discharges of infection, and foreign bodies from the ear canal.

Otic suspensions can be used when a long duration of drug effect is desired or when the drug is not soluble in the vehicles commonly used in otic preparations.

Otic ointments are seldom used. Any ointment base can be used in their preparation, however, and they can include antibacterial, antifungal, or corticosteroid ingredients. These ointments are applied directly to the exterior portions of the ear.

Fine powders used as insufflations can contain an antibacterial and/or an antifungal agent that will create a repository for the drug. A small rubber or plastic bulb insufflator (powder blower or puffer) can be used to blow, or insufflate, the powder into the ear.

Composition

Categories of medications commonly used in the ear include local anesthetics, cleansing agents (peroxides), anti-infectives, and antifungals. Also included are liquids for cleaning, warming, or drying the external ear and for removing any fluids that can be entrapped by a local waxy buildup.

Vehicles used most often in otic preparations are glycerin, propylene glycol, and the lower molecular weight polyethylene glycols (PEGs), especially PEG 300. These vehicles are viscous and will adhere to the ear canal. Water and alcohol (ethanol and isopropyl) can be used as vehicles and solvents for some medications but are used primarily for irrigation because they moisten the ear canal and a therapeutic aim of these preparations is to keep the ear canal dry to minimize bacterial/fungal growth. Alcohol can be used full strength. Vegetable oils, especially olive oil, are good vehicles. Mineral oil has been used as a vehicle for some antibiotics and anti-inflammatory medications. Otic ointments primarily contain petrolatum as a vehicle, whereas otic powders can contain talc or lactose as a vehicle.

Preparation

The method of formulating otic preparations is similar for all four dosage forms. The box "Preparation of Otic Products" lists the specific steps involved in preparing otic solutions, suspensions, ointments, and powders.

Preparation of Otic Products

Solutions

1. Accurately weigh or measure each of the ingredients.
2. Dissolve the ingredients in about three fourths of the quantity of the vehicle and mix well.
3. Add sufficient vehicle to volume and mix well.
4. Take a sample of the solution and determine the pH, clarity, and other quality control factors.
5. Package and label.

Suspensions

1. Accurately weigh or measure each of the ingredients.
2. Dissolve or mix the ingredients in about three fourths of the quantity of the vehicle and mix well.
3. Add sufficient vehicle to volume and mix well.
4. Take a sample of the suspension and determine the pH, and other quality control factors.
5. Package in a suitable container.
6. Label.

Ointments

1. Accurately weigh or measure each of the ingredients.
2. Mix each of the ingredients with the vehicle.
3. Take a sample of the ointment and determine the quality control factors.
4. Package and label.

Powders

1. Accurately weigh or measure each of the ingredients.
2. Geometrically mix the powders together, starting with the powders present in the smallest quantity.
3. Take a sample of the powder and determine the quality control factors.
4. Package and label.

Physicochemical Considerations

Physicochemical considerations in developing otic preparations include solubility, viscosity, tonicity, surfactant properties, and preservatives. Although sterility is not generally a consideration, the products need to be "clean."

Many drugs are soluble in the vehicles commonly used in these preparations. If a drug is insoluble in these vehicles, the preparation can be prepared as a suspension. Because most of these vehicles are relatively viscous agents, the addition of suspending agents may not be necessary.

The viscosity of the preparation is important in keeping the medication in the ear canal. If the preparation is too thin, the medication will drain out of the ear. However, if the medication is too thick, it may not reach the inner recesses of the ear.

Hygroscopicity and tonicity are important in the product's ability to aid in withdrawing fluids from the immediate area of the ear. If the product is hypertonic, some fluid can be withdrawn from the ear, thereby releasing some of the pressure. If the product is hypotonic, however, some fluid may flow into the area.

Because many ear conditions are related to the difficulty in cleaning the ear, the presence of a surfactant in the preparation helps the medication spread out and aids in breaking up earwax. This action makes it easier to remove any foreign material.

Many otic preparations are self-preserving because of the high concentration of glycerin, propylene glycol, and the like. If these agents are not present, it may be wise to add a preservative to minimize the chance of introducing bacteria that might grow in an unpreserved product.

Quality Control

The compounding pharmacist should follow standard quality control procedures. These procedures include checking the volume/weight, pH, viscosity, appearance, and odor of these products.

Packaging/Storage/Labeling

Otic preparations should be packaged in dropper containers (Figure 20-2), puffers, or tubes appropriate for the product and method of administration. Generally, otic preparations should be stored at either room or refrigerated temperatures. They should not be frozen. These preparations should be labeled "For the Ear," "Discard after [appropriate date]," and "Use Only as Directed."

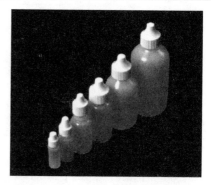

Figure 20-2. Dropper containers in various sizes (3 mL, 7 mL, 15 mL, 30mL, 60 mL, 125 mL).

Stability

Beyond-use dates for water-containing formulations are no later than 14 days, when stored at cold temperatures, for products prepared from ingredients in solid form. If nonaqueous liquids are prepared with a manufactured product, the beyond-use recommendation is no later than 25% of the time remaining on the product's expiration date or 6 months, whichever is earlier. For all other products, the beyond-use recommendation is the intended duration of therapy or 30 days, whichever is earlier. These beyond-use recommendations can be extended if valid scientific information is available to support the stability of the product, as discussed in Chapter 4, "Stability of Compounded Products."

Patient Counseling

Patients should be instructed on how to apply drops to the ear from dropper bottles. They should be told to place a cotton or gauze pad in the ear to keep the liquid from escaping.

Sample Formulations

R℣ **Benzocaine Otic Solution**

Benzocaine		200 mg
Glycerin	qs	15 mL

1. Calculate the quantity of each ingredient required for the prescription.
2. Accurately weigh or measure each ingredient.
3. Dissolve the benzocaine in sufficient glycerin to make 15 mL of solution.
4. Package and label.

Nasal Preparations

Definitions

Nasal solutions are solutions prepared for nasal administration either as drops or as sprays. *Nasal suspensions* are liquid preparations containing insoluble materials for nasal administration. *Nasal gels* and *ointments* are semisolid preparations prepared for nasal application that can be for either local or systemic use. The gels are generally water soluble.

Historical Use

Collunaria is the term for early nasal preparations that originally contained various oils as the vehicles. As it became apparent that spraying or dropping mineral oil into the nose could be harmful, preparation shifted to using aqueous vehicles. Aqueous vehicles with some modifications are used today in these preparations. In recent years, the trend in vehicle preparation has been toward developing isotonic, preserved vehicles that do not interfere with the action of nasal cilia.

Applications

A number of drug substances can be prepared as nasal solutions to be administered either as drops or as sprays; other dosage forms include nasal gels, jellies, or ointments. Some drugs are sufficiently volatile that they can be carried into the nose through an inhaler.

Composition

In addition to the active drugs, nasal preparations contain a number of excipients, including vehicles, buffers, preservatives, tonicity-adjusting agents, gelling agents, and, possibly, antioxidants. Ingredients used in the formulation process must be nonirritating and compatible with the nose.

Preparation

The methods used to formulate the four dosage forms of nasal preparations are similar. The box "Preparation of Nasal Products" lists the steps to be followed when preparing nasal solutions, suspensions, ointments, and gels.

Preparation of Nasal Products

Solutions

1. Accurately weigh or measure each of the ingredients.
2. Dissolve the ingredients in about three fourths of the quantity of sterile water for injection and mix well.
3. Add sufficient sterile water for injection to volume and mix well.
4. Take a sample of the solution and determine the pH, clarity, and other quality control factors.
5. Filter through a sterile 0.2-μm filter into a sterile nasal container.
6. Package and label.
7. If a large number of solutions are to be prepared, select a random sample to be assayed and checked for sterility.

Suspension (Method 1)

1. Accurately weigh or measure each ingredient.
2. Dissolve/mix the ingredients in about three fourths of the quantity of sterile water for injection and mix well.
3. Add sufficient sterile water for injection to volume and mix well.
4. Take a sample of the suspension and determine the pH and other quality control factors.
5. Package in a suitable container for autoclaving.
6. Autoclave, cool, and label.
7. If a large number of suspensions are to be prepared, select a random sample to be assayed and checked for sterility.

Suspension (Method 2)

1. Accurately weigh or measure each ingredient.
2. Sterilize each ingredient using a suitable method.
3. Using aseptic technique, dissolve/mix the ingredients in about three fourths of the quantity of sterile water for injection and mix well.
4. Add sufficient sterile water for injection to volume and mix well.
5. Take a sample of the suspension and determine the pH and other quality control factors.
6. Package and label.
7. If a large number of suspensions are to be prepared, select a random sample to be assayed and checked for sterility.

Ointments

1. Accurately weigh or measure each ingredient.
2. Sterilize each ingredient using a suitable method.
3. Using aseptic technique, mix each ingredient with the sterile vehicle.
4. Take a sample of the ointment and determine the quality control factors.
5. Package and label.
6. If a large number of ointments are to be prepared, select a random sample to be assayed and checked for sterility.

Gels

1. Accurately weigh or measure each ingredient.
2. Dissolve the ingredients in about three fourths of the quantity of sterile water for injection and mix well.

Preparation of Nasal Products (cont.)

3. Filter through a sterile 0.2-μm filter into a sterile container.
4. Add the gelling agent (previously sterilized) and mix well.
5. Add sufficient sterile water for injection to volume/weight and mix well.
6. Take a sample of the gel and determine the pH, clarity, and other quality control factors.
7. Package and label. (Note: Sterile 1-mL syringes that are preloaded with individual doses work well.)
8. If a large number of gels are to be prepared, select a random sample to be assayed and checked for sterility.

Physicochemical Considerations

A vehicle for a nasal solution should have a pH in the range of 5.5 to 7.5 and a mild buffer capacity. It should be isotonic, stable, preserved, and compatible with normal ciliary motion and ionic constituents of nasal secretions, as well as with the active ingredient. It should not modify the normal mucus viscosity.

pH and Buffering

Nasal preparations are ordinarily buffered at the pH of maximum stability for the drug(s) they contain. The buffers are included to minimize any change in pH that can occur during the storage life of the drug. This change in pH can affect the solubility and stability of drugs; consequently, it is important to minimize such fluctuations. The buffer system should be designed to maintain the pH throughout the expected shelf life of the product but with a low buffer capacity. Generally, pH in the range of 4 to 8 is considered optimum. pH and buffer-phosphate buffer systems are usually compatible with most nasal medications.

Tonicity Adjustment

The preferred agents for adjusting the tonicity of nasal solutions are sodium chloride and dextrose. Severely hypertonic solutions should be avoided. Nasal fluid has an isotonicity value similar to a 0.9% sodium chloride solution. If the isotonicity is beyond the proper range, the nasal ciliary movement can slow or even stop. Tonicity values ranging from 0.6% to 1.8% sodium chloride equivalency are generally acceptable. If the solution of the active drug is hypotonic, it may be necessary to add a substance to attain the proper tonicity range. Sodium chloride, boric acid, and dextrose are commonly used for this purpose. A tonicity of 300 mOsm/L is ideal, although a range of 200 to 600 mOsm/L is acceptable.

Sterility

Nasal preparations should be sterile. Sterility is best achieved through sterile filtration, which involves using a sterile membrane filter with a pore size of 0.45 μm or 0.2 μm and filtering into a sterile container. Other methods of sterilizing ingredients include dry heat, steam under pressure (autoclaving), and gas sterilization with ethylene oxide.

Antioxidants

Antioxidants may be required for selected active drug ingredients. Table 20-3 contains antioxidants that can be used in nasal preparations.

Other Excipients

Because most nasal preparations are prepared in multiuse containers, they must be preserved. The preservative used must be compatible with the active drug as well as with all other excipients in the product. Common preservatives that can be used for nasal products are shown in Table 20-2.

Quality Control

The compounding pharmacist should follow standard quality control procedures. These procedures include checks for sterility, clarity (for solutions), pH, and volume/weight. Sterility can be checked by plating a sample of the product on an agar plate and checking for microbial growth. If this procedure is not feasible, product samples can be sent to a laboratory for testing.

Packaging/Storage/Labeling

Containers for dispensing nasal preparations include dropper bottles, spray bottles (Figure 20-3), and syringes (for gels and ointments). Generally, these preparations should be stored either at room temperature or refrigerated. They should not be frozen. These preparations should be labeled "For the Nose" and "Discard after [appropriate date]."

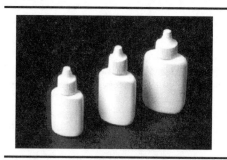

Figure 20-3. Nasal spray bottles in various sizes (15 mL, 20 mL, 30 mL).

Stability

Beyond-use dates for water-containing formulations are no later than 14 days, when stored at cold temperatures, for products prepared from ingredients in solid form. If nonaqueous liquids are prepared with a manufactured product, the beyond-use recommendation is no later than 25% of the time remaining on the product's expiration date or 6 months, whichever is earlier. For all other products, the beyond-use recommendation is the intended duration of therapy or 30 days, whichever is earlier. These beyond-use recommendations can be extended if valid scientific information is available to support the stability of the product, as discussed in Chapter 4, "Stability of Compounded Products."

Patient Counseling

When systemic therapeutic drugs, such as dihydroergotamine mesylate or morphine sulfate, are to be administered, the pharmacist should calibrate a dropper or spray container to deliver a consistent and uniform dose. The patient should be taught how to use the dosage device properly.

Sample Formulations

Vehicle

General Nasal Solution Vehicle

(pH 6.5 and isotonic)

Sodium acid phosphate, hydrous		0.65 g
Disodium phosphate, hydrous		0.54 g
Sodium chloride		0.45 g
Benzalkonium chloride		0.05–0.01 g
Distilled water	qs ad	100 mL

1. Calculate the quantity of each ingredient required for the vehicle.
2. Accurately weigh or measure each ingredient.
3. Dissolve the ingredients in about 75 mL of the distilled water.
4. Adjust the pH to 6.5 if necessary.
5. Add sufficient distilled water to make 100 mL.
6. Filter through a 0.2-μm filter.
7. Package and label.

Ingredient-Specific Preparations

℞ **Atropine Sulfate 0.5% Nasal Solution**

Atropine sulfate		500 mg
Sodium chloride		835 mg
Sterile water for injection	qs	100 mL

1. Calculate the quantity of each ingredient required for the prescription.
2. Accurately weigh or measure each ingredient.
3. Dissolve the atropine sulfate and the sodium chloride in about 95 mL of sterile water for injection.
4. Add sufficient water for injection to make 100 mL.
5. Filter through a 0.2-μm filter into a sterile container.
6. Package and label.

℞ Desmopressin Acetate Nasal Solution 0.033 mg/mL

Desmopressin solution 0.1 mg/mL	2.5 mL
0.9% Sodium chloride solution	5 mL

1. Calculate the quantity of each ingredient required for the prescription.
2. Accurately weigh or measure each ingredient.
3. Mix the two solutions together and mix well.
4. Filter through a 0.2-µm filter into a sterile container.
5. Package and label.

℞ Saline Nasal Mist

Sodium chloride	650 mg
Monobasic potassium phosphate	40 mg
Dibasic potassium phosphate	90 mg
Benzalkonium chloride	10 mg
Sterile water for injection qs	100 mL

1. Calculate the quantity of each ingredient required for the prescription.
2. Accurately weigh or measure each ingredient.
3. Dissolve the ingredients in sufficient sterile water for injection to make 100 mL of solution.
4. Filter through a 0.2-µm filter into a sterile solution.
5. Package in a nasal spray bottle.

℞ Xylometazoline Hydrochloride Nasal Drops

Xylometazoline hydrochloride	100 mg
Sodium chloride	850 mg
Benzalkonium chloride	10 mg
Sterile water for injection qs	100 mL

1. Calculate the quantity of each ingredient required for the prescription.
2. Accurately weigh or measure each ingredient.
3. Dissolve all the ingredients in sufficient sterile water for injection to make 100 mL.
4. Filter through a sterile 0.2-µm filter into a sterile container.
5. Package and label.

℞ Progesterone 2 mg/0.1 mL Nasal Solution

Progesterone	20 mg
Dimethyl-β-cyclodextrin	62 mg
Sterile water for injection	1 mL

1. Calculate the quantity of each ingredient required for the prescription.
2. Accurately weigh or measure each ingredient.
3. Dissolve the dimethyl-β-cyclodextrin in 0.9 mL of sterile water for injection.
4. Add the progesterone and stir until dissolved.
5. Adjust the pH to 7.4 using either dilute hydrochloric acid or dilute sodium hydroxide solution.
6. Add sufficient sterile water for injection to make 1 mL.
7. Package and label.

℞ Scopolamine Hydrobromide 0.4 mg/0.1 mL Nasal Solution

Scopolamine hydrobromide		400 mg
Buffer solution (pH 5)		5 mL
0.9% Sodium chloride solution	qs	100 mL

1. Calculate the quantity of each ingredient required for the prescription.
2. Accurately weigh or measure each ingredient.
3. Dissolve the scopolamine hydrobromide in about 50 mL of the 0.9% sodium chloride solution.
4. Add the pH 5 buffer and mix well.
5. Add sufficient 0.9% sodium chloride solution to volume and mix.
6. Filter through a 0.2-μm sterile filter into a sterile container.
7. Package in a metering nasal spray container and label.

℞ Buprenorphine Hydrochloride 150 μg/100 μL Nasal Spray

Buprenorphine hydrochloride	150 mg
Glycerin	5 mL
Methylparaben	200 mg
0.9% Sodium chloride injection	95 mL

1. Calculate the quantity of each ingredient required for the prescription.
2. Accurately weigh the buprenorphine hydrochloride and methylparaben powders.
3. Dissolve the methylparaben in the glycerin.
4. Add the buprenorphine hydrochloride to the sodium chloride injection.
5. Add the methylparaben in glycerin to the sodium chloride injection.
6. Sterilize by filtering through a sterile 0.2-μm filter into a sterile container.
7. Package and label.

Rx Fentanyl 25 µg/0.1 mL Nasal Spray (10 mL)

Fentanyl citrate	2.5 mg
Methylparaben	10 mg
Propylparaben	10 mg
Propylene glycol	0.2 mL
0.9% Sodium chloride solution qs	10 mL

1. Calculate the quantity of each ingredient required for the prescription.
2. Accurately weigh or measure each ingredient.
3. Dissolve the methylparaben and propylparaben in the propylene glycol.
4. Dissolve the fentanyl citrate in about 9 mL of 0.9% sodium chloride solution.
5. Add the paraben mixture and mix well.
6. Add sufficient 0.9% sodium chloride solution to volume and mix well.
7. Sterilize by filtering through a sterile 0.2 m filter into a sterile metered spray bottle.
8. Package and label.

Rx Meperidine Hydrochloride 50 mg/mL Nasal Solution

Meperidine hydrochloride	5 g
Phenol	200 mg
Sterile water for injection qs	100 mL

(Note: Metacresol 100 mg can be used in place of phenol as a preservative.)

1. Calculate the quantity of each ingredient required for the prescription.
2. Accurately weigh the meperidine hydrochloride powder and phenol crystals and place in a graduate.
3. Add sufficient sterile water for injection to volume and mix well.
4. Sterilize by filtering through a sterile 0.2-µm filter into a sterile container.
5. Package and label.

Rx Methyl Sulfonylmethane (MSM) 16% Nasal Solution (100 mL)

Methyl sulfonylmethane	16 g
Benzalkonium chloride	20 mg
Purified water qs	100 mL

1. Calculate the quantity of each ingredient required for the prescription.
2. Accurately weigh or measure each ingredient. Dilutions may be required to obtain the correct quantity of benzalkonium chloride.
3. Dissolve the methyl sulfonylmethane and benzalkonium chloride in sufficient purified water to make 100 mL and mix well.
4. Package and label.

℞ Mupirocin 0.5% Nasal Drops (30 mL)

Mupirocin ointment (2%)		15 g
0.9% Sodium chloride solution	qs	30 mL

1. Calculate the quantity of each ingredient required for the prescription.
2. Empty the contents of a 15-g tube of mupirocin (Bactroban) ointment into an appropriate graduated cylinder.
3. Add sufficient 0.9% sodium chloride solution to 30 mL.
4. Mix until uniform.
5. Package and label.

Hints for Administration of Ophthalmic Preparations

1. The normal volume of the fluid in the eye is about 10 μL. The volume of an average drop ranges between 25 and 50 μL. Consequently, only one drop should be administered to the eye at one time.
2. If more than one drop or more than one drug is to be administered, one should wait at least 5 minutes between doses to allow the drug to be distributed and absorbed.
3. Immediately after instilling a drop into the eye, placing pressure on the lacrimal sac for a minute or two will help decrease "systemic" absorption of the drug that occurs when the drug is removed by the nasolacrimal duct and swallowed, thereby entering the gastrointestinal tract.
4. An advantage to ophthalmic suspensions is that they dissolve slowly and remain in the cul-de-sac longer.
5. Ophthalmic ointments provide maximum contact between the drug and the eye because they are cleared quite slowly (0.5% per minute) from the eye.
6. The size of a drop delivered can vary with the angle of the dropper and the size of the dropper orifice.

Chapter 21

Inhalation Products

Definitions/Types

Inhalation is a method of drug delivery that has been used throughout history in forms such as aromatic perfumes/oils, burned incenses, smoked leaves and herbs, and so forth. Drugs can be introduced into the lungs quite easily with this method. The patient simply inhales a dose of a drug incorporated in a properly designed dosage form. The drug is then caught up in the flow of air and carried into the deep recesses of the pulmonary environment, that is, into the respiratory bronchioles and the alveolar region. Drugs can take the form of a vapor, a very fine powder, or a solution in the form of an aerosol. An *aerosol* is a dispersed system consisting of a solid or liquid internal phase in an outer gaseous phase. Examples of natural aerosols are mist (i.e., water/air) and dust (i.e., solid/air). Products administered by inhalation can produce either a local or a systemic effect. Drugs commonly administered for respiratory purposes include bronchodilators, corticosteroids, antitussives, expectorants, surfactants, respiratory stimulants, and therapeutic gases.

Aromatherapy is a contemporary term used to describe one of the age-old methods of drug administration. Today, the term *aromatherapy* primarily refers to the use of volatile or aromatic oils that serve as room sprays, massage products, room fresheners, and even inhalants when placed in hot water.

Oral inhalation products have numerous advantages, including the following:

- Rapid onset of action.
- Bypass of the first-pass effect.
- Absence of drug degradation in the gastrointestinal tract.
- Low dosages to minimize adverse reactions.
- Dose titration capability.
- Good dosage form for as-needed dosing.
- An alternate route when other drugs may chemically or physically interact with concurrent drugs.
- An alternate route for drugs with erratic oral or parenteral administration pharmacokinetics.

The ultimate deposition of inhalation aerosols depends on (1) the product's formulation; (2) the design of the components, the packaging, and the container; (3) the administration skills and techniques of the product user; and (4) the anatomic and physiologic status of the respiratory system.

A wide range of dosage forms and methods of administering drugs by inhalation is available. They include aerosols, atomizers, inhalations, insufflations, metered-dose inhalers (MDIs), nebulizers, and vaporizers.

By definition, an *aerosol* is a colloidal dispersion of a liquid or a solid in a gas. Both oral inhalation and nasopharyngeal medications can be administered in the form of an aerosol. These products are commonly administered by manual sprays or from pressurized packages. Aerosol use has become so widespread that the term has come to mean a self-contained product that is sprayed, through the propelling force of either a liquefied or a compressed gas. In pharmacy, these pressure-packaged products consist of the active drug dissolved, suspended, or emulsified in a propellant or a mixture of a solvent and a propellant. These aerosols are generally designed either for topical administration or for inhalation into the nasopharyngeal region or bronchopulmonary system. For pulmonary delivery, particles greater than 60 μm are usually deposited in the trachea; those greater than 20 μm are deposited between the trachea and the bronchioles but not into the bronchioles. Particles about 1 μm often remain airborne and are exhaled. Consequently, particles ranging between about 5 μm and 20 μm would be needed to reach the bronchioles. The largest group of oral aerosol products formulated as either solutions or suspensions is inhalation aerosols.

An *atomizer* is an instrument used to disperse a liquid in a fine spray. Many of the older pressure-type atomizers used Bernoulli's principle. When a stream of air moves at a high velocity over the tip of a dip tube, the pressure is lowered, which causes the liquid to be drawn into the airflow. The liquid is broken up into a spray as it is taken up into the air stream. To produce smaller droplets, a baffle, bead, or other device can be put in the flow to break the droplets into smaller droplets as they collide with the stationary device. These smaller droplets are then carried by the airflow into the inhaled stream of air. Many different configurations are available that use Bernoulli's principle. A finer spray can be obtained if a pressure atomizer is used. Today's plastic spray bottles are similar to the pressure atomizers. When the plastic bottle is squeezed, the air inside is compressed, forcing the liquid up a dip tube into the tip. The liquid stream is mixed with air as it is emitted from the nozzle, thereby producing a spray.

Inhalations are preparations designed to deliver the drug into the respiratory tree of the patient for local or systemic effect. Rapid relief is obtained when the vapors or the mist/droplets reach the affected area. The *United States Pharmacopeia 25/National Formulary 20* definition of *inhalations* states that "inhalations are drugs or solutions or suspensions of one or more drug substances administered by the nasal or oral respiratory route for local or systemic effect." The drugs can be nebulized to produce droplets sufficiently fine and uniform in size to reach the bronchioles. The patient can breathe the mist directly from the nebulizer of a face mask or tent. An intermittent positive-pressure breathing machine can be used to produce a contained environment to maximize the quantity of drug available in the breathing environment to be delivered into the lungs.

According to the *British Pharmacopoeia (BP)*, inhalations are solutions or suspensions of one or more active ingredients that can contain an inert, suspended diffusing agent. These liquids are designed to release volatile constituents for inhalation, either when placed on a pad or when added to hot water. An example of the latter is adding 1 teaspoonful of benzoin inhalation BP to 1 quart of hot water and inhaling the vapors.

Inhalants are drugs that are characterized by a high vapor pressure and can be carried by an air current into the nasal passage where the drugs generally exert their effect. The device or the container from which the inhalant is generally administered is called an inhaler. An inhalant consists of cylindrical rolls of a fibrous material that has been impregnated with the drug, usually containing an aromatic substance in addition to an active substance. These devices are often cylindrical in nature, with a cap in place to retard the loss of the medication. The patient removes the cap and inserts the inhaler into a nostril. When the patient inhales, the air passes through the inhaler and carries the vapor of the medication into the nasal passage. An actual "drug vapor" is being delivered to the patient. For example, menthol, camphor, propylhexedrine, and tuaminoheptane inhalants are of this type. Another type, the amyl nitrite inhalant, is packaged with the drug contained in a thin glass ampule encased in gauze netting. When the product is squeezed and the glass ampule broken, the amyl nitrite is released and is absorbed on the gauze netting and inhaled by the patient.

Insufflations are powders administered with the use of a powder blower (or puffer) or insufflator. These devices can consist of a rubber bulb connected to a container and a delivery pipe. As the bulb is squeezed, air is blown into the container creating turbulence. This turbulence causes the powder to fly around. As the air leaves the container, some of the fine particles are carried out with the air through the delivery tube and are ready for inhalation. The puffer device consists of a plastic accordion-shaped container with a spout on one end. The powder is placed in the puffer, and, as the puffer is sharply squeezed, a portion of the powder is ejected from the spout into the air, where it is available for inhalation or application. Contemporary delivery systems include powders that can be delivered by various mechanical devices designed so that the patient can breathe deeply to inhale the powder particles. The inspiration step provides the energy to spin a propeller that serves to break up and distribute the particles as they are inhaled.

Metered-dose inhalants are propellant-driven drug products, either in the form of solutions or suspensions, which contain the drug and a liquified gas propellant with or without a cosolvent. MDIs are designed to deliver a metered dose of the drug and commonly deliver a volume from 25 to 100 μL of liquid drug for inhalation.

Nebulae, or spray solutions, are intended for spraying into the throat and nose. Generally, these are simple solutions. Plastic spray bottles work in much the same way as pressure atomizers. When the flexible plastic container is squeezed, the air is compressed, forcing the liquid in the container up through a dip tube into the tip where it mixes with a stream of air. Droplets are formed depending on the geometry of the device and the pressure exerted by the person squeezing the bottle.

A *nebulizer* was formerly described as a small, vacuum-type atomizer inside a chamber. Large droplets would strike the walls of the chamber, fall back, and be reprocessed. The smaller particles would be carried out of the unit in the air stream. The nebulizer would be placed in the mouth of the patient who would inhale while simultaneously squeezing the bulb. Electrically powered nebulizers are now used; the solution (usually less than 5 mL) is placed in the reservoir, and the mouthpiece/nosepiece is placed in position for administration. For nebulizers to be suitable for administering inhalation solutions, they must produce droplets sufficiently fine and uniform in size (optimally 0.5 to 7 μm) that the mist will reach the bronchioles. An advantage to the newer pressurized aerosols is that they produce a fine mist and more uniform doses than the older manual nebulizers.

A *vaporizer* is an electrical device producing moist steam, either with or without medication, for inhalation. It is often used to soothe upper respiratory irritations but is relatively ineffective in providing medications to the deeper areas of the respiratory tract.

Historical/Future Use

One of the earliest ways to inhale drug products was to burn the material and inhale the smoke. In some cases, a natural vegetable product was dried, broken up, and burned; in others, an oil or another material was burned and its vapors were inhaled. Until recently, an asthma "cigarette" (Asthmador) containing the drug was available. The cigarette was smoked and inhaled, delivering the bronchodilator to the lungs. This principle is still used by recreational drug users for substances such as tobacco, marijuana, and opium. Some recreational drugs are simply inhaled in the powder form, resulting in a rapid onset of action. There is no question about the effectiveness of this route of administration for drugs.

One problem encountered with the use of an inhaler to deliver drugs to the patient was the inability to determine the accuracy of the dose. This problem has been partly overcome with the advent of the newer MDIs, because the same volume of drug will be administered every time. Not addressed, however, is the variability in the rate of inspiration, breath holding, and expiration, which means that varying quantities of the drug can be absorbed.

In the past, inhalations were simple solutions of volatile medications, usually volatile oils, in alcohol or an alcoholic preparation. Often compound benzoin tincture was used. A sample formulation is as follows:

Pine oil	5 mL
Eucalyptus oil	5 mL
Compound benzoin tincture	30 mL

Sig: Add 1 teaspoonful to 1 pint of hot water; inhale the vapor.

Other inhalations designed to be added to hot water were aqueous preparations containing a volatile oil, water, and light magnesium carbonate. The light magnesium carbonate served as a distributive or dispersing agent. The volatile material was distributed on the light magnesium carbonate, which was then mixed with the water. This mixture ensured that the oil was uniformly dispersed on shaking because it was distributed throughout the mixture rather than remaining as a globule or being dispersed as large globules. The presence of the light magnesium carbonate did not interfere with the free volatilization of the oil when the product was added to hot water. If the oil would emulsify, it would actually retard volatilization. An approximate ratio of 100 mg of light magnesium carbonate to 0.2 mL of oil was used. A sample formulation is as follows:

Menthol		325 mg
Eucalyptus oil		3.7 mL
Light magnesium carbonate		2 g
Purified water	qs	30 mL

Sig: Add 1 teaspoonful to 1 pint of hot water (not boiling). Inhale the vapor. Shake the bottle before using.

In the early 1950s, Riker Laboratories introduced the first contemporary pressurized aerosol dosage form. The Medihaler Epi consisted of epinephrine hydrochloride in a hydroalcoholic solvent system containing sorbitan trioleate as a dispersing agent and a fluorinated hydrocarbon propellant system. Today, these small, self-contained aerosol propellant systems generally contain up to about 30 mL of product in a small, stainless steel container fitted with a metered-dose valve. The four components include a product concentrate, propellant, container, and suitable dispensing/metering valve. Products available in this dosage form have included epinephrine bitartrate, isoproterenol hydrochloride, albuterol, triamcinolone acetonide, dexamethasone sodium phosphate, beclomethasone dipropionate, isoetharine mesylate, and metaproterenol sulfate.

Oral and nasal inhalation products are a promising means of administering many local and systemic drugs. Thus, pharmacists may have many opportunities to compound these products in the future. With their rapid onset of action, generally good stability profiles, easy titration, and simple formulation development, these products will continue to meet patient needs and their use will continue to grow.

Applications

Oral inhalants are most commonly used to deliver drugs directly to the airways and the lungs in the treatment of pulmonary disorders. Gases are administered by this method to provide anesthesia during surgery. Oral inhalants used for local treatment include products that suppress coughing, break up mucus, and treat fungal infections. Systemic agents administered by oral inhalation include antiasthmatics, anti-inflammatories, and respiratory stimulants.

Composition

Solution aerosols are fairly simple to formulate if the active drug is soluble in the propellant system. If not, a suspension or an emulsion aerosol can be prepared. For oral inhalation, either solution or suspension aerosols are used. Table 21-1 lists example ingredients used in oral inhalations or nasal aerosol solutions.

Suspension aerosols have been used to formulate antiasthmatic aerosols, steroids, antibiotics, and others. Potential problems include caking, agglomeration, particle size growth, and clogging of the valve systems. Table 21-2 lists example ingredients used in nasal aerosol solutions or suspensions.

Citric acid is often used in these formulations as an acidifying agent. Polysorbate 80 is used as an emulsifying and solubilizing agent. Sodium chloride and dextrose are used as tonicity-adjusting agents.

Table 21-1. General Formula Components for Oral, Inhalation, and Nasal Aerosol Solutions

Component	Example
Active ingredient	Ingredient appropriate for condition; soluble in vehicle
Solvents	Ethyl alcohol, propylene glycol, purified water
Surfactants	Polysorbate 80
Antioxidants	Ascorbic acid
Flavor	Aromatic oils
Propellants	As needed

Table 21-2. General Formula Components for Nasal Aerosol Solutions or Suspensions

Component	Example
Active ingredient	Solubilized or suspended forms of appropriate ingredient for condition
Antioxidants	Ascorbic acid, bisulfites
Preservatives	Benzalkonium chloride
Buffers	Phosphate buffer
Tonicity adjustment	Sodium chloride
Surfactants	Sorbitan esters
Vehicle	Purified water

Preparation

The steps that follow should be used when preparing most inhalation products in solution form. All formulations in the section "Sample Formulations" are solutions; therefore, these steps are appropriate for use in their preparation.

1. Calculate the quantity of the individual ingredients required for the prescription.
2. Accurately weigh or measure each of the ingredients.
3. Dissolve the solids in about two thirds of the volume of vehicle.
4. Add the liquid ingredients and mix well.
5. Add sufficient vehicle to volume and mix well.
6. Sterilize by filtering through a sterile 0.2-μm filter system into sterile containers.
7. Package and label.

Physicochemical Considerations

When compounding, or formulating, products for oral or nasal inhalation, the variables to consider include particle size, solubility, vehicles, tonicity, pH, sterility, preservatives, viscosity, buffers, surfactants, and moisture content.

Particle Size

Generally, the particle size should be within the range of about 0.5 to 10 μm. The range should preferably be between about 3 and 6 μm, if the inhaled drug is intended to penetrate to the small bronchioles and the lung alveoli and to provide a rapid effect. This size range of particles will deposit in the lung by gravitational sedimentation, inertial impaction, and diffusion into terminal alveoli by Brownian motion. For inhalation aerosols, particles of 5 to 10 μm are common, whereas for topical sprays, the range of 50 to 100 μm is typical.

Solubility

Active drugs that are soluble in the matrix and in the pulmonary fluids will have a rapid onset of action and ordinarily a shorter duration of action, compared with drugs that are somewhat less soluble in the matrix and in the pulmonary fluids. Drugs that are poorly soluble in the pulmonary fluids can cause problems by irritating the lung tissue. When a pharmacist is preparing a suspension, it is best to select a vehicle in which the drug is not very soluble to minimize the phenomenon of particle size growth. This growth results when the drug in solution crystallizes out onto the crystals that are present. Polymorphic forms of crystalline drugs should not be used for suspension aerosols. To enhance the stability of a suspension aerosol, the compounding pharmacist should select a liquid phase with a density similar to that of the suspensoid, which will minimize the tendency to settle.

Vehicles

Sterile water for inhalation and 0.9% sodium chloride inhalation solution are commonly used vehicles to carry the drugs in inhalations. Some inhalations are simple solutions of nonvolatile or volatile medications in water or cosolvent mixtures. Small quantities of alcohol or glycerin can be used to solubilize ingredients.

Tonicity

Generally, it is best to have inhalation solutions that are isotonic with physiologic fluids, that is, equivalent to 0.9% sodium chloride or an osmolality of about 290 mOsm. The solution should be slightly hypotonic to enhance the movement of the fluid and drug through the alveoli. If it is hypotonic, the administered drug solution may have a greater tendency to move into the tissue for more rapid absorption and therapeutic effect. However, if the solution were hypertonic, the fluids would tend to move from the alveoli into the pulmonary space to reach an isotonic equilibrium.

pH

A pH in the neutral range, similar to body fluids, should minimize any cough reflex that might occur if the pH were too low. However, the solubility and stability characteristics of the drug must be taken into consideration when establishing the pH.

Sterility

Inhalation solutions are required to be sterile. Compounded oral inhalation solutions should be sterilized to ensure that patients get the best products available. Sterility can be easily accomplished by using 0.2-μm filtration systems designed for extemporaneous compounding (Figure 21-1).

Preservatives

Any preparation that is not in unit-dose containers should contain a preservative, especially with the sterility requirement for this class of dosage

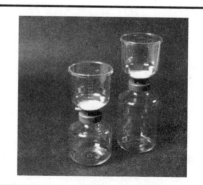

Figure 21-1. Sterile disposal vacuum filters (0.2-μm filter; 500 mL volume).

forms. The minimum amount of preservative that is still effective should be used. Incorporating too high a concentration can initiate a cough reflex in the patient. If the concentration of certain preservatives that are also surfactants is too high, foaming can result, which could interfere with the delivery of the complete dose.

Viscosity

The viscosity of the external phase for most aerosol products is quite low; consequently, they are very sensitive systems. Evaporation, sedimentation, and an increase in particle size are processes that can occur and change rapidly.

Buffers

A buffer, if used, should be at low buffer strength to maintain the desired pH. It should not induce pH changes in a microenvironment in the pulmonary cavity.

Surfactants

Surfactants can be used as dispersing agents for suspensions, as solubilizing agents to enhance the solubility of the drug, and as spreading agents when the drug is deposited in the lungs. The sorbitan esters, especially sorbitan trioleate, can be used, as well as lecithin derivatives, oleyl alcohol, and others. One should be cautious and keep the surfactant concentration as low as possible to minimize foaming that might interfere with proper administration.

Moisture Content

The moisture content for inhalation dispersion aerosols should be kept extremely low for all active and inactive ingredients. The ingredients should be anhydrous to minimize caking.

Quality Control

The compounding pharmacist should follow standard quality control procedures. Solutions should be checked for precipitation, discoloration, haziness, gas formation resulting from microbial growth, and final volume.

Packaging/Storage/Labeling

Oral inhalation products should be packaged in individual, sterile, unit-of-use containers. Generally, these preparations should be stored at either room or refrigerated temperatures. These products should be labeled "Oral Inhalation Use Only. Not for Injection." Labeling should also contain detailed instructions for proper use of the product.

Stability

Beyond-use dates for water-containing formulations prepared from ingredients in solid form are no later than 14 days, when stored at cold temperatures. These dates are extended if valid scientific information supports the stability of the product, as discussed in Chapter 4, "Stability of Compounded Products."

Patient Counseling

The patient or caregiver should be thoroughly instructed on how to administer oral inhalation solutions. If the solution does not include a preservative, the patient should be instructed to discard any remaining solution in the individual dosage vials and in the device used for aerosolization.

Sample Formulations

The sample formulations illustrated here are preservative free. They should be packaged as single-use or unit-dose products. Formulations are provided for 100-mL quantities for ease of calculations. The formulas should be reduced or expanded based on the total quantity to be compounded. These solutions can be preserved by adding 4 mg of benzalkonium chloride per 100 mL of solution. (This amount would be 3 mL of a benzalkonium chloride 1:750 solution.) The steps listed in the section "Preparation" apply to all the formulations given here.

 Albuterol Sulfate 0.5% Inhalant Solution (Preservative free)

Albuterol sulfate	500 mg
Citric acid, anhydrous	100 mg
Sodium chloride	800 mg
Sterile water for inhalation qs	100 mL

 Albuterol Sulfate 2.7% Inhalant for Hand Nebulizer (Preservative free)

Albuterol sulfate	2.7 g
Citric acid, anhydrous	100 mg
Sterile water for inhalation qs	100 mL

 Beclomethasone Dipropionate 0.042% Nasal Solution (Preservative free)

Beclomethasone dipropionate, monohydrate	43 mg
Dextrose	5.4 g
Polysorbate 80	1 mL
Hydrochloric acid (3%–5%)	Adjust to pH 7
Ethanol, 95%	13 mL
0.9% Sodium chloride solution qs	100 mL

 Cromolyn Sodium 1% Inhalation Solution (Preservative free)

Cromolyn sodium	1 g
Sterile water for inhalation qs	100 mL

 Cromolyn Sodium 4% Inhalation Solution (Preservative free)

Cromolyn sodium	4 g
Sterile water for inhalation qs	100 mL

 Flunisolide 0.025% Inhalation Solution (Preservative free)

Flunisolide	25 mg
Ethanol, 95%	2 mL
0.9% Sodium chloride solution qs	100 mL

℞ Ipratropium Bromide 0.02% Solution (Preservative free)

Ipratropium bromide		20 mg
Citric acid, anhydrous		50 mg
0.9% Sodium chloride solution	qs	100 mL

℞ Metaproterenol Sulfate 0.3% Solution (Preservative free)

Metaproterenol sulfate		300 mg
Citric acid, anhydrous		250 mg
0.9% Sodium chloride solution	qs	100 mL

℞ Metaproterenol Sulfate 0.6% Solution (Preservative free)

Metaproterenol sulfate		600 mg
Citric acid, anhydrous		500 mg
0.9% Sodium chloride solution	qs	100 mL

℞ Metaproterenol Sulfate 5% Concentrate (Preservative free)

Metaproterenol sulfate		5 g
Citric acid, anhydrous		500 mg
0.9% Sodium chloride solution		50 mL
Sterile water for inhalation	qs	100 mL

℞ Terbutaline Sulfate 0.1% Inhalant Solution (Preservative free)

Terbutaline sulfate		100 mg
Citric acid, anhydrous		100 mg
0.9% Sodium chloride solution	qs	100 mL

℞ Albuterol–Cromolyn–Betamethasone for Inhalation (Preservative free)

Albuterol sulfate		500 mg
Cromolyn sodium		1 g
Betamethasone sodium phosphate		250 mg
Citric acid, anhydrous		100 mg
Sodium chloride		800 mg
Sterile water for inhalation	qs	100 mL

Adjust pH to 6.8–7.0.

R₂ **Albuterol–Ipratropium for Inhalation (Preservative free)**

Albuterol sulfate	100 mg
Ipratropium bromide	20 mg
Citric acid, anhydrous	50 mg
Sterile water for inhalation qs	100 mL

R₂ **Ipratropium–Metaproterenol–Betamethasone for Inhalation Concentrate (Preservative free)**

Ipratropium bromide	125 mg
Metaproterenol sulfate	5 g
Betamethasone sodium phosphate	250 mg
Citric acid, anhydrous	100 mg
Sterile water for inhalation qs	100 mL

Chapter 22

Parenteral Preparations

Definitions/Types

A parenteral is a product that is administered to the body by injection. Because an injection bypasses the normal body defense mechanisms, it is essential that these products be prepared with a higher degree of care and skill than is present in preparing routine oral or topical products. The finished product must be sterile, nonpyrogenic, and free from extraneous insoluble materials. Because of their critical nature, sterile products must be prepared under strict environmental conditions, thus providing a challenge to the compounding pharmacist.

Classification Systems

Two organizations have developed standards and technical assistance bulletins on the preparation of sterile products. These publications are the ASHP Technical Assistance Bulletin on Quality Assurance for Pharmacy-Prepared Sterile Products (ASHP-TAB), published by the American Society of Health-System Pharmacists (Bethesda, Md) and Chapter ⟨1206⟩, "Sterile Drug Products for Home Use," in the *United States Pharmacopeia 25/National Formulary 20 (USP 25/NF 20)*, published by the United States Pharmacopeial Convention (Rockville, Md).

ASHP-TAB Risk Levels

The ASHP-TAB describes three different risk levels, with risk level 1 posing the least risk to the patient and risk level 3 posing the greatest risk. The reader is advised to obtain a copy of the bulletin.

Risk Level 1

Risk level 1 applies to compounded sterile products that exhibit characteristics 1, 2, or 3, as described below. All risk level 1 products should be prepared with sterile equipment (e.g., syringes, vials), sterile ingredients and solutions, and sterile contact surfaces for the final product. Of the three risk levels, risk level 1 requires the least amount of quality assurance. Risk level 1 includes the following:

1. Products
— Stored at room temperature and completely administered within 28 hours from preparation.

— Stored under refrigeration for 7 days or less before complete administration to a patient over a period not to exceed 24 hours.

— Frozen for 30 days or less before complete administration to a patient over a period not to exceed 24 hours.

2. Unpreserved sterile products prepared for administration to one patient, or batch-prepared products containing suitable preservatives prepared for administration to more than one patient.

3. Products prepared by closed-system aseptic transfer of sterile, nonpyrogenic, finished pharmaceuticals obtained from licensed manufacturers into sterile final containers (e.g., syringe, minibag, portable infusion-device cassette) obtained from licensed manufacturers.

Risk Level 2

Risk level 2 applies to sterile products that exhibit characteristics 1, 2, or 3, as stated next. All risk level 2 products should be prepared with sterile equipment, sterile ingredients and solutions, and sterile contact surfaces for the final product and by using closed-system transfer methods. Risk level 2 includes the following:

1. Products stored beyond 7 days under refrigeration, stored beyond 30 days frozen, or administered beyond 28 hours after preparation and storage at room temperature.

2. Batch-prepared products without preservatives that are intended for use by more than one patient. (Note: Batch-prepared products without preservatives that will be administered to multiple patients carry a greater risk to the patients than products prepared for a single patient because of the potential effect of product contamination on the health and well-being of a larger patient group.)

3. Products compounded by combining multiple sterile ingredients, which have been obtained from licensed manufacturers, in a sterile reservoir, which has been obtained from a licensed manufacturer, by using closed-system aseptic transfer before subdividing into multiple units to be dispensed to patients.

Risk Level 3

Risk level 3 applies to sterile products that exhibit either characteristic 1 or characteristic 2, as follows:

1. Products compounded from nonsterile ingredients or compounded with nonsterile components, containers, or equipment.

2. Products prepared by combining multiple ingredients—sterile or nonsterile—by using an open-system transfer or open reservoir before terminal sterilization or subdivision into multiple units to be dispensed.

USP 25/NF 20 Risk Levels

Chapter ⟨1206⟩, "Sterile Drug Products for Home Use," describes two risk levels: low and high.[1]

Low Risk Level

Low-risk products are those with the following characteristics:

1. The finished product is compounded with commercially available, sterile drug products.

2. Compounding involves only basic, and relatively few, aseptic manipulations that are promptly executed.
3. Closed-system transfers are used. The container-closure system remains essentially intact throughout the aseptic process, compromised only by the penetration of a sterile, pyrogen-free needle or cannula through the designated stopper or port to effect transfer, withdrawal, or delivery in accordance with the labeled instructions for the pertinent, commercially available devices.

High Risk Level

High-risk products are classified as either Category I or Category II. Category I high-risk products have the following characteristics:

1. Compounding involves the pooling of sterile drug products in an intermediate closed system.
2. Compounding includes complex and/or numerous aseptic manipulations executed over a prolonged period.
3. An individual finished product is administered as a multiday infusion by a portable pump or reservoir.

Category II high-risk products have the following characteristics:

1. A nonsterile drug substance or an injectable drug product prepared in-house from a nonsterile substance is used to compound the product.
2. Open systems are used, for example, when combining ingredients in a nonsealed reservoir before filling or when fluid passes through the atmosphere during a fill-seal operation.

The reader should obtain a copy of the complete chapter for more detailed explanations. Also, some states have additional definitions and procedures that must be followed.

Historical Use

In 1656, Sir Christopher Wren, a professor of surgery and a mathematician, used a syringe and pipe to inject opium, which had been dissolved in wine, into a dog. Two years later, in 1658, a solution was injected into a human by using a pig's bladder and a goose quill. Few advancements were made over the next 200 years, but, by the middle of the 19th century, analgesics were being injected with greater frequency. When an antisyphilitic was found to be effective by injection but not by mouth, the use of injections expanded rapidly. In the mid-1920s, the need for sterility was recognized, and it became a requirement for injections. Today, parenterals must be free of both microorganisms and their byproducts and endotoxins. Over the past 50 years, the use of parenteral products and their preparation by pharmacists has dramatically increased. This growth is due to the increase in available products, clean rooms, laminar airflow (LAF) hoods, automated compounding equipment, and, especially, the home health care movement, which has led to more patients being treated at home.

Applications

Parenteral preparations are used in the form of standard injections (e.g., intravenous [IV], intramuscular, intradermal, subcutaneous, intrathecal, epidural), parenteral admixtures (i.e., combinations of two or more preparations mixed together), and parenteral nutrition products (i.e., products containing caloric sources such as carbohydrates, proteins, and fats). Parental preparations are also used in hospital and home health care products (including patient-controlled analgesia, chemotherapy, and antibiotic therapy). As one of the fastest-growing segments in health care today, home health care offers many opportunities for aseptic compounding.

Composition

When compounding parenteral admixtures, one must be aware of the presence of various adjuvants. These adjuvants include the vehicles, cosolvents, buffers, preservatives, antioxidants, inert gases, surfactants, complexation agents, and chelating agents.

Water is the most common vehicle used today. If a drug is not very water soluble, a number of cosolvents (ethyl alcohol, 1%–50%; glycerin, 1%–50%; polyethylene glycol [PEG], 1%–50%; propylene glycol, 1%–60%) can be used.

So that a desired pH in a solution for both solubility and stability can be maintained, many preparations contain buffer systems. The buffer capacity (i.e., the resistance to change on the addition of either an acid or a base) is generally low, so that these systems will not alter the pH of the body fluids on injection. They are sufficiently strong, however, to resist changes in pH under normal storage and use.

Products that are packaged in multiple-dose vials are required to contain a preservative to prevent the growth of microorganisms that may be introduced when the container is manipulated. However, these preservatives may not always be compatible with other drugs to which they may be added. For example, benzyl alcohol is incompatible with chloramphenicol sodium succinate, and the parabens and phenol preservatives are incompatible with nitrofurantoin, amphotericin B, and erythromycin. When one is reconstituting with bacteriostatic water for injection, it is important to select a product with a preservative that will be compatible with the solution. Preservatives must be compatible with the container and the closure to which they are added. Table 22-1 provides a list of the preservatives used in parenteral products.

Table 22-1. Preservatives Used in Parenteral Products

Agents	Usual Concentration (%)
Benzalkonium chloride	0.01
Benzethonium chloride	0.01
Benzyl alcohol	1.0–2.0
Chlorobutanol	0.25–0.5
Chlorocresol	0.1–0.3
Cresol	0.3–0.5
Metacresol	0.1–0.3
p-Hydroxybenzoate esters	
Butyl	0.015
Methyl	0.1–0.2
Propyl	0.02–0.2
Phenol	0.25–0.5
Phenylmercuric nitrate	0.002
Thimerosal	0.01

Antioxidants and inert gases are used to enhance stability. Table 22-2 cites a variety of antioxidants used in parenteral products, along with their usual concentrations.

Table 22-2. Antioxidants Used in Parenteral Products

Agents	Usual Concentration (%)
Ascorbic acid	0.01–0.5
Butyl hydroxyanisole	0.005–0.02
Cysteine	0.1–0.5
Monothioglycerol	0.1–1.0
Sodium bisulfite	0.1–1.0
Sodium metabisulfite	0.1–1.0
Thiourea	0.005
Tocopherol	0.05–0.5

Surfactants can be used to increase the solubility of a drug in an aqueous system. It is possible that the presence of a surfactant can result in an increase or decrease in the rate of drug degradation. Some examples of surfactants include polyoxyethylene sorbitan monooleate (0.1%–0.5%) and sorbitan monooleate (0.05%–0.25%). Others are listed in Table 22-3.

Table 22-3. Solubilizing, Wetting, and Emulsifying Agents for Parenteral Products

Agents	Usual Concentration (%)
Dimethylacetamide	0.01
Dioctyl sodium sulfosuccinate	0.015
Ethyl alcohol	0.61–0.49
Ethyl lactate	0.1
Glycerin	14.6–25
Lecithin	0.5–2.3
PEG-40 castor oil	7–11.5
PEG 300	0.01–50.0
Polysorbate 20	0.01
Polysorbate 40	0.05
Polysorbate 80	0.04–4.0
Povidone	0.2–1.0
Propylene glycol	0.2–50.0
Sodium desoxycholate	0.21
Sorbitan monopalmitate	0.05

Complexation and chelating agents can also be used to enhance solubility and stability. Ethylenediaminetetraacetic acid salts (0.01%–0.075%) are an example of these agents.

Preparation

All aseptic manipulations should be carried out in a class 100 LAF hood (horizontal or vertical) enclosed within a class 10,000 clean room by validated aseptic compounding pharmacists. Only pharmacists who have been adequately trained should attempt to prepare sterile parenteral products. Personnel should be properly gowned with the appropriate attire for the risk level of product to be prepared. Study the Standard Operating Procedures (SOPs) titled "General Aseptic Procedures Used at a Laminar Airflow Workbench," "Maintenance of a Horizontal Laminar Airflow Hood," and "Maintenance of the Clean Room."

All items should be removed from their outer cartons before being placed on a clean cart or being manually carried into the clean room. A nonlinting wiper should be used to wipe the surfaces of the materials before their placement in the hood. At no time should any object come between the airflow of the high-efficiency particulate air cleaner (HEPA) filter and the critical site or the critical area. The critical site is the point of entry into a container, and the immediate environment surrounding the critical site is the critical area. Anything placed upstream from the critical area can contaminate the critical site. This situation occurs when the airflow washes over the item, removes any foreign material, and carries it into the critical site.

To prepare sterile parenteral products, the compounding pharmacist should carefully follow each step in the box "Preparation of Parenteral Products."

When withdrawing a drug from an ampule, the pharmacist should place the beveled side of the needle against the ampule wall to reduce the possibility of aspirating glass fragments along with the solution. The glass fragments will ordinarily be at the bottom of the ampule or floating on the surface of the drug. If the needle tip is placed at a position halfway down the ampule during withdrawal and the ampule is slowly rotated, the larger glass particles will often stick to the bottom of the ampule as it is turned more horizontally. If one slowly moves the needle bevel down the side of the ampule to the shoulder and continues to rotate the ampule a little more, the remainder of the solution can be withdrawn, with the larger particles adhering to the bottom of the ampule and the smaller ones floating on the surface of the remainder of the solution. The pharmacist should then remove the needle from the ampule, replace it with a filter and a new needle, and inject the solution into the new container.

Withdrawing a solution from a vial can be easily done by injecting an equivalent amount of clean air into the vial. It may be necessary to do this stepwise by injecting a small portion of the air in the syringe into the vial, aspirating a portion of the liquid, rotating the vial and syringe so that the needle is pointing up, and injecting another portion of air into the vial. This process should be continued until all of the solution is withdrawn.

When one is reconstituting a drug, it is advisable to inject the reconstitution fluid slowly into the vial and rotate or rock the vial for dissolution. If this process is done too rapidly, foaming can result, making it difficult to measure the desired volume of the drug. The drug solutions should be immediately labeled after reconstitution.

Preparation of Parenteral Products

1. Clean the work area thoroughly with a suitable sanitizing agent. A 70% iso-propyl alcohol spray or another equally effective disinfectant or cleaner should be used to wipe the internal surfaces. A water-based preparation should be used for the plastic side panels, because alcohol may discolor the plastic. Cleaning should begin at the innermost surface and advance outward (toward the opera-tor) in a uniform line of movement. Nonlinting cloths should be used for this pro-cedure. No solutions should ever be directed at the HEPA filter. After cleaning, the pharmacist should allow the surface to dry before proceeding.

2. Place the items for one prescription at a time in the work space of the LAF; avoid both bunching and placing any item in the direct airflow pathway of another item.

3. Remove the packaging/wrapping from the necessary syringes, needles, bags, and the like and place them on the work area, also being cognizant of the air path-way and the critical site.

4. Remove the protective aluminum or plastic cap or seals from the containers. Using an appropriate sanitizing agent, such as 70% isopropanol or ethanol, clean the tops, stoppers, and ampule necks of the individual items.

5. Move the plungers on the syringes back and forth to loosen them.

6. If ampules are used, break off the neck by breaking away the body.

7. Withdraw the medications from the ampules or vials. If vials are used, it may be necessary to inject a volume of air equal to that of the medication to be removed.

8. Filter the solution(s) during the withdrawal phase or the injection phase.

9. Use separate needles for the injection and withdrawal phases.

10. Place the medications in the appropriate container, vial, bag, or syringe.

11. Swirl to mix the medications after each addition.

12. After all medications are added and mixed, place an additive cap on the syringe or seal on the bag.

13. Label.

14. If necessary, place an overwrap or an amber overwrap on the product. Label the overwrap with a second, identical label.

Physicochemical Considerations

Freezing Products

In facilities that do a lot of sterile compounding, a common practice is to recon-stitute and prefill syringes and additive bags or vials. This process saves time; some manufacturers even provide frozen antibiotics that are ready to thaw and use. However, one should not indiscriminately freeze drugs and assume they are stable. One should check the manufacturer's literature, drug information services, and sta-bility literature to ensure that a product is stable before freezing the additives. Because different freezers are set at different temperatures, it is important to moni-tor the temperature. Some freezers can be set at −5°C to −20°C, but some products may require an ultrafreezer that reaches temperatures as low as −70°C to −80°C.

If the drugs are frozen, they must be thawed and returned to room temperature before compounding. This process should be done by hanging the bags or placing the vials or containers in a clean area and forcing room temperature air over the units. Microwave thawing should generally not be used, nor should the bags be placed in hot or warm water baths or sinks. A second LAF hood works well for thawing products.

Sorption and Leaching

Another consideration in compounding parenteral products is sorption of the drug to the container, filters, stopper, administration sets, and the like. For example, clomethiazole edisylate, chlorpromazine hydrochloride, diazepam, hydralazine, insulin, promazine hydrochloride, promethazine hydrochloride, thiopental sodium, thioridazine hydrochloride, trifluoperazine dihydrochloride, and warfarin sodium have been shown to be lost from aqueous solutions during infusion through plastic IV administration sets.

In some circumstances, the drug product itself can extract substances from the container (i.e., leaching). For example, Taxol contains a solvent system that extracts diethylhexylphthalate from plastic containers. Other types of containers and administration sets are available for administering Taxol.

Incompatibilities

pH, solubility, concentration, complexation, and light are among the factors that contribute to compatibility and stability of drug substances.

pH

The most important factor responsible for parenteral incompatibilities is a change in the acid-base environment of the drug. The solubility and stability profiles of a drug can be critically related to pH. As a solution goes away from the pH of maximum solubility, the drug can precipitate out of solution. As the solution goes away from the pH of maximum stability, the drug can degrade more rapidly and have a short beyond-use date. The pH range of 5% dextrose in water varies from 3.5 to 6.5, depending on the free sugar acids present and formed during the sterilization process and product storage. This low pH must be considered to avoid incompatibilities with additives. For example, sodium, potassium, or related salts are usually more soluble at higher pH levels, but the free acids are formed at lower pH values and can be less soluble. Acid salts (e.g., hydrochlorides, sulfates) are more soluble at lower pH values, and the basic drugs can precipitate out at higher pH levels. Generally, solutions of high pH are incompatible with solutions of low pH because of the relatively poor solubility of the free bases or free acids that are formed.

Solubility

Water is the most commonly used solvent in parenterals. When a compound is not soluble in water or is degraded in water, it can be dissolved in a nonaqueous solvent. A nonaqueous solvent must be nontoxic, nonirritating, nonsensitizing, and pharmacologically inactive to be used. Also, the solvent must be in the proper viscosity range to permit easy injection. Propylene glycol, glycerin, low molecular weight PEGs, and ethanol have been used, among others. The effect of these cosolvent systems can be complicated and difficult to predict. In some cases, fixed oils (e.g., corn oil, cottonseed oil, peanut oil, sesame oil) can be used as solvents for parenterals, and these vehicles should be considered. Any preparation containing oils may be incompatible with the water-based parenterals.

Concentration

Some drug products are stable and compatible at certain concentrations but not at others. Detailed stability information should be consulted.

Complexation

Some materials, such as tetracycline in the presence of calcium ions, will complex and reduce the activity of the drug. Complexation can also be used to enhance the solubility of a drug (e.g., caffeine and sodium benzoate).

Light

Light-sensitive drugs, such as amphotericin B, vitamin K, furosemide, Adriamycin, cisplatin, daunomycin, B complex vitamins, and NephrAmine, should be protected from light. In the case of admixtures, the drugs are removed from their protective environment and mixed in a new medium and new environment. They must be protected from light through use of a light barrier, such as foil or an amber overwrap, during both storage and administration.

Precautions

A number of precautions can be taken to decrease the occurrence of incompatibilities. These precautions include the following:

- Always use freshly prepared solutions. Solutions, if not used, should be discarded after 24 hours, or earlier as indicated.
- Store the solutions at room temperature during preparation, unless advised otherwise.
- Reconstitute solutions according to the manufacturers' instructions, unless advised otherwise. Some products may not be soluble or stable if not reconstituted as instructed.
- Use as few additives as possible in infusion fluids. Incorporating more additives increases the possibility of incompatibilities.
- Mix thoroughly after each addition. This task will distribute the drugs throughout the entire solution and minimize the possibility of any interaction between areas of high concentrations of drugs.
- If one particular additive is a problem, dilute it before incorporating any other additives.
- Check all containers first for clarity of solution and complete dissolution of reconstituted products.
- During filtration, make sure that an active drug or an important excipient is not being removed. For example, if a drug precipitates out of solution because of pH or solvent problems, it can be filtered out; also, some preservatives, such as benzalkonium chloride, can be retained on membrane-type filters.
- Be aware of potential incompatibilities in advance. Use published compatibility charts and prepare a compatibility notebook, adding observations as they occur.

If an incompatibility problem cannot be prevented, use a different administration technique such as (1) administering the problem drugs at staggered intervals so that they are physically separated, (2) using a heparin lock for administration, (3) selecting an alternative site or route of administration, and (4) using a Y-site administration set and thoroughly flushing the line between the drugs so that the problem drugs do not come into actual contact with each other.

Quality Control

Quality control of parenterals can include tests for sterility, pyrogens, particulate matter, and pH. It also includes visual observations for particulate matter and checks for the volume or weight prepared.

According to the USP 25/NF 20 Chapter ⟨788⟩, "Particulate Matter in Injections,"

> Particulate matter consists of mobile, randomly-sourced, extraneous substances, other than gas bubbles, that cannot be quantitated by chemical analysis due to the small amount of material that it represents and to its heterogeneous composition. Injectable solutions, including solutions constituted from sterile solids intended for parenteral use, should be essentially free from particles that can be observed on visual inspection.[2]

Chapter ⟨1206⟩, "Sterile Drug Products for Home Use," states, "All finished home-use sterile drug products should be individually inspected in accordance with written procedures after compounding and, if not distributed promptly, prior to leaving the pharmacy."[1] Common sources of particulates include chemicals (undissolved substances, trace contaminants), solvent impurities, packaging components (glass, plastic, rubber, IV administration sets), environmental contaminants (air, surfaces, insect parts), processing equipment (glass, stainless steel, rubber, rust), fibers, and people (skin, hair). Particulate matter can be detected with a light or dark background as described in the box "Visual Check for Particular Matter."[3,4] See the SOPs "Quality Assessment of Injectable Solutions," "Particulate Testing for Sterile Products," and "Quality Assessment of Parenteral Nutrition Products."

Visual Check for Particulate Matter

1. Inspect the product immediately after preparation. If the product is not dispensed immediately, it should be inspected again just before dispensing.
2. Inspect the contents, container, and closure during this procedure.
3. Make sure the container is free of any labels or attachments.
4. Remove any external particles with a dampened nonlinting wiper.
5. Place clean, talc-free gloves on the hands.
6. Hold the container by its top and carefully swirl its contents by rotating the wrist in a circular motion. Avoid vigorous swirling.
7. Discount any air bubbles that rise to the top.
8. Hold the container horizontally about 4 in. below the light source against the white and black background; slowly move the container back and forth between the white and the black background.
9. If no particles are noted, slowly invert the container and observe whether any heavy particles are on the bottom of the container or are sliding down the container walls.

Packaging

Packaging materials should not interact, physically or chemically, with the contained drug product to ensure that the drug concentration, quality, and purity are not altered. An ideal container should do the following:

- Allow visual inspection of the contents.
- Be chemically inert.
- Not interact with the drug or drug additives.
- Not contribute to particulate contamination.
- Not allow for loss of the drug or solution.
- Maintain the sterility of the contents before and during administration.

▸ Maintain the nonpyrogenicity of the contents before and during administration.

IV bags and bottles do not meet all the criteria for an ideal container, but they are the only commercially available containers that come close to meeting these criteria.

Storage/Labeling

The recommended storage temperature is an important element that will vary, depending on the product. Recommended storage temperatures can be room temperature (15°C–25°C), refrigerator temperature (2°C–8°C), frozen (−20°C), or ultrafrozen (down to −80°C).

Labeling for parenterals should, as a minimum, include the following:

▸ Patient's name and other appropriate identification information.
▸ Solution and ingredient names, amounts, strengths, and concentrations.
▸ Expiration or beyond-use date.
▸ Administration instructions.
▸ Auxiliary labeling.
▸ Storage requirements.
▸ Identification of the responsible pharmacist.
▸ Other information as required.

Stability

In the past, a beyond-use time of 24 hours was routinely placed on parenteral products due in large part to the potential for microbiological contamination. Today, with the use of clean rooms, LAF hoods, and the like, the concern over maintaining sterility has largely been addressed. Also, the 24-hour time limits were routine procedure in hospitals, where it was relatively simple to remove the product from the nursing units if it had not been used. With home health care, however, medications are dispensed to the patient or caregiver and can remain in the home for a few days before their actual administration. This practice has altered the way beyond-use times are assigned. Emphasis now appears to be placed on whether the drug is chemically and physically stable for the projected time of dispensing, storage, and administration, assuming that the product is prepared in a sterile manner. Manufacturers' literature, the published literature, and other sources can be used to obtain information on the stability of a drug in a certain situation. It should be emphasized that simply because a drug was found to be stable in 1000 mL of 5% dextrose in water does not mean that the drug will be stable when the same quantity of it is placed in 50 mL of 5% dextrose in water in an ambulatory drug-delivery device. The storage and administration conditions are different and must be considered. According to Chapter ⟨795⟩, "Pharmacy Compounding," beyond-use dates for water-containing formulations are no later than 14 days when stored at cold temperatures, unless otherwise documented.[5]

Patient Counseling

Patients should be instructed as to the proper storage and use of any parenteral products placed under their care. They should be informed about the proper method of maintaining a sterile administration site and the handling of administration sets and equipment. It may be necessary to train them in how to program the ambulatory pumps, if used, and how to deal with emergencies. Also, the correct disposal of parenteral products, needles, syringes, and tubing should be discussed in detail, so that the patient is aware of the potential harm that can occur if appropriate procedures are not followed.

Sample Formulations

℞ Antiemetic Injection for Cancer Chemotherapy

Reglan (5 mg/mL)	30 mL	150 mg
Ativan (2 mg/mL)	0.5 mL	1 mg
Mannitol 25%	50 mL	12.5 g
Compazine (5 mg/mL)	2 mL	10 mg
5% Dextrose injection	50 mL	

(Note: This procedure should be carried out in an LAF hood in a clean room by a qualified, aseptic compounding pharmacist.)

1. Calculate the quantity of each ingredient required for the prescription.
2. Accurately measure each ingredient.
3. Add each ingredient in sequence to a 50-mL IV partial-fil piggyback bag of 5% dextrose injection, mixing thoroughly after each addition.
4. Label.

℞ Fentanyl and Bupivacaine Injection for Ambulatory Pump Reservoirs

Fentanyl citrate		20 µg/mL
Bupivacaine hydrochloride		0.125%
0.9% Sodium chloride injection	qs	100 mL

(Note: All procedures should be carried out in a clean air environment by a qualified, aseptic compounding pharmacist.)

1. Calculate the quantity of each ingredient required for the prescription.
2. Aseptically, withdraw 40 mL of fentanyl citrate injection (Sublimaze) and introduce into a reservoir.
3. Aseptically, withdraw 25 mL of 0.5% bupivacaine hydrochloride injection, introduce into the reservoir, and mix well.
4. Aseptically, withdraw 35 mL of 0.9% sodium chloride injection and introduce into the reservoir, along with a few milliliters of air.
5. Rotate the reservoir so that the air bubble will mix the contents.
6. Position the reservoir so that the air bubble is near the exit port; remove the air in the reservoir and tubing by withdrawing the solution up to the end of the port.
7. Clamp, package, and label.

℞ Doxorubicin Hydrochloride and Vincristine Sulfate Injection

Doxorubicin hydrochloride, 2 mg/mL		83.5 mL
Vincristine sulfate, 1 mg/mL		3.5 mL
0.9% Sodium chloride injection	qs	100 mL

(Note: All procedures should be carried out in a clean air environment by a qualified, aseptic compounding pharmacist.)

1. Calculate the quantity of each ingredient required for the prescription.
2. Reconstitute the doxorubicin hydrochloride, if necessary, according to the manufacturer's directions.
3. Carefully measure the required volumes of the reconstituted doxorubicin hydrochloride solution and the vincristine sulfate injection.
4. Add the measured volumes of doxorubicin hydrochloride and vincristine sulfate injections to a sterile container.
5. Add 13 mL of 0.9% sodium chloride injection to the container and mix well.
6. Withdraw the solution into a sterile syringe and fill the required reservoir/administration device container.
7. Expel any excess air and seal.
8. Package and label.

℞ Hydromorphone Hydrochloride 50 mg/mL Injection

Hydromorphone hydrochloride		2.5 g
Bacteriostatic 0.9%		22.2 mL
sodium chloride injection		
Bacteriostatic water for injection	qs	50 mL

(Note: All procedures should be carried out in a clean air environment by a qualified, aseptic compounding pharmacist.)

1. Check the calibration on the balance to be used for weighing the hydromorphone hydrochloride.
2. Accurately weigh the 2.5 g of hydromorphone hydrochloride.
3. Place the powder in a previously sterilized graduated cylinder.
4. Accurately measure the required volume of bacteriostatic 0.9% sodium chloride injection, add to the hydromorphone hydrochloride powder, and mix well.
5. Add sufficient bacteriostatic sterile water for injection to make 100 mL and mix well. (Note: The same bacteriostatic agents should be used in both the bacteriostatic 0.9% sodium chloride solution and the bacteriostatic water for injection to maintain a proper bacteriostatic agent concentration.)
6. Withdraw the solution into a sterile 60-mL syringe.
7. Affix a sterile 0.22-μm filter to the end of the syringe.
8. Filter the solution into the desired reservoir for administration.
9. Package and label.

General Injection

 Hyaluronidase Injection

Hyaluronidase		15,000 U
Sodium chloride		850 mg
Edetate disodium		100 mg
Calcium chloride dihydrate		53 mg
Thimerosal		10 mg
Sodium phosphate monobasic, anhydrous		170 mg
Sterile water for injection	qs	100 mL
Sodium hydroxide 1% solution	qs	to pH 6.4–7.4

(Note: This preparation should be prepared in an aseptic working environment by a validated aseptic compounding pharmacist using aseptic technique.)

1. Calculate the quantity of each ingredient required for the prescription.
2. Accurately weigh or measure each ingredient.
3. Dissolve the sodium chloride, edetate disodium, calcium chloride dihydrate, and thimerosal in about 80 mL of sterile water for injection.
4. Add the hyaluronidase and stir until dissolved.
5. Add the sodium phosphate monobasic and stir until dissolved.
6. Dropwise, adjust the pH by using the sodium hydroxide 1% solution until a pH in the range of 6.4 to 7.4 has been obtained.
7. Add sufficient sterile water for injection to volume and mix well.
8. Filter through a sterile 0.2-μm filter into sterile vials.
9. Package and label.

Sclerotherapy Injections

Sodium Chloride 20% Hypertonic Injection

Sodium chloride		20 g
Sterile water for injection	qs	100 mL

(Note: This preparation should be prepared in an LAF hood by a validated aseptic compounding pharmacist using aseptic technique.)

1. Calculate the quantity of each ingredient required for the prescription.
2. Accurately weigh or measure each ingredient.
3. Dissolve the salts in sufficient sterile water for injection to volume.
4. Filter through a sterile 0.2-μm filter into sterile vials.
5. Package and label.

℞ Sodium Chloride 20% with Lidocaine Hydrochloride 0.5% Injection

Sodium chloride		20 g
Lidocaine hydrochloride		500 mg
Sterile water for injection	qs	100 mL

(Note: This preparation should be prepared in an LAF hood by a validated aseptic compounding pharmacist using aseptic technique.)

1. Calculate the quantity of each ingredient required for the prescription.
2. Accurately weigh or measure each ingredient.
3. Dissolve the salts in sufficient sterile water for injection to volume.
4. Filter through a sterile 0.2-μm filter into sterile vials.
5. Package and label.

℞ Phenol 5% Aqueous Injection

Phenol		5 g
Glycerin		5 mL
Edetate disodium		50 mg
Sodium bisulfite		100 mg
Sterile water for injection	qs	100 mL

(Note: This preparation should be prepared in an LAF hood by a validated aseptic compounding pharmacist using aseptic technique.)

1. Calculate the quantity of each ingredient required for the prescription.
2. Accurately weigh or measure each ingredient.
3. Dissolve the edetate disodium in about 30 mL of the sterile water for injection.
4. Dissolve the sodium bisulfite in about 30 mL of the sterile water for injection.
5. Dissolve the phenol in the glycerin, followed by adding about 30 mL of the sterile water for injection.
6. Combine the first two solutions and add them to the phenol solution.
7. Add sufficient sterile water for injection to volume and mix well. (If cloudy, gentle heat will clear the solution.)
8. Filter through a sterile 0.2-μm filter into sterile vials (or package in vials and autoclave).
9. Package and label.

℞ Phenol 2.5%, Dextrose 25%, and Glycerin 25% Aqueous Injection

Liquified phenol	2.8 g (2.6 mL)
Dextrose	25 g
Glycerin	25 g
Sterile water for injection	qs 100 mL

1. Calculate the quantity of each ingredient required for the prescription.
2. Accurately weigh or measure each ingredient.
3. Dissolve the dextrose in about 50 mL of the sterile water for injection.
4. Mix the liquified phenol with the glycerin and add about 25 mL of the sterile water for injection.
5. Add step 3 to step 4 with mixing, followed by a sufficient quantity of sterile water for injection to volume and mix well.
6. Filter through a sterile 0.2-μm filter into sterile vials (or package in vials and autoclave).
7. Package and label.

℞ Phenol 10% in Glycerin

Phenol	10 g
Glycerin	qs 100 mL

1. Calculate the quantity of each ingredient required for the prescription.
2. Accurately weigh or measure each ingredient.
3. Dissolve the phenol in the glycerin and mix well.
4. Filter through a sterile 0.2-μm filter into sterile vials.
5. Package and label.

Standard Operating Procedures (SOPs)

General Aseptic Procedures Used at a Laminar Airflow Workbench

Purpose of SOP

The purpose of the procedure is to provide guidelines for personnel working at a laminar airflow workbench (LAFW).

Equipment/Supplies

The following items are used for this procedure:

- Laminar airflow workbench.
- Nonlinting gauze sponges.
- Disinfectant (70% alcohol or other, as required by facility SOP).
- Materials for compounding.

Procedure

1. Before beginning work, (all personnel) scrub and gown (including rescrubbing and regowning) according to the specific SOPs of the facility. Wear clean apparel that is appropriate for the level of aseptic compounding to be done.
2. Operate the hood blower continuously if the hood is used on a daily basis. If the hood is not used daily, turn it off but start it at least 30 minutes before use.
3. Clean the entire interior surface of the workbench, except for the filter grill, with a nonlinting gauze sponge dampened with distilled water; then clean the entire interior surface of the workbench, except for the filter grill, with a nonlinting gauze sponge dampened with a suitable disinfectant (Note: Disinfectants may be rotated, depending on the SOPs of the facility).
4. Do not spray disinfectant solutions at or on the filter or filter grill.
5. If any spills occur, immediately wash the area with sterile water for injection; then clean the area with a nonlinting gauze sponge dampened with the disinfectant.
6. Plan the work for a certain time period to minimize movement within the hood and in the immediate work area surrounding the hood.
7. Remove all supplies from their outer cartons, boxes, and the like before bringing the supplies into the clean room or immediate work area.
8. Clean each vial or ampule to be placed in the LAFW by wiping the outer surface with a suitable disinfectant, such as 70% alcohol.
9. Remove syringes, needles, and the like from their immediate wrapper and place them in the aseptic work area.
10. Place only the necessary supplies for the immediate preparation in the LAFW at one time. (Do not use the LAFW to store items.)
11. Organize all materials to enhance efficiency of work and to maintain the integrity of the critical sites for all materials in accordance with the flow of air, horizontal or vertical.
12. All work shall be done at least 6 in. into the LAFW.
13. Be careful not to touch the critical sites of any of the items with the gloved hands, as the hands are not sterile.
14. Periodically use an alcohol wipe on the gloved hands, as necessary.
15. Immediately before opening, clean the necks of ampules with a nonlinting gauze sponge and a disinfectant (e.g., 70% alcohol).
16. Clean all rubber stoppers of vials and other containers, before opening or penetrating with a needle, with a nonlinting gauze sponge and a disinfectant (e.g., 70% alcohol).
17. Filter all solutions removed from glass ampules to remove possible glass particles before adding the solutions to a vehicle or to another component.
18. During addition of drugs, gently swirl or rotate the solutions to speed mixing and minimize the occurrence of an incompatibility.
19. During preparation, constantly observe the preparation for precipitation, cloudiness, leakage, and gas formation as indicated by a stopper bulging outward, cracks in the container, and particulates.
20. As appropriate, sterile-filter products through a 0.22-μm filter into sterile containers.
21. After completion, observe the final product for any evidence of an incompatibility, and visually inspect for particulate matter.
22. Place a tamper-evident cap or seal on the finished product, as appropriate.

23. Label the product, remove it from the LAFW, and place it in an overwrap, if required, and seal.
24. Remove the empty containers, used syringes and needles, and other materials from the LAFW, and wipe area by using a clean, nonlinting sponge dampened with a suitable disinfectant.

Maintenance of a Horizontal Laminar Airflow Hood

Purpose of SOP

The purpose of this procedure is to document the maintenance of a horizontal LAF hood.

Principle

An aseptic working environment is required for any pharmacy preparing sterile products. It is recommended that a class 100 horizontal LAF hood located within a class 10,000 clean room be used for aseptic processing. The procedure describes how to conduct nonroutine, thorough cleaning; filter replacement; and lubrication for the LAF.

Materials

The following items are used in one or more of the maintenance steps:

- Mild detergent or suitable disinfectant.
- Prefilter.
- Plastic bag.
- HEPA filter.
- Sticker.
- Lubricant.

Procedure

Cleaning.

1. Clean the exterior surfaces of the LAF hood with a mild detergent or suitable disinfectant, according to the disinfectant rotation program. (Note: Do not use 70% isopropyl alcohol or any other liquid that may damage the hood's clear plastic surfaces. Check with the manufacturer to determine which substances should not be used.)
2. Remove access panel(s) and clean all accessible interior surfaces with a suitable mild detergent or disinfectant solution. (Note: Do not touch the HEPA filter unit.)
3. Replace the access panel cover(s).
4. Document the required information on the "Laminar Airflow Hood Maintenance Log" (Figure 22-1).

Prefilter Changes.

1. Change the prefilter(s) every _____ months. (Change on a regular basis, depending on level of use.)
2. Clean exterior surfaces of access panel with a mild detergent or suitable disinfectant.
3. Open the access panel to expose the filter and filter housing.
4. Clean the exterior of the filter housing with the detergent or disinfectant.
5. Remove the soiled prefilter, place it in a new plastic bag, and close tightly.

6. Clean the interior of the filter housing with the detergent or disinfectant.
7. Insert a new prefilter, observing the airflow direction indicator, and lock in place.
8. Close the access panel and lock in place.
9. Document the required information on the "aminar Airflow Hood Maintenance Log" (Figure 22-1).

Laminar Airflow Hood Maintenance Log

Date	Procedure	Cleaning Agent	Initials

Procedures:
    Filter   Filter replacement
    Cleaning   Nonroutine, thorough cleaning and disinfection
    Lube   Lubrication of motor and fan bearings
    Other   Describe

Figure 22-1. Sample documentation form for LAF hood maintenance.

HEPA Filter Changes.

1. Change the HEPA filter(s) every _____ months. (Change on a regular basis, depending on level of use.)
2. Ensure that a qualified contractor changes the HEPA filter.
3. Document the required information on the "Laminar Airflow Hood Maintenance Log" (Figure 22-1).
4. Ensure that a qualified pharmacist conducts media fills to document hood performance.

Certification.

1. Ensure the LAF hood is certified by a qualified contractor at least every 6 months, or when it is relocated, to ensure operational efficiency and integrity.
2. Obtain a copy of the procedures used by the contractor and place in an SOP notebook.
3. Document the required information on the "Laminar Airflow Hood Maintenance Log" (Figure 22-1).
4. Affix a sticker to the LAF hood, indicating that service has been done and giving a date when it should be repeated.
5. Ensure that a qualified pharmacist conducts settle plate or other appropriate tests and media fills to document hood performance.

Lubrication (if recommended by the manufacturer).

1. Clean the exterior surface of the hood containing the access panel(s) to the motor and blowers with a mild detergent or suitable disinfectant.
2. Remove the access panel(s) and clean the accessible surfaces.
3. Lubricate the motor and blower bearings, if recommended by the manufacturer.
4. Replace the access panel cover(s).
5. Document the required information on the "Laminar Airflow Hood Maintenance Log" (Figure 22-1).
6. Perform air velocity and other quality control checks, as recommended.

Maintenance of the Clean Room

Purpose of SOP

The purpose of this procedure is to establish appropriate guidelines and documentation for the maintenance of the clean room.

Regulatory Requirements

Chapter ⟨1206⟩, "Sterile Drug Products for Home Use,"[1] states that:

> The cleaning, sanitizing and organizing of the LAFW (Laminar Air Flow Workspace) should be the responsibility of trained operators (pharmacists and technicians) following written procedures and should be performed at the beginning of each shift.

Work surfaces near the LAFW in the Buffer Room should be cleaned in a similar manner, including counter tops and supply carts. Storage shelving should be emptied of all supplies and then cleaned and sanitized at least weekly, using approved agents.

Floors in the Buffer Room should be cleaned by mopping once daily when no aseptic operations are in progress.

Equipment/Materials

The following items are used in one or more of the cleaning steps:

- Sponge mop and bucket (appropriately labeled for the floors of the clean room, separate from the anterooms/auxiliary rooms).
- Bucket, sponges, and squeegee (appropriately labeled for the walls, cabinets, sink, and so forth).
- Disinfectants.
- Graduated cylinders and/or other measuring devices.
- Tacky roll mop or equivalent.

Procedure

General Considerations.

1. No cleaning operations are to occur during compounding.
2. Areas will be cleaned immediately after any repairs.
3. Order of cleaning rooms is as follows: The immediate vicinity of the LAFW will be cleaned first, followed by anterooms and auxiliary rooms.
4. The order within each room is as follows:
   —Clean the ceiling first (when scheduled), starting at a point farthest from the door and working toward the door.
   —Clean the walls next, starting on the wall farthest from the door and working toward the door.
   —Clean the floor last, starting from a far corner and working toward the center from each side wall toward the door.
   —The sponge mop should be damp, not dripping wet. The mop should be rinsed frequently during cleaning.
5. Maintain all cleaning/maintenance records in a logbook.
6. Do not combine disinfectants or use in concentrations other than those outlined in the SOPs.

Preparation of Cleaning Solutions.

1. Prepare cleaning solutions the day of use. Discard after completing work.
2. Alternate cleaning disinfectants on a monthly basis, and document on the maintenance record (according to SOPs).

Daily Cleaning Schedule.

1. Empty all waste receptacles.
2. Clean countertops with cleaning solution.
3. Clean windows and communication devices.
4. Clean floor with a tacky roll mop.
5. Damp mop floor with the cleaning solution.

Weekly Cleaning Schedule.

1. Using a long-handled squeegee or sponge, clean all accessible wall space.
2. A nonshedding lint-free wiper can be dampened and used to wash and disinfect the ceiling surface.

Quality Assessment of Injectable Solutions

Purpose of SOP

The purpose of this procedure is to provide a method of documenting quality assessment tests and observations on injectable solutions. Additional tests can be done as appropriate.

Materials

The following items are used in one or more of the assessment tests:

- Balance.
- pH meter.
- Pycnometers/refractometer (optional).
- Light/dark background.
- Sterility test supplies/kit (optional).
- Pyrogen test kit (optional).
- Osmometer (optional).

Procedure

The appropriate tests should be conducted and the results/observations recorded on the "Quality Assessment Form for Injectable Solutions" (Figure 22-2).

pH. The pH meter should be calibrated, and the pH of the product determined.

Specific Gravity.

Method I.

1. If a pycnometer is available, make sure it is clean and dry.
2. Weigh the empty pycnometer.
3. Fill it with the prepared solution, being careful not to entrap air bubbles.
4. Weigh it a second time.
5. Subtract the first weight from the second weight to obtain the net weight of the solution.
6. Divide this weight (grams) by the volume (milliliters) of the pycnometer to obtain the density/specific gravity of the solution:

$$SG = W \text{ (g)}/V \text{ (mL)}$$

Method II.

1. Tare the balance by using an empty container–closure system.
2. Accurately weigh a measured volume of the solution.
3. Calculate the specific gravity by dividing the weight (grams) by the volume (milliliters).

Method III.

1. For the specific solution being prepared, calibrate a refractometer to read specific gravity.
2. Determine the refractive index (related to specific gravity) of the solution.

Osmolality. This test can also be done by sending a sample of the compounded solution to a contract analytical laboratory.

1. Calibrate the osmometer according to the manufacturer's instructions.
2. Determine the osmolality of the solution.

Quality Assessment Form for Injectable Solutions

Product _____ Date _____

Lot/Rx Number _____

Characteristic	Theoretical	Actual	Normal Range
pH	_____	_____	_____
Specific gravity	_____	_____	_____
Osmolality	_____	_____	_____

Active drug assay results (ingredient tested _____)

	Theoretical	Actual	Normal Range
Initial assay	_____	_____	_____
After storage No. 1	_____	_____	_____
After storage No. 2	_____	_____	_____
Color	_____		
Clarity	_____		
Particulate matter	Yes	No	
Sterility test, passed	Yes	No	
Pyrogen test, passed	Yes	No	(endotoxin level _____ e.u.)

Sample set aside for physical stability observation: Yes No

If yes, results: Date Observations

Date	Observations
_____	_____
_____	_____
_____	_____
_____	_____
_____	_____
_____	_____
_____	_____
_____	_____
_____	_____
_____	_____
_____	_____
_____	_____
_____	_____
_____	_____
_____	_____

Figure 22-2. Sample worksheet for quality assessment of injectable solutions.

Active Drug Assay Results. As appropriate, have representative samples of the solution assayed for active drug content by a contract analytical laboratory. Stability can be assessed by storing the solution at room or refrigerated temperatures and having the assay repeated on the stored samples.

Color. It may be advisable to use a color chart to determine the actual color of the solution.

Clarity. Clarity is evaluated by visual inspection.

Particulate Matter. The compounding pharmacist should follow the procedure to assess particulate matter described in the SOP published elsewhere.[3]

Sterility Test. This test can also be done by sending a sample of the compounded solution to a contract analytical laboratory.

1. Conduct a sterility test by using a sample of the solution and a method such as the QTMicro System, which involves filtering a sample of up to 120 mL of the solution through a specially housed, 0.2-μm filter.
2. Add the growth media and incubate the unit, observing it daily for not less than 7 days.

Pyrogen Test. This test can also be done by sending a sample of the compounded solution to a contract analytical laboratory.

1. Conduct a pyrogen test by using an endotoxin test kit, such as the PyroTest kit (Q.I. Medical).
2. Have a well-trained person conduct the test, following the instructions provided in the kit.

Particulate Testing for Sterile Products

Purpose of SOP

The purpose of this procedure is to determine the presence or absence of particulates in compounded sterile drug products.

Materials

The following items are used to test for particulates:

- White/black background that is well illuminated.
- Nonlinting wipers.
- Talc-free gloves.

Procedure

1. Inspect the product (i.e., contents, container, and closure) immediately after preparation. If the product is not dispensed immediately, it should be inspected just before leaving the pharmacy.
2. The container should be free of any labels or attachments.
3. Remove any external particles by using a dampened nonlinting wiper.
4. Place clean, talc-free gloves on the hands.
5. Hold the container by its top and carefully swirl contents by rotating the wrist in a circular motion. Avoid vigorous swirling. (Note: Air bubbles will rise to the top and can be discounted.)

6. Hold the container horizontally about 4 in. below the light source against the white/black background; move the container slowly back and forth between the white and the black backgrounds.
7. If no particles are observed, slowly invert the container and observe for heavy particles that may be on the bottom of the container and that may slide down the container walls.
8. Record results of the observation on the formulation worksheet or prescription.

Note: A white/black background can be constructed as follows:

1. Obtain a single piece of Masonite or similar hard-surfaced material, approximately 24 in. by 24 in.
2. Paint one half flat black and the other half flat white. (Do not use a glossy finish paint.)
3. Affix to a wall at eye-level in the immediate vicinity of product preparation.
4. Above the white/black background, install a 2-ft long, 2-tube fluorescent fixture with a covering such that the light does not shine directly in the operator's eyes.

Quality Assessment of Parenteral Nutrition Products

Purpose of SOP

The purpose of this procedure is to provide a method of documenting quality assessment tests on and observations of parenteral nutrition products.

Materials

The following items are used in one or more of the assessment tests:

- Balance.
- pH meter.
- Pycnometers/refractometer (optional).
- Light/dark background.
- Microscope.
- IV solution sterility test kit (QTMicro).
- Pyrogen test kit.

Procedure

The appropriate tests should be conducted and the results/observations recorded on the "Quality Assessment Form for Parenteral Nutrition Products" (Figure 22-3).

Weight/Volume.

1. Tare the balance with an empty bag.
2. Place a filled bag on the balance and accurately weigh.
3. Calculate the volume from the specific gravity of the product.

pH. The pH meter should be calibrated, and the pH of the product determined.

Specific Gravity.

1. If a pycnometer is available, make sure it is clean and dry.
2. Weigh the empty pycnometer.

Quality Assessment Form for Parenteral Nutrition Products

Product _____   Date _____

Lot/Rx Number_____   Form: Solution   Emulsion (contains lipids)

Characteristic	Theoretical	Actual	Normal Range
Weight/Volume	_____	_____	_____
pH	_____	_____	_____
Specific gravity	_____	_____	_____

Active drug assay results (ingredient tested _____)

Initial assay	_____	_____	_____
After storage No. 1	_____	_____	_____
After storage No. 2	_____	_____	_____
Color	_____		
Clarity	_____		
Particulate matter	Yes	No	

Globule size range (estimate, mm)_____

Sterility test, passed	Yes	No	
Pyrogen test, passed	Yes	No	(endotoxin level _____e.u.)

Sample set aside for physical stability observation: Yes   No

If yes, results: Date   Observation

_____	_____
_____	_____
_____	_____
_____	_____
_____	_____
_____	_____
_____	_____
_____	_____
_____	_____
_____	_____
_____	_____
_____	_____
_____	_____

Figure 22-3. Sample worksheet for quality assessment of parenteral nutrition products.

3. Fill it with the prepared product, being careful not to entrap air bubbles.
4. Weigh it a second time.
5. Subtract the first weight from the second weight to obtain the net weight of the product.
6. Divide this net weight (grams) by the volume (milliliters) of the pycnometer to obtain the density/specific gravity of the product:

$$SG = W\,(g)/V\,(mL)$$

7. Alternatively, calibrate a refractometer to read specific gravity and determine the refractive index (related to specific gravity) of the product.

Active Drug Assay Results. As appropriate, representative samples of the product should be assayed by a contract analytical laboratory for amino acid content, dextrose content, or any other active drug content. Stability can be assessed by storage of the product at room or refrigerated temperatures and repeating the respective assays on the stored samples.

Color of Product. It may be advisable to use a color chart to determine the actual color of the product.

Clarity. Clarity is evaluated by visual inspection.

Particulate Matter. The compounding pharmacist should follow the procedure to assess for particular matter described in the SOP published elsewhere.[3]

Globule Size Range (for solutions containing a lipid).

1. Place a drop of the product on a glass plate (microscope slide) and illuminate from the bottom.
2. Using a microscope, estimate the globule size range of the product.

Sterility Test. A sterility test should be conducted by using a sample of the product and a method such as the QTMicro System. This method involves filtering a sample of up to 120 mL of the product through a specially housed, 0.2-μm filter. The growth media is added, and the unit is incubated and observed daily for not less than 7 days.

Pyrogen Test. A pyrogen test should be conducted by using an endotoxin test kit, such as the PyroTest kit. The commercial kit instructions must be carefully followed, and the test should be performed by a well-trained person.

References

1. Sterile drug products for home use. In: *United States Pharmacopeia 25/National Formulary 20.* Rockville, Md: United States Pharmacopeial Convention; 2001.
2. Particulate matter in injections. In: *United States Pharmacopeia 25/National Formulary 20.* Rockville, Md: United States Pharmacopeial Convention; 2001.
3. Allen LV Jr. Standard operating procedure for particulate testing for sterile products. *Int J Pharm Compound.* 1998;2(1):78.
4. Turco, SJ. *Sterile Dosage Forms: Their Preparation and Clinical Application.* 4th ed. Philadelphia: Lea & Febiger; 1994:30–1, 77.
5. Expert Advisory Panel on Pharmacy Compounding Practices. Pharmacy compounding. In: *United States Pharmacopeia 25/National Formulary 20.* Rockville, Md: United States Pharmacopeial Convention; 2001.

Chapter 23

Biotechnology Preparations

Definitions/Types

The world of pharmaceuticals is changing rapidly as biotechnology continues to grow and the era of nanotechnology appears on the horizon. For now, we will look at biotechnology, because it is gaining in importance in extemporaneous pharmaceutical compounding. The term *biotechnology* has varied meanings: (1) a science that applies the techniques of engineering and technology to the study of any living organism; (2) the use of living organisms and their cellular, subcellular, and molecular components to produce useful substances; or (3) any technique that uses living organisms (or parts of organisms) to make or modify products or to improve plants or animals for beneficial use. As is evident, definitions of biotechnology are numerous. In one sense, biotechnology involves the use of living organisms to produce products with beneficial use, including antibiotics, alcohol, and dairy products. More specifically, it can even involve the cloning of a specific gene with subsequent insertion into a host cell and cloning in a cell culture or in a microorganism.

Historical Use

Use of biotechnology techniques has been traced back more than 5000 years. People of ancient civilizations, such as the Mesopotamians and the Egyptians, added yeast to food substances and nutrients to produce beer.[1] Similar techniques were used later to produce wines, cheeses, and various other fermented products. However, biotechnology health care products were not developed until the 19th century.

DNA, the basic component for developing these health care products, was first isolated in 1869; its chemical composition was delineated in the early 1900s. In 1953, James D. Watson and Francis H. C. Crick proposed that the structure of DNA was a double helix; that is, two strands of sugar and phosphate molecules coiled around each other, similar to the structure of a spiral staircase. The strands are connected by four bases: adenine, guanine, cytosine, and thymine. Adenine and thymine always pair up opposite each other; the same is true for guanine and cytosine. In each DNA molecule, the sequence of the paired bases has a specific pattern. The pattern constitutes the DNA message for maintaining cells and organisms and for developing the next generation of organisms.

DNA duplicates by cloning itself. By altering the cloning process and using DNA probes, lysing agents, strands, and other materials to recombine the various parts, scientists can modify DNA to produce a different protein than the one it was originally programmed to produce. This "life technology," or biotechnology, results in products that can be used to diagnose and treat disease. A number of different approaches to biotechnology that are of interest to industry may ultimately involve the compounding pharmacist, including (1) the production of pharmacologically active recombinant proteins or modified proteins; (2) the use of recombinant proteins to design pharmacologically active, smaller molecules; (3) the manipulation of cells and tissues to accomplish a therapeutic effect; and (4) the production of transgenic bacteria or animals that can be used as "factories" to produce human and animal pharmaceuticals. In the last case, the bacteria can possibly be encapsulated and implanted in a human, where it will derive nutrients, grow, and produce a specific compound of interest.

Applications

Human insulin, which is used to treat diabetes, and somatrem, which is used to treat human growth hormone deficiency in children, were the first proteins to be developed by recombinant DNA technology. These products became available in October 1982 and October 1985, respectively. In June 1986, two major biotechnology products came onto the market: interferon alfa, which is used to treat hairy cell leukemia, and muromonab-CD3, which is used to treat acute allograft rejection in patients who have received renal transplantations. In the 1980s, about 12 recombinant DNA products were approved for marketing. Since then, more than 50 biotechnologically derived medications have been approved.[2]

Potential routes of delivery for these products include parenteral (intravenous, subcutaneous, intramuscular), oral (mucosal, sublingual, buccal), nasal, oral inhalation, and transdermal. Most biotechnology drug products cannot be administered orally (swallowed) because of their instability in the strong acid environment of the stomach and their low systemic absorption through the gastrointestinal mucosa.

Biotechnology presents compounding pharmacists with an exceptional, lucrative, new source of therapeutic agents that require their special expertise. This situation is especially true because these biotechnologically derived products are not the same as conventional drugs.

Composition

Most of the biotechnology products are proteins, but some may soon be smaller peptidelike molecules. Proteins are inherently unstable molecules, and their degradation profiles can be quite complex. Biotechnology products differ in their method of preparation and in the potential problems they present in their formulation. Pharmacists involved in compounding with biologically active proteins will be interested in their stabilization, formulation, and delivery.

In working with biotechnologically derived drugs, one must be cognizant of both the active drug constituent and the total drug-delivery system, or carrier. Protein drugs are extremely potent and are generally used in quite low concentrations. The bulk of most compounded products can be the excipients. In addition to the vehicle, buffers, and the like, stabilizers are often incorporated in these products. A number of different stabilizers can be used, including surfactants, amino acids, polyhydric alcohols, fatty acids, proteins, antioxidants, reducing agents, and metal ions. Table 23-1 lists specific agents used as stabilizers and their mechanisms of action.

Proper pH adjustment is important because it is one of the key factors in developing a stable product. pH can be controlled by the proper selection of physiologic buffers for the optimal pH range for the specific product. Generally, the buffer

Table 23-1. Stabilizing Agents for Biotechnology Preparations

Class	Agent	Action
Amino acids	Alanine	Serves as a solubilizer
	Arginine	Serves as a buffer
	Aspartic acid	Inhibits isomerism
	Glycine	Serves as a stabilizer
	Glutamic acid	Serves as a thermostabilizer
	Leucine	Inhibits aggregation
Antioxidants	Ascorbic acid, cysteine hydrochloride, glutathione, thioglycerol, thioglycolic acid, thiosorbitol	Help stabilize protein conformation
Chelating agents	EDTA salts	Inhibit oxidation by removing metal ions, glutamic acid, and aspartic acid
Fatty acids	Choline, ethanolamine, phosphotidyl	Serve as stabilizers
Proteins	Human serum albumin	Prevents surface adsorption; stabilizes protein conformation; serves as a complexing agent and cryoprotectant
Metal ions	Ca^{++}, Ni^{++}, Mg^{++}, Mn^{++}	Help stabilize protein conformation
Polyhydric alcohols	Ethylene glycol	Serves as a stabilizer
	Glucose	Strengthens conformation
	Lactose	Serves as a stabilizer
	Mannitol	Serves as a cryoprotectant
	Propylene glycol	Prevents aggregation
	Sorbitol	Prevents denaturation and aggregation
	Sucrose	Serves as a stabilizer
	Trehalose	Serves as a stabilizer
Polymers	Polyethylene glycol, povidone	Prevent aggregation
Surfactants	Poloxamer 407	Prevents denaturation and stabilizes cloudiness
	Polysorbate 20 and polysorbate 80	Retard aggregation

Source: Bontempo JA. Development of Biopharmaceutical Parenteral Dosage Forms. New York: Marcel Dekker; 1997:112–13.

concentrations are in the range of 0.01 to 0.1 M. It should be noted that as the buffer concentration is increased, there is generally an increase in pain on injection.

Chelating agents can be incorporated to bind trace metals such as copper, iron, calcium, manganese, and others. Ethylenediaminetetraacetic acid (EDTA) is commonly used at a concentration of about 0.01% to 0.05%.

Antioxidants are often incorporated because oxidation is one of the major factors in protein degradation. Ascorbic acid, sodium disulfide, monothioglycerol, and a-tocopherol are frequently used at a concentration of about 0.05% to 0.1%.

Preservatives can be required and could include phenol (0.3% to 0.5%), chlorobutanol (0.3% to 0.5%), and benzyl alcohol (1.0% to 3.0%).

Polyols are good stabilizers and are commonly used in concentrations from 1% to 10%.

Tonicity-adjusting agents include sodium chloride and dextrose in a concentration necessary for the tonicity equivalent of a 0.9% sodium chloride solution, or approximately 290 mOsm/L.

Preparation

A general rule of thumb when working with biotechnology-type formulations is to keep procedures as simple as possible. Most manipulations are the same as those involved in Chapter 22, "Parenteral Preparations," and Chapter 8, "Preservation, Sterilization, and Depyrogenation." Sterility must be maintained in any preparation of parenteral products because most do not contain a preservative. It is recommended that only one dose be prepared from each vial or container to minimize contamination. This arrangement is not practical in many situations, however, when specific manipulations are required to meet the special needs of patients. Facilities should be clean, and proper techniques should be used. A kit for testing aseptic technique in preparing formulations is available from equipment suppliers (Figure 23-1). Preparation, at a minimum, requires a laminar airflow hood and appropriate attire. All equipment must be sterile. Any additive used to compound parenteral drug products must be free from pyrogens. If the product becomes contaminated with pyrogens, it should be discarded.

Only two other special considerations concerning biotechnologically derived products will be discussed in this chapter, namely, the use of filters and the sorption of these drugs to containers. Filters used in manipulating biotechnology products can result in some loss of the drug available to the patient. For example, muromonab-CD3 (Ortho-clone OKT3) injection should be filtered with a low protein-binding filter of 0.2 to 0.22 μm. Many biotechnology products should not be filtered at all. If a filtration device is part of the intravenous apparatus, biotechnology drugs should generally be administered distal to the site of the filter. Filters that have been

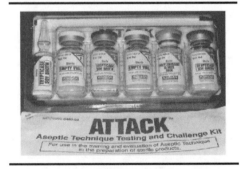

Figure 23-1. Aseptic technique testing and challenge kit.

shown to minimize protein adsorption are those made from polyvinylidene difluoride, polycarbonate, polysulfone, and regenerated cellulose. As a precaution, low protein-binding filters should be used.

Sorption of proteins to containers can result in drug loss. This loss can be minimized either by the use of albumin or by siliconization. Adding about 0.1% albumin to the product can decrease the sorption of proteins to containers. If glass mixing vessels are used, the albumin solution should be added before the drug. If siliconization is used, the compounding pharmacist should prepare a silicon solution or emulsion and soak or rinse the glass vials in it. The drained vials should then be placed in an oven at about 250°C for 5 to 6 hours. This procedure will minimize protein adsorption to glass and can be used for both the preparation equipment and the packaging containers.

Physicochemical Considerations

One must be aware of the factors involved in handling proteins to retain a drug's biologic activity up to the time when it is administered to the patient. Procedures that are involved include selecting an appropriate vehicle for drug delivery, individualizing dosages, administering drugs through novel drug-delivery systems, preparing drugs for delivery through these systems, monitoring their efficacy, and counseling patients on their use.

Some of the issues distinctive to protein pharmaceuticals include the following:

- Their high molecular weight and potential for aggregation (i.e., a small change in structure may or may not result in a change in activity).
- Their immunogenic potential because some are produced by a fermentation-type process and proteins can co-purify with proteins.
- The assignment of potency to the reference standards (when traditional pharmaceuticals are about 98% pure, these materials may be only 0.1% to 1% active, with their activity assigned by potentially variable assays).
- The use of micropipets, which can require frequent calibration.
- The concern that constituted products can be less stable than lyophilized products.
- The effects of the agitation of the product on its stability.
- The possible interaction of the product with the inner wall of the glass vial and with the elastomeric closure.
- The effectiveness of the preservative if a multidose product is mixed with other products.

Some of the physicochemical factors to be considered in compounding protein drug products include the structure of the protein drug; isoelectric point; molecular weight; solubility and factors affecting solubility (e.g., surfactants, salts, metal ions, pH); stability and factors affecting stability (e.g., pH, temperature, light, oxygen, metal ions, freeze-thaw cycles, mechanical stress); polymorphism; stereoisomers; filtration media compatibility; shear; and surface denaturation.

Solubility depends on a number of factors, including chemical structure, pH, and temperature. Proteins are generally more soluble in their native environment or medium or in a matrix that mimics their native environment, such as sodium chloride, trace elements, lipids, and other proteins in an aqueous medium. Before compounding these products, pharmacists must consider the ingredients' effects on the solubility of the active drug, especially because most of the products are currently administered parenterally. This task is especially critical because the actual drug is present in a small quantity and can go unnoticed if it precipitates. Generally, sterile water for injection and 0.9% sodium chloride solution are good vehicles with which to begin working with a formulation.

The pH of the compound should be maintained close to the pH of the original product because alterations caused by changes in pH can affect proteins in numerous ways. Chemical degradation rate constants are pH related, and hydrogen ion concentration can affect the actual structure of proteins (i.e., quaternary structure). Buffer systems may be needed for compounding, and they should be prepared at the minimum buffer strength required to produce the most stable drug product.

Chemical instability of proteins is defined as the modification of protein structures by bond formation or cleavage to yield a new compound. *Physical instability* generally involves changes in structure, conformation, or behavior in a particular environment. Stability, both chemical and physical, depends on pH, temperature, and agitation, as well as on the overall environment in which the drug is contained.

Sorption is a problem with colony-stimulating factors and with aldesleukin (Proleukin) at low concentrations. To minimize the "sticking" of the protein to the glass, it may help to add about 0.1% albumin to the product to occupy the potential binding sites in the container. Pharmacists must consider this problem before making any changes in packaging.

Agitation, which is frothing created by the physical decomposition of the protein, can adversely affect the product in two ways. First, frothing can cause difficulties in using a syringe to withdraw the required amount of drug from a vial. To avoid this problem, the formulator should mix the product by rolling the vial in the hands or gently swirling it. Second, excessive agitation can cause changes in a protein's quaternary structure, which often reduce or eliminate a drug's therapeutic activity. Some products, such as filgrastim (Neupogen) and sargramostim (Leukine), are reconstituted by directing a soft stream of diluent against the inside of the container wall. Others, such as recombinant tissue plasminogen activator (tPA; alteplase), are reconstituted by directing a stream of diluent directly into the product at the bottom of the vial.

Quality Control

The compounding pharmacist should follow standard quality control procedures. Tests that can be done on these compounded preparations include pH, final volume, sterility, pyrogenicity, and physical observations for clarity, presence of gas bubbles and particulate matter, and change in color.

Packaging

The container used for storage after compounding must be chosen carefully. For example, the manufacturer's directions for interleukin-2 (aldesleukin) suggest the use of a plastic bag because that type of dilution container enhances consistent drug delivery. Unless otherwise specified, USP type I glass should be used for packaging when storage for extended time periods is indicated. The compounding pharmacist should be aware of the potential for sorption of the drug to the glass walls. Closures and stoppers should be selected that are compatible and flexible, have low levels of particulates, and have few problems with adsorption, absorption, and permeation.

Storage/Labeling

The recommended storage temperature is an important element that will vary, depending on the product. Recommended storage temperatures can be room temperature (15°C–25°C), refrigerator temperature (2°C–8°C), frozen (−20°C), or ultrafrozen (down to −80°C). Freezing does affect the activity of certain products. For instance, the activity of filgrastim decreases if it is frozen. Some products can retain potency at room temperature after reconstitution. Sargramostim retains potency for up to 30 days at 25°C. However, most manufacturers recommend refrigeration at 2°C to 8°C, regardless of the product's potency at room temperature.

The short shelf-life of these products after reconstitution can be due to chemical or physical instability or to the fact that most do not contain preservatives. The manufacturer's recommendations or those validated by the published literature should be followed for products after they are reconstituted and manipulated. One example is tPA, which has been used in treating intraocular fibrin formation after a vitrectomy and in managing subconjunctival hemorrhage after glaucoma filtration surgery. The prepared solution is stable in a pH range of 5 to 7.5 and is incompatible with bacteriostatic agents. For compounding, the commercial product is reconstituted according to the manufacturer's directions, using sterile water for injection without preservatives, which yields a concentration of 1 mg/mL. This solution is further diluted with 0.9% sodium chloride injection to yield a concentration of 25 µg/100 µL. Aliquots of 0.3 mL are withdrawn into 1-mL tuberculin syringes and capped. The syringes are stored in an ultrafreezer at −70°C. This product has been shown, by both bioassay and clinical use, to retain its activity for at least 1 year. This type of specific product information is not included in the manufacturer's label information and is usually obtained from the literature or by asking the manufacturer directly.

Stability

Physically, biotechnology products can degrade by aggregation, denaturation, and precipitation. Aggregation can be the result of covalent or noncovalent processes and can be either physical or chemical in nature. Aggregate formation can actually begin when primary particles are formed from protein molecules, resulting from brownian movement.

Denaturation can result from heat, cold, extreme pH values, organic solvents, hydrophilic surfaces, shear, agitation, mixing, filtering, shaking, freeze-thaw cycles, ionic strength, and other factors. Denaturation can be quite complex and can be either reversible or irreversible.

Precipitation can result from shaking, heating, filtration, pH, and chemical interactions. The first step in a precipitation process is generally aggregation. When the aggregates gain a sufficient size, they precipitate out of solution and are clearly evident. Precipitation can actually occur on membrane filters, in equipment, in tubing, and in contact with other equipment and supplies. According to Chapter <795>, "Pharmacy Compounding,"[3] water-containing formulations (prepared from ingredients in solid form) can have a beyond-use date of no longer than 14 days when stored at cold temperatures, unless otherwise documented.

Patient Counseling

Patients should be aware of the importance of proper and careful handling of these drugs. Thus, they should be instructed on the proper preparation, administration, and disposal of the product.

Sample Formulation

℞ **Tissue Plasminogen Activator (tPA) 25 μg/100 μL Ophthalmic Solution**

Tissue plasminogen activator	20-mg vial
Sterile 0.9% sodium chloride injection	60 mL
Sterile water for injection	20 mL

1. Reconstitute a commercial 20-mg vial of tissue plasminogen activator (alteplase) according to the manufacturer's directions by adding 20 mL of sterile water for injection, without preservatives, to result in a 20 mg/20 mL (1 mg/mL) concentration.
2. Dilute this solution by adding 60 mL of sterile 0.9% sodium chloride injection to yield a concentration of 250 μg/mL, or 25 μg/100 μL.
3. Mix thoroughly, using gentle swirling and/or slow inversion of the container.
4. Withdraw 0.3-mL aliquots into the desired number of 1-cc syringes and cap.
5. Place the syringes that are not going to be used immediately in a –70°C ultrafreezer.

References

1. Bush, Peggy. Overview of technology. *J Pharm Practice.* 1998;11(1):6.
2. Ansel HC, Allen LV Jr, Popovich NG. *Pharmaceutical Dosage Forms and Drug Delivery Systems.* Baltimore: Lippincott Williams & Wilkins; 1999.
3. Expert Advisory Panel on Pharmacy Compounding Practices. Pharmacy compounding. In: *United States Pharmacopeia 25/National Formulary 20.* Rockville, Md: United States Pharmacopeial Convention; 2001.

Compounding for Special Populations and Special Products

The uniqueness of pharmacy compounding is the ability to prepare individualized medications, that is, medications for special populations. These populations can include pediatric and hospice patients, patients experiencing pain, patients with diabetes, patients of advanced age, and many other types of special populations. This chapter gives a brief presentation of the opportunities that are present and some sample compounded formulations for natural, herbal, and dietary supplement products and iontophoresis solutions. A Standard Operating Procedure (SOP) is included for pharmacies that offer compounding for environmentally sensitive patients.

This chapter is divided into sections according to specialized population or specialized compounded product.

Dental Patients

Many opportunities are available for working with dentists. Special oral hygiene products, preoperative medications, and preparations used in dental surgical areas are only a few of the mixtures needed. A number of disease states can result in oral ulceration. Compounding dental mouth rinses from bulk powders (anti-inflammatory agents, antibiotics, and the like) has numerous advantages over using commercial dosage forms. Each manufactured product has numerous ingredients that can contribute to compatibility or stability problems. Therefore, fewer stability and compatibility problems will complicate the administration of the product. Also, if a preservative is present but the commercial product is diluted as a result of mixing it with other products, then the preservative can be below its effective concentration. Active drugs can be incorporated into toothpastes and gels. For gum disease, antibiotics can be incorporated into a poloxamer gel (a reverse thermal gel) and applied to the gum line between the gum and the tooth. The poloxamer will thicken and release the drug over a longer time period than if a rinse or irrigation were used. Many options are available depending on the patient's conditions and needs.

Sample Formulations

℞ Mouthwash/Gargle

Cetylpyridinium chloride		100 mg
Polysorbate 20		1 mL
Spearmint oil		0.25 mL
Ethanol 95%		10 mL
Sodium saccharin		100 mg
Sodium benzoate		200 mg
Sorbitol 70% solution		10 mL
Purified water	qs	100 mL

1. Calculate the quantity of each ingredient required for the prescription.
2. Accurately weigh or measure each ingredient.
3. Add the spearmint oil to the polysorbate 20 and mix well.
4. Add the ethanol and mix well.
5. Separately, add the cetylpyridinium chloride, sodium saccharin, and sodium benzoate to about 70 mL of purified water, followed by the sorbitol solution.
6. Combine the two solutions together and mix well.
7. Add a few drops of food color if desired.
8. Add sufficient purified water to volume and mix well.
9. Package and label.

℞ Tooth Gel Vehicle

Glycerin	22 g
Carbopol 934	500 mg
Purified water	25.2 mL
Tetrasodium pyrophosphate	250 mg
Sodium saccharin	200 mg
Sodium benzoate	500 mg
Sodium hydroxide 50% solution	0.4 mL
Dicalcium phosphate dihydrate	48.76 g
Sodium lauryl sulfate	1.2 g
Flavor	1 mL

℞ Tooth Gel Vehicle (cont.)

1. Calculate the quantity of each ingredient required for the prescription.
2. Accurately weigh or measure each of the ingredients.
3. Add the tetrasodium pyrophosphate, sodium saccharin, sodium benzoate, sodium lauryl sulfate, and flavor to the purified water.
4. Mix the Carbopol 934 with the glycerin.
5. Mix the two mixtures until uniform.
6. Add the sodium hydroxide solution and mix well.
7. Geometrically, incorporate the dicalcium phosphate dihydrate into the gel vehicle.
8. Package and label.

℞ Toothpaste Vehicle

Calcium pyrophosphate	45 g
Sorbitol 70% solution	20 mL
Sodium lauryl sulfate	1.2 g
Sodium carboxymethylcellulose	600 mg
Sodium saccharin	100 mg
Peppermint oil	0.75 mL
Purified water	32.35 mL

1. Calculate the quantity of each ingredient required for the prescription.
2. Accurately weigh or measure each of the ingredients.
3. Add the sodium lauryl sulfate, sodium saccharin, and peppermint oil to the purified water.
4. Add the sodium carboxymethylcellulose to the sorbitol solution.
5. Mix the two preparations until uniform.
6. Geometrically, incorporate the calcium pyrophosphate to form a paste.
7. Package and label.

℞ Dental Cavity Varnish

Camphor	70 g
Prednisolone	1 g
Parachlorophenol	26.5 g
Metacresol acetate	2.5 g

1. Calculate the quantity of each ingredient required for the prescription.
2. Accurately weigh or measure each ingredient.
3. Mix the camphor with the parachlorophenol.
4. Add the metacresol acetate.
5. Add the prednisolone and mix well.
6. Package and label.

℞ Dental Chemical Curettage Agent

Sodium hydroxide	7.8 g
Sodium hypochlorite solution	100 mL
Sodium carbonate	19 g (approximate)

1. Calculate the quantity of each ingredient required for the prescription.
2. Accurately weigh or measure each ingredient.
3. Using an ice bath to keep the solution cool, slowly dissolve the sodium hydroxide in the sodium hypochlorite solution.
4. Allow the solution to warm to room temperature.
5. Add the sodium carbonate solution until the solution is saturated. It may not take all of the sodium carbonate.
6. Package and label.

℞ Dental Pressure-Indicating Paste

Zinc oxide ointment	53 g
White petrolatum	17 g
Mineral oil	25 g
White wax	5 g
Flavoring	qs

1. Calculate the quantity of each ingredient required for the prescription.
2. Accurately weigh each ingredient.
3. Reduce the white wax to a fine state by grating.
4. Heat the grated wax until it melts, using a double boiler to eliminate scorching.
5. Heat the mineral oil and white petrolatum in a separate double boiler to a temperature near that of the melted wax.
6. Add the mineral oil/petrolatum combination slowly, in small increments, with continuous stirring to the melted wax.
7. After the two oleaginous liquids are thoroughly mixed, and while constantly stirring the mixture, add the zinc oxide ointment in small increments.
8. When the mixture is completely melted and displays a uniform creamy white appearance, remove the heat and allow the mixture to cool.
9. If a volatile flavoring agent is used, such as lemon oil or peppermint oil, add it during cooling, just before solidification occurs.
10. Pour the paste while it is still slightly warm into the desired ointment jars, or allow it to solidify and place with a spatula into appropriate containers.
11. Package and label.

Patients with Diabetes

Compounding for patients with diabetes can provide for an enhanced lifestyle for these patients. The following few formulas can increase the quality of life for these patients.

Sample Formulations

℞ **Foot Care Ointments for Patients with Diabetes**

	Formula 1 (g)	Formula 2 (g)	Formula 3 (g)
Aquabase/Aquaphor	4		
Lanolin	1		1
Glycerin	1		
Wheat germ oil	1	1	
Cocoa butter		2	
Olive oil		1	
Cod liver oil			1
White petrolatum			2

Formula 1

1. Calculate the quantity of each ingredient required for the prescription.
2. Accurately weigh or measure each ingredient.
3. Blend the wheat germ oil and glycerin with the lanolin.
4. Incorporate the mixture into the Aquabase/Aquaphor and mix well.
5. Package and label.

Formula 2

1. Calculate the quantity of each ingredient required for the prescription.
2. Accurately weigh or measure each ingredient.
3. Blend the wheat germ oil with the olive oil and mix well.
4. Incorporate the mixture into the cocoa butter by using mild heat, if necessary, and mix well to yield a thick, fluid preparation.
5. Package and label.

Formula 3

1. Calculate the quantity of each ingredient required for the prescription.
2. Accurately weigh or measure each ingredient.
3. Blend the cod liver oil with the lanolin.
4. Incorporate the white petrolatum and mix well.
5. Package and label.

℞ Skin Ulcer Cream for Patients with Diabetes

Misoprostol	2.5 mg	
Phenytoin	2 g	
Ketoprofen	2 g	
Lidocaine	2 g	
Propylene glycol	qs	
Oil-in-water emulsion base	qs	100 g

1. Calculate the quantity of each ingredient required for the prescription.
2. Accurately weigh or measure each ingredient.
3. Comminute 12.5 of the 200 g misoprostol tablets to a very fine powder.
4. Add sufficient propylene glycol to make a smooth paste.
5. Mix and comminute the other powders to a very fine powder.
6. Add sufficient propylene glycol to make a smooth paste and combine with step 4.
7. Incorporate the paste into a sufficient quantity of an oil-in-water emulsion base to make 100 g.
8. Package and label.

Patients of Advanced Age

One of the greatest challenges in compounding is individualizing dosage forms for patients of advanced age. More than 85% of the older adult ambulatory population and more than 95% of the older adult institutionalized population receive prescription drugs. The average number of prescriptions for persons 65 years of age and older is approximately 13. Most dosage forms are created for adults and pediatric patients with little thought given to the segment of the population that takes a significant portion of drug products. The most common dosage form today is the tablet, which tends to "hang" on the back of the tongue or throat; capsules and coated tablets have less tendency to do so. For bedridden patients or patients with swallowing difficulties, other dosage forms must be considered. For example, liquids, lozenges, frozen ices, lollipops, gummy gels, puddings, flavored gelatins, ointments, creams, gels, sprays, baths, washes, suppositories, and others can be used.

Even though the patient is an adult, physical, emotional, and/or social difficulties can affect compliance. Although patients of advanced age experience changes relative to the skin, transdermal administration is still a reasonable alternative. For masking taste, mint and fruit flavors continue to be popular among this population. Because the older adult patient does not remember everything said during a counseling session, it is important to provide written instructions on each and every prescription. It may be necessary to develop patient leaflets for the more commonly compounded preparations for older adults.

Commonly compounded preparations can include oral liquids, gummy-type preparations, and soft lozenges.

Hospice Patients and Patients Experiencing Pain

Hospice is a multidisciplinary program that provides health, psychological, and social services to terminally ill patients and their families. Hospice is designed to provide these services for patients who can no longer benefit from curative treatment, with most patients having a life expectancy of less than 6 months. The concept of hospice can be traced back to early Western civilization when the term was used to describe a place of shelter and rest for weary or sick travelers on long journeys. It was first applied to specialized care for dying patients in 1967 at St. Christopher's Hospice in a residential suburb of London. The first hospice program began in the United States in 1974; today there are more than 2500 hospice programs that serve more than 250,000 patients.

About 60% or 70% of hospice patients have cancer and experience intractable pain, severe anxiety, and depression and have social, psychological, and financial concerns. The current thought is that there should be no ceiling for maximum use of analgesics for these patients. Analgesics should be provided on a scheduled basis with supplemental doses as needed to continue providing adequate blood levels until the patients start feeling comfortable again. Antidepressants and anxiolytics are sometimes given to help relieve a patient's symptoms of depression and anxiety.

Hospice care deals with grief and grieving and can be accomplished either in an institutional environment or at home through home care. Advantages of home hospice care include logistical, psychological, social, emotional, and financial benefits, which are provided in the comfort of patients' homes. Commonly provided services include wound care, pain management, palliative care, and other services to maintain activities of daily living and basic functional skills.

Sample Formulations

℞ Morphine Sulfate 10-, 25-, and 50-mg/mL Injections (Preservative free)

	10 mg/mL	25 mg/mL	50 mg/mL
Morphine sulfate	0.5 g	1.25 g	2.5 g
0.9% Sodium chloride injection	42.2 mL	30.6 mL	11.1 mL
Sterile water for injection qs	50 mL	50 mL	50 mL

1. Calculate the quantity of each ingredient required for the prescription.
2. Accurately weigh the required quantity of morphine sulfate powder.
3. Place the morphine sulfate in a previously sterilized graduated cylinder.
4. Accurately measure the required volume of 0.9% sodium chloride injection, add to the morphine sulfate powder, and mix well.
5. Add sufficient sterile water for injection to volume and mix well.
6. Filter through a sterile 0.22-μm filter into the desired sterile reservoir/container for administration.
7. Package and label.

℞ Morphine Sulfate and Clonidine Hydrochloride Epidural Injection

Morphine sulfate	2 g
Clonidine hydrochloride	1 mg
0.9% Sodium chloride injection	69 mL
Sterile water for injection	qs 100 mL

(Note: This preparation should be prepared in a laminar airflow hood in a clean room by a validated, aseptic compounding pharmacist using strict aseptic technique.)

If the source of the ingredients is commercially available, preservative-free injectable products, compound as follows:

1. Calculate the quantity of each ingredient required for the prescription.
2. Accurately measure the volume of each ingredient and pour into the sterile reservoir or container. An air bubble can be injected and used to thoroughly mix the solution.
3. Remove the air from the reservoir and tightly seal/close the outlet.
4. Package and label.

If the source of the ingredients is other than commercially prepared injections, compound as follows:

1. Calculate the quantity of each ingredient required for the prescription.
2. Accurately weigh the solid ingredients, preparing dilutions if necessary.
3. Accurately measure the volume of the liquid ingredients.
4. Place in a clean graduated cylinder or suitable measuring vessel/device that has been suitably depyrogenated.
5. Add sufficient sterile 0.9% sodium chloride to volume.
6. Filter through a 0.2-μm sterile filter into a sterile reservoir and tightly seal/close the outlet.
7. Package and label.

℞ Ketamine Hydrochloride 10%, Gabapentin 6%, Baclofen 2%, Amitriptyline Hydrochloride 2%, and Clonidine Hydrochloride 0.1% in Pluronic Lecithin Organogel

Ketamine hydrochloride	10 g
Gabapentin	6 g
Baclofen	2 g
Amitriptyline hydrochloride	2 g
Clonidine hydrochloride	100 mg
Diethylene glycol monoethyl ether	10 mL
Polysorbate 80 (Tween 80)	1–2 mL
Sorbitan oleate (Span 80)	1–2 mL
Lecithin:isopropyl palmitate solution	22 mL
Pluronic F-127 30% gel	qs 100 mL

(Note: The lecithin:isopropyl palmitate solution can be prepared by mixing 0.2 g of sorbic acid, 50 g of soy lecithin, and 50 g of isopropyl palmitate.

The Pluronic F-127 gel can be prepared by mixing 0.2 g of potassium sorbate, 30 g of Pluronic F-127, and sufficient purified water to make 100 mL. Pluronic F-127 gel [30%; 100 mL] can be prepared by mixing 0.2 g of sorbic acid, 30 g of Pluronic F-127, and sufficient purified water to make 100 mL. The pH should be adjusted to about 4.5 for maximum effectiveness of the sorbic acid as a preservative. Dissolution is accomplished by placing the gel in a sealed container in a refrigerator, with periodic agitation that does not incorporate air into the gel.)

1. Calculate the quantity of each ingredient required for the prescription.
2. Accurately weigh or measure each ingredient.
3. Mix the powders together.
4. Add the diethylene glycol monoethyl ether and mix to form a smooth paste.
5. Add the lecithin:isopropyl palmitate solution and the sorbitan oleate; mix well.
6. Add the polysorbate 80, previously blended with about 20 mL of Pluronic F-127 30% gel, followed by sufficient additional Pluronic F-127 30% gel to volume and mix thoroughly, using a mechanical shearing force.
7. Package and label.

℞ Promethazine Hydrochloride 50 mg/mL in Pluronic Lecithin Organogel

Promethazine HCl	5 g
Purified water	4 mL
Lecithin: isopropyl palmitate solution	22 mL
Pluronic F-127 30% gel	qs 100 mL

(Note: Pluronic F-127 gel [30%; 100 mL] can be prepared by mixing 0.2 g of sorbic acid, 30 g of Pluronic F-127, and sufficient purified water to make 100 mL. The pH should be adjusted to about 4.5 for maximum effectiveness of the sorbic acid as a preservative. Dissolution can be easily accomplished by placing the gel in a sealed container in a refrigerator, with periodic agitation that does not incorporate air into the gel.)

1. Calculate the quantity of each ingredient required for the prescription.
2. Accurately weigh or measure each ingredient.
3. Dissolve the promethazine hydrochloride in the purified water.
4. Add this solution to about 70 mL of the Pluronic F-127 30% gel and mix well.
5. Incorporate the lecithin: isopropyl palmitate solution with shear mixing.
6. Add additional Pluronic F-127 30% gel to volume and continue shear mixing.
7. Package and label.

Pediatric Patients

Oral liquids, including solutions, suspensions, and emulsions, are the most commonly used dosage forms for pediatric patients. Other dosage forms commonly used include lozenges, flavored ices, gummy gels, chewing gums, lollipops, puddings, flavored gelatins, and topical formulations.

Variables that must be considered in preparing pediatric formulations include dose (concentration and quantity to be administered), stability (chemical, physical, and microbiological), taste, color, packaging, storage, and administration devices/techniques that may be required.

The primary factor influencing patient compliance is probably taste. Taste includes factors such as flavor, sweetener, pH, color, and mouth feel. In some cases, it can be advantageous to prepare some placebo "taste samples" for the child and ask the child to select the one he or she likes best, putting the child in a more active role in decision-making in his or her therapy.

Sample Formulations

℞ Nystatin Frozen Ices (for 10 frozen ices)

Nystatin powder		2.5×10^6 U
Sorbitol 70% solution		20 mL
Syrup NF		50 mL
Flavoring (banana or other to taste)		5 mL
Purified water	qs	300 mL

(Note: Because ice cube trays and molds vary, it may be necessary to calibrate the specific tray or mold being used and adjust the formula before actual preparation.)

1. Calculate the quantity of each ingredient required for the prescription.
2. Accurately weigh or measure the ingredients.
3. Add the nystatin powder to the sorbitol 70% solution and mix thoroughly.
4. Add the syrup, flavoring, and purified water and mix well.
5. Pour 30 mL into each cavity in an ice cube tray (with deep cubes) or an appropriate plastic sleeve and place in a freezer for 1 or 2 hours.
6. Insert a stick (junior tongue depressor) into each frozen ice to serve as a handle and continue freezing until frozen firmly.
7. Remove each frozen ice and package in a 6-in. × 9-in. sealable plastic bag and label.

℞ Malathion 0.5% Topical Lotion for Head Lice

Malathion		500 mg
Isopropyl alcohol 70%		68 mL
Fragrances		
Lavender oil		30 drops
Bay/pine oil		3 drops
Ethyl alcohol 95%	qs	100 mL

(Note: Malathion fumes can be irritating to the mucous membranes of the nasal passages; therefore, this product should be prepared in a well-ventilated area or under an exhaust hood. Wear disposable gloves to prevent retaining the odor on the hands. This preparation can be used for treatment of resistant head lice, as well as scabies.)

1. Calculate the quantity of each ingredient required for the prescription.
2. Accurately weigh or measure the ingredients.
3. Disperse the Malathion in the isopropyl alcohol.
4. Add the fragrances and mix well.
5. Add sufficient ethyl alcohol to volume and mix well.
6. Package and label.

Natural, Herbal, and Dietary Supplement Products

The use of nutraceuticals continues to increase in our society. *Nutraceuticals* are defined by the American Nutraceutical Association as "naturally occurring dietary substances in pharmaceutical dosage forms," thus including dietary supplements as defined by the Dietary Supplement Health Education Act (DSHEA) of 1994, as well as comparable substances unintended for oral ingestion. The popularity of nutraceuticals is consumer driven, and pharmacists are often asked about the composition and use of the substances. Nutraceuticals covered under DSHEA have no real published standards. USP monographs are being developed for some of the substances, so any preparation bearing the USP designation must meet certain prescribed standards. Because many of the commercial products do not meet USP standards, patients cannot be sure of their quality. However, some of the bulk drug substances are available as USP quality, so the compounding pharmacist can assure patients of the quality of the compounded nutraceuticals they are receiving.

Most compounding of natural preparations and nutraceuticals involves the capsule dosage form. When capsules are not desired, extracts can be prepared, such as alcoholic and/or aqueous extracts. These extracts can be flavored.

Sample Formulations

℞ Compounded Coenzyme Q10 100 mg Capsules

Coenzyme Q10	10 g
Lactose	30 g

1. Calculate the quantity of each ingredient required for the prescription.
2. Accurately weigh each of the ingredients.
3. Reduce particle size, if necessary, so both products have a similar particle size.
4. Thoroughly mix until uniform.
5. Encapsulate into 100 capsules, each weighing 400 mg.
6. Package and label.

Iontophoresis Solutions

Iontophoresis is a method of administering medications through the skin by using a small electric current. Analgesics, anesthetics, and so forth can be administered transdermally by iontophoresis for a local/systemic effect. The solutions used for this procedure should contain only the active drug and sterile water for injection. Any additional agents would compete for the current and decrease the efficacy of the iontophoresis process. These formulations are simple to prepare and should be sterile and packaged in single-use containers.

Sample Formulations

 Dexamethasone Sodium Phosphate 4 mg/mL for Iontophoresis

Dexamethasone sodium phosphate		400 mg
Sterile water for injection	qs	100 mL

1. Calculate the quantity of each ingredient required for the prescription.
2. Accurately weigh the dexamethasone sodium phosphate powder.
3. Place in a suitable graduated cylinder and add sufficient sterile water for injection to volume.
4. Mix well and filter through a 0.2-μm sterile filter into a sterile container.
5. Package and label.

 Estriol Solution for Iontophoresis for Acne Scars

Estriol	300 mg
Citric acid	100 mg
Sterile water for injection	100 mL

1. Calculate the quantity of each ingredient required for the prescription.
2. Accurately weigh the required quantity of estriol and citric acid.
3. Accurately measure the required quantity of sterile water for injection.
4. Dissolve the citric acid and the estriol in the sterile water for injection.
5. Filter through a 0.2-μm sterile filter into a sterile container.
6. Package and label.

 Ketorolac Solution for Iontophoresis

Ketorolac tromethamine	600 mg
Sterile water for injection	100 mL

1. Accurately obtain the required quantity of ketorolac tromethamine (from tablets as necessary).
2. Accurately measure the required volume of sterile water for injection.
3. Mix/dissolve the ketorolac tromethamine powder in the sterile water for injection.
4. Filter to remove tablet excipients.
5. Filter through a 0.2-μm sterile filter into a sterile container.
6. Package and label.

Environmentally Challenged Patients

Some patients seem to be allergic or sensitive to almost anything in the environment. Consequently, they lead a limited lifestyle and have great difficulty obtaining pharmaceuticals they can use. Some pharmacies specialize in compounding for these environmentally challenged patients.

Standard Operating Procedure (SOP)

Compounding for Environmentally Challenged Patients

Purpose of SOP. The purpose of this procedure is to provide guidance for pharmacists compounding for patients who are environmentally challenged. The pharmacist must pay special attention to details related to the product composition and the compounding procedures to minimize the possibility of inducing an adverse patient response. It may be advisable to have a specially designated area for this purpose. The pharmacist should select the specific procedures that relate to the products being compounded and the patients being served. Additional procedures may be required because of the specific needs of products being prepared and stimuli to which patients may react.

Facility Guidelines.

- Do not use wallpaper or paneling; wood or metal is preferred.
- Paint with a water-base latex paint. Baking soda can be added at the rate of 250 g to 1 gal of paint immediately before painting to reduce paint odors.
- Keep area free of carpets, rugs, and draperies. (Use plastic or aluminum blinds; if draperies must be used, they should be made of cotton or natural fibers.)
- Avoid dust-catching areas such as flat tops of shelving units (use slanted tops that are easy to clean or recessed cabinets that are flush with the wall).
- Do not hang items that might catch dust on walls.
- Keep area free of stuffed furniture, pillows, and the like; use simple wooden or metal furniture.
- Keep air-handling system clean.
- Change air filters frequently, and preferably use electrostatic filters or high-quality pleated filters.
- Use a portable room air cleaner as indicated.
- Prevent moisture buildup in the air-handling units and ductwork.
- Keep the area clean and dry.
- If plants are in the area, do not overwater because overwatering leads to mold growth.
- Discard old magazines and newspapers.
- Do not allow pets in the facility.
- Remove sources of strong, offensive odors.
- Use activated charcoal to adsorb odors in the work area; replace frequently.
- Keep the area clean; remove damp towels from the area as quickly as feasible.
- For pest control, use boric acid, a baking soda/powdered sugar mixture, a plaster of paris/flour mixture, or other nonvolatile pesticide in the area.

Equipment Guidelines.

- Clean area and equipment frequently with a solution of borax or benzalkonium chloride.
- If possible, avoid aluminum and copper equipment that may come in contact with the product.

Materials Guidelines.

- Use stainless steel, glass, or other hard-surface materials as much as possible.
- Avoid the use of dyes, flavors, and preservatives, as appropriate, in formulating products for these patients.
- Avoid the use of soft plastic materials such as plastic wrap, plastic bags, and the like.
- Use oxygenating bleaches that contain hydrogen peroxide for cleaning.
- Use baking soda for cleaning.
- Use vinegar (15 mL/L of water) for cleaning windows and surfaces.
- Use borax (1.5 cups/gal of water) as a disinfectant.
- Use benzalkonium chloride solution as a fungicide and germicide.

Procedure Guidelines.

- Wash area, equipment, windows, and the like on a routine schedule.
- Remove all outer packaging material in a location that is not in the clean working area.
- Do not allow smoking in the building, especially in the area around vent intakes.
- Wear freshly laundered clothing free of scent.
- Do not wear perfume, scented deodorant, or scented hair products. Do not use lotions.

Chapter 25

Veterinary Pharmaceutical Compounding

Historically, veterinarians dispensed most of the drugs they used in practice. Over the past few years, this tradition has changed, and pharmacists are developing working relationships with local veterinarians. Pharmacists who become involved in veterinary compounding should develop a basic knowledge of veterinary pharmacology to be able to choose the appropriate vehicle, preservative, flavoring agents, and the like to meet the patients' needs. Some of the reasons veterinary compounding is necessary include the following:

1. Need for multiple injections in the absence of a compounded product.
2. Rapid changes in management and disease problems in veterinary medicine.
3. Problems associated with the treatment of a large number of animals with several drugs in a short period of time.
4. Cost-prohibitive factors associated with the extremely large volume of some parenterals required for large animals.
5. Need for previously prepared antidotes for use in cases of animal poisoning.
6. Need to minimize suffering, harmful stress, and mortality in animals.
7. Need to combat multiple and concurrent disease processes.
8. Desire to achieve an additive therapeutic effect when simultaneously administering two or more products.
9. Encouragement of compliance by animal owners or their agents who are instructed to administer two or more products as part of a treatment regimen.
10. Need to achieve an appropriate treatment regimen for the species, age, or size of the animal patient.

The Relationship Between Pharmacists and Veterinarians

Veterinary pharmaceutical compounding presents unusual challenges and rewards. The veterinarian and the compounding pharmacist must use professional judgment and work hand-in-hand when deciding to compound a medication for an animal. The reader is urged to become thoroughly familiar with veterinary laws and regulations before attempting to compound for milk- or food-producing animals because some of the compounded medications can inadvertently find their way to the dining table. Done properly, veterinary compounding provides a service to the consumer and many opportunities for the professionals involved.

Some pharmacists have become extensively involved in working hand-in-hand with veterinarians in the treatment of animals, large and small, regular and exotic. Animals are usually categorized as companion pets (dogs, cats, parakeets, parrots, and the like); pocket pets; household, recreational, and work animals (horses, oxen); and food animals (cattle, hogs, poultry). Some veterinarians have the opportunity of working with such animals as varied as mink, alligators, llamas, alpacas, vicuña, ostriches, elephants, gorillas, tigers, sharks, and poisonous snakes, among others.

Marketing to veterinarians is generally quite easy: most do not realize the potential for working with a compounding pharmacist and need only some vision and assistance. Most veterinarians have a "wish list" of medications and dosage forms they would like to have. The compounding pharmacist can adjust the concentration of drugs and offer various routes of administration. This flexibility is invaluable. Attending veterinary meetings is an excellent way to become acquainted with veterinarians in an area. It is helpful to understand that some animals have greater tendencies to develop certain disorders than others, including guinea pigs (vitamin C deficiencies), ferrets (cancer), reptiles (respiratory problems), and birds (respiratory problems). One interesting opportunity for compounding pharmacists is that of working with zoos. In recent years, pharmacists have developed preparations such as raspberry jam-containing metronidazole (for a chimp), a cored apple containing a paste of drug and ground apple, raspberry-flavored Carbopol gel, a capsule or tablet placed inside the rectum of a live anesthetized mouse (for a boa constrictor), a peanut butter-flavored gel, the use of processed cheese spread to cover bitter or tart-tasting medications like methimazole (for cats), and the application of prednisone in a Pluronic lecithin organogel to the inner ear of a cat. Other preparations have been beef- and fish-flavored troches (a blank is given first followed by a medicated troche), banana cream-flavored troches for ferrets, and a fish-flavored paste applied to a cat's paw (tuna in oil or water is blended and then the drug is incorporated).

Veterinary Compounding Guidelines

To ensure that compounded medications are safe and therapeutic for animals but do not inadvertently enter the food chain, compounding pharmacists need to be aware of some of the guidelines under which veterinarians practice. The Drug Compounding Task Force of the American Veterinary Medical Association (AVMA) drafted guidelines for pharmaceutical compounding, which were approved by the AVMA House of Delegates in July 1991 and amended by the AVMA Executive Board in November 1991. The following information from the article "Guidelines for Pharmaceutical Compounding" is intended to provide enough background material to acquaint pharmacists with the guidelines.[1] For ease of reference, the guidelines are presented in outline form.

I. The resulting medicament is a restricted product that

A. Must be used only by or on the order of a licensed veterinarian;

B. Must be used only within the confines of a valid veterinarian-client-patient relationship and must follow the *AVMA Guidelines for Supervising Use and Distribution of Veterinary Prescription Drugs;*[2]

C. May be used or dispensed only for the treatment or prevention of disease or to improve the health and/or welfare of the animal(s); and

D. May be used only when a need has been established and products approved by the Food and Drug Administration (FDA) are not available or clinically effective.

II. The veterinarian must use professional judgment consistent with currently acceptable veterinary medical practice to ensure the safety and efficacy of the medicament, including

A. The safety for the target animal; and

B. The avoidance of violative residues in meat, milk, or eggs when administered to a food-producing animal.

III. The veterinarian must use professional judgment consistent with proper pharmaceutical and pharmacologic principles when compounding medicaments. The following points should be considered:

A. The stability of the active ingredients.

B. The physical and chemical compatibility of the ingredients.

C. The pharmacodynamic compatibility of the active ingredients.

D. The composition of the active ingredients and diluents to ensure that they are not contaminated with harmful substances or agents.

IV. The prepared medicament must be properly labeled before being dispensed. Labeling practices include the following:

A. When the medicament is administered by the veterinarian or is administered under his or her direct supervision, no label is required.

B. When the medicament is dispensed according to the veterinarian's order, the product must have a complete, indelible, legible label attached. A complete label requires the following items:

(1) Name and address of the attending veterinarian.

(2) Date dispensed.

(3) Medically active ingredients.

(4) Identity of animal(s) to be treated (i.e., species, class, group, or individual animal[s]).

(5) Directions for use.

(6) Cautionary statements, if needed.

(7) Slaughter withdrawal times and/or milk-withholding times, if needed.

These requirements are consistent with the *AVMA Guidelines for Supervising Use and Distribution of Veterinary Prescription Drugs*, the *1993 Pasteurized Milk Ordinance*,[3] and section 615.100 of the FDA *Compliance Policy Guides*.[4] The following additional information can be included on a label:

(8) Disease conditions to be treated.

(9) Expiration date.

V. Compounded medicaments must not be advertised or displayed to the public.

VI. When compounded medicaments are used, appropriate patient records must be maintained.

VII. When compounded medicaments are used in food-producing animals, appropriate drug residue tests, when available and practical, and other procedures for ensuring violative residue avoidance should be instituted.

Regulatory Issues

From a regulatory standpoint, there are basically two types of veterinary compounding. First, compounding from FDA-approved veterinary and human drugs is covered under the Animal Medicinal Drug Use Clarification Act of 1994 (AMDUCA). This act legalized the "extra-label" (not in accordance with labeling) use of drugs in animals under certain circumstances and likewise legalized this form of compounding. Second, the compounding from bulk drugs is not covered under AMDUCA. A *bulk drug* is defined as ". . . an active ingredient (in unfinished form) intended for manufacture into finished dosage form drug products." FDA considers the use of bulk drugs illegal but exercises discretion if the provisions of the Compliance Policy Guide (CPG) for the Compounding of Drugs for Use in Animals are followed.

The CPG states that veterinary compounding from raw chemicals must meet the following conditions. The veterinarian is responsible for ensuring that these conditions exist:

1. A legitimate medical need is identified.
2. A need exists for an appropriate dosage regimen for the species, age, size, or medical condition of the patient.
3. No marketed, approved animal or human drug can be used as labeled or in an extra-label manner; or some other rare extenuating circumstance is present (e.g., the approved drug cannot be obtained in time to treat the animal[s] in a timely manner, or there is a medical need for different excipients).

After those three determinations are made, the following criteria should be met:

1. The compounded product can be dispensed by the veterinarian in the course of his or her practice or by a pharmacist, who must have a prescription from a veterinarian.
2. The veterinarian should take measures to ensure that no illegal residues occur when a compounded product is used in food animals, an extended time period is assigned for withdrawal, and steps are taken to ensure assigned time frames are observed.
3. A pharmacist compounding for a veterinary patient must adhere to the National Association of Boards of Pharmacy Good Compounding Practices (GCP), or to equivalent state GCP regulation, except where provisions conflict with this CPG.
4. The label of a compounded veterinary prescription should contain the following information when filled by a pharmacist:
   ‣ Name and address of the veterinary practitioner.
   ‣ Active ingredient(s).
   ‣ Date dispensed and expiration date (not to exceed length of prescribed treatment unless the veterinarian can establish the rationale for a later expiration date).

- Directions for use, including the class/species to identify the animal(s), and the dose, frequency, route of administration, and duration of therapy.
- Cautionary statements specified by the veterinarian and/or the pharmacist, including all appropriate warnings to ensure safety of humans handling the drugs.
- Veterinarian's specified withdrawal/discard time(s) for meat, milk, eggs, or any food that might be derived from the treated animal(s) (Although the veterinarian is responsible for setting the withdrawal time, he or she can use relevant information provided by a pharmacist in setting the time).
- Name and address of the dispenser, serial number, and date of order or its filling.
- Any other applicable requirements of state or federal law.

Veterinary prescription drugs are drugs restricted by federal law to use by or on the order of a licensed veterinarian. Any other drugs used in animals in a manner not in accordance with their labeling should be subjected to the same supervisory precautions that apply to veterinary prescription drugs. Veterinary prescription drugs can be prescribed only within the context of a valid veterinarian-client-patient relationship. Any veterinary prescription filled by a pharmacist requires a prescription from a veterinarian.

Veterinary prescription medication labels read "Caution: Federal law restricts this drug to use by or on the order of a licensed veterinarian." This statement is the veterinary counterpart to the human legend and must appear on the label of all manufactured veterinary prescription products. Phrases such as "For veterinary use only" and "Sold to veterinarians only" do not refer to the drug's prescription status but rather to sales policies of companies.

Applications and Other Factors

Compounding can be considered when no effective FDA-approved products exist for treatment of the disease or condition diagnosed by the veterinarian and when the failure to treat would result in patient suffering or death. Even if dosage forms are available, they can be inappropriate for one or more of the following reasons:

- Patient size.
- Patient anatomy.
- Patient physiology.
- Patient safety.
- Individual patient sensitivity or idiosyncrasy.
- Patient stress or suffering from formulations that require multiple injections or administration of large volumes.
- Danger to personnel who must deal with animals difficult to restrain.

Veterinarians also may consider compounding to minimize side effects or to increase the effectiveness of therapy. For example, combining specific anesthetic agents increases the analgesic and muscle relaxant effects while reducing the total dose of anesthetics used. This practice lessens the adverse cardiac and respiratory effects. Combining intra-articular medications for single injection minimizes both the discomfort to the patient and the probability of introducing pathogenic microorganisms into the animal.

Finally, compounding can be considered in extreme situations wherein economic realities would preclude treatment with the approved product. In such situations, pain, suffering, or even death would result from failure to treat.

It is virtually inconceivable that there will ever be FDA-approved veterinary drugs labeled for every therapeutic need, and it appears that compounding for veterinary medicine will become more prevalent, as it has in human medicine, especially with the future introduction of biotechnologically derived products with limited stability.

Considerations in Deciding to Compound

The veterinary compounding pharmacist must ask the following questions when considering whether to compound a prescription for an animal:

- What is known about the physical and chemical compatibility of the drugs?
- What is known about the stability of these drugs—before, during, and after the compounding process?
- What is known about the pharmacodynamic compatibility of the active ingredients?
- What is the overall goal of the treatment of this animal?
- Are any similar products available commercially to treat the animal?
- What regulatory concerns may be involved?
- Is this animal a food animal?
- Will the drug treatment cause a residue problem?
- Is there any risk to personnel who handle the drug during compounding or during administration of the compounded form?

Devices for Administering Medications

As with humans, a variety of dosage forms can be prepared for animals, using several different routes of administration. Except for the intramammary route of administration, the administration routes used in animals are the same as those for humans. A multitude of devices are available for delivering a specified dose of a medication or for administering the medication by one of the routes used most frequently in veterinary medicine: oral, topical, parenteral, and nasal.

Oral Administration

Oral dosage forms present the greatest challenge in administering medications to animals. Some ingenious devices have been developed to meet this challenge. A brief description of the most commonly used devices is presented here.[5] For more detailed information, the reader is referred to Blodinger's *Formulation of Veterinary Dosage Forms* as well as the other veterinary references listed in "Additional References."

Balling guns are relatively simple devices that have a barrel through which passes a plunger capable of dislodging the bolus(es) into the gullet of the animal.

Esophageal delivery devices are syringes and tubes that are usually designed to deliver the medication directly into the stomach.

Drench syringes are either single- or multiple-dose devices that are capable of delivering preset volumes of liquid into the gullet.

Liquid drench guns are either single- or multiple-dose devices that are capable of delivering oral solutions or suspensions of an aqueous or oily nature relatively quickly.

Powder drench guns are devices, usually spring loaded, that are capable of delivering the required amount of powder into the back portion of the mouth, where it usually adheres and is subsequently swallowed.

Paste dispensers include devices such as paste guns, paste syringes, squeeze bottles, and squeeze tubes that are capable of delivering a specified dose to an animal.

Water medication-metering devices provide a method of adding a medication to the water supply of numerous animals. The amount of medication released in the water depends on the average daily water intake of the animals. These devices are often used to administer medications, vaccines, wormers, electrolytes, disinfectants, and antibloating surfactants.

Miscellaneous oral dose dispensers include pump-type dispensers, nursers, droppers, mineral dispensers, and mouthpieces.

Rumen-lodging devices are incorporated into medications that have a controlled-release delivery system. These devices aid the product in sticking to the mucosal surface and allowing the medication to be released at the desired rate.

Hollow bits have a hollowed-out area in which medications that have a heat-sensitive release matrix are placed. Saliva causes the medication to be released slowly through perforations in the surface of the bit. A confection is often included in the matrix. Hollow bits are used to administer medications to horses.

Buoyant devices, which resemble large, floating tablets, allow the dosage form to float in the intestine and release the medication over an extended period of time. To allow it to float, the dosage form must have a specific gravity somewhat less than that of the animal's intestinal contents. Some of these devices also release carbon dioxide, which aids in keeping the dosage form afloat.

Topical Administration

Several devices have been developed to aid in ridding animals of parasites such as lice and fleas, protecting the animals from biting or stinging insects, and treating skin conditions caused by these organisms or other environmental factors. The following descriptions of topical administration devices were adapted from Blodinger.[5]

Pour-on, spot-on applicators are ordinarily used to treat skin conditions or surface (horns, hooves) conditions of animals.

Dust bags are used to apply powders to cattle as they brush up against or walk underneath the bags. These devices are especially useful for the topical application of insecticide powders to control flies and lice. The pore size of the bag allows for ease of application of the product.

Spray race and dip applicators are long troughs with deep sides that are commonly used for dipping treatments. To be safe and effective, the length, width, and depth of the dipping bath must be adequate to immerse the animal completely without injuring it.

Teat dip applicators are cups in which medication is added to a depth sufficient to immerse the lower extremity of the teat. The cups are filled with medication and then lifted to the teat.

Aerosol dispensers are a convenient and effective means of applying medications.

Flea and tick collars generally use slow-release generators containing medications that either have a high vapor pressure or are designed as a solid solution so that the product will migrate from the collar over the body.

Percutaneous absorption drug-reservoir devices are drug-containing matrices that allow the drug to diffuse from the device into the animal's skin or onto the skin surface. These devices can be attached to the skin by an adhesive, clips, pins, or staples. Drug-impregnated bandages, films, and ear tampons have also been used.

Parenteral Administration

Because injections can often be administered quickly from a safe distance, they are often the easiest method of administering medications to animals. Several devices are available that allow administration of the therapeutic agents from a safe distance. Further, using a syringe to administer a medication through an orifice or to place a sustained-release medication in a body cavity is often the only viable option for long-term treatment of some conditions. Several devices have been developed for administering these types of injections. The following descriptions of these and other parenteral administration devices were adapted from Blodinger.[5]

Single-dose syringes are often used when treating only one animal at a time. Disposable syringes as well as resterilizable syringes made of nylon, polypropylene, or glass are available. Both types of syringes are available in numerous sizes. Prefilled syringes in sterilized packs are also available.

Multiple-dose syringes are generally used to treat small herds when an automatic syringe is not required. As the name implies, the syringe barrel, which has a stepping plunger, can contain several doses, allowing the veterinarian to treat several animals without stopping to reload the syringe.

Automatic syringes, which are used to treat large herds, include the adaptable, chamber-fill, handle-fill, and specialized varieties.

Multi-compartment syringes are used for unstable drug products that require the diluent to be added to the dry powder just before injection.

Pole-mounted syringes allow injectable formulations to be administered from a safe distance.

Mastitis syringes are used to insert a drug formulation directly into the mammary gland through the teat canal.

Jet injectors contain orifices through which a liquid can be administered under extremely high pressure onto or near the skin of the animal.

Projectile delivery systems include arrows and darts that can be propelled by bows or blowguns. The drug can be placed on the tip of the arrow or dart, or in a special syringe that will expel the contents on contact with the animal.

Implants are sterile dosage forms designed so that a depot of drug can be placed at a site in the body for prolonged release of the drug.

Implanting devices are used to insert pellets, balls, and molten and ballistic types of implants at the chosen site in the body.

Intrauterine drug dispensers are designed to stay in the uterine cavity for a period of days, weeks, or months to deliver a sustained-release drug. Some of these devices will even self-destruct at the end of the drug delivery period.

Vaginal drug dispensers are used to deliver drug-containing sponges and suppositories.

Nasal Administration

Nasal administration of drugs results in a rapid onset of action that is almost as fast as the onset of action of intravenous injections. Nasal administration, which does not involve piercing, has the advantage of avoiding some of the problems associated with parenteral administration. Vaccines for a number of diseases, including Newcastle disease and infectious bronchitis, and antibiotics are often administered through the nasal passageways. The following types of dispensers are used most often to administer these agents to animals.

Dropper dispensers are generally used to deliver a single dose of a medication. This type of dispenser can be as simple as a plastic dropper attached to a rubber bulb; the dropper must be properly calibrated to deliver the required dose. A syringe without a needle or a syringe with a plastic tip can also be used. These types of syringes will not cause injury to mucosal membranes.

Spray dispensers are used to immunize small chicks against a number of poultry viral pathogens. The chicks pass through a closed chamber and inhale vaccine solutions that are dispensed as an aerosol spray. These devices can also dispense a vaccine as a powder mist. Metered-spray dispensers are also available.

Pharmacologic Considerations

Each species of animal has distinguishing features that contribute to the variability in the way it handles drugs. In many pharmacologic studies, species variations have been shown to be attributable for differences in systemic availability, accessibility to the site of action, and the rate of elimination.

Pharmacokinetics

As in humans, the effect of a drug on an animal depends on the drug's movement throughout the body and the concentration that builds up at the specific site of action. The extent of the response of the individual animal's receptors is important. Factors that influence the concentration of a drug in the plasma include the size of the dose, formulation of the drug, route of administration, extent of distribution and plasma protein binding, and rate of elimination. These factors can differ from animal to animal, but they involve the same four basic processes: absorption, distribution, metabolism, and excretion.

Absorption

Gastric emptying is an important physiologic factor controlling the rate of drug absorption. Some animals, such as the horse, are continuous feeders, and their stomachs are seldom empty. The emptying rate of multi-stomach animals can vary as greatly as the consistency of the material in each of the stomachs.

Distribution

The distribution of drugs to the various tissues and organs will differ between animals because they have different body compositions. Table 25-1 provides a comparison of the body composition of several animals, including humans.

Metabolism

The rate at which drugs are metabolized differs from animal to animal. For example, cats have a slow rate of glucuronide synthesis, acetylation is absent in the dog, and sulfate conjugation is present in the pig only to a limited extent. The slow rate of glucuronide conjugation in cats means that compounds such as aspirin and phenols, which undergo glucuronide formation, appear to be relatively more toxic in cats.

Excretion

The urinary pH of herbivores is alkaline (pH 7–8), but the urinary pH of carnivores is acidic (pH 5.5–7). This difference obviously can affect the excretion rate of drug products, especially those with pKa values in the close vicinity of these ranges. The half-lives of drugs vary between animals, as is shown in Table 25-2.

Table 25-1. Body Composition (% of Live Weight) of Various Animals, Including Humans

Anatomical Component	Horse	Dog	Goat	Human
Blood	8.6	—	—	7.8
Brain	0.2	0.5	0.3	2.0
Heart	0.7	0.8	0.5	0.5
Lung	0.9	0.9	0.9	1.4
Liver	1.3	2.3	2.0	2.6
Kidney	0.4	0.6	0.4	0.4
Gastrointestinal tract	12.7	0.7	13.9	1.4
Skin	7.4	9.3	9.2	3.7
Muscle	40.1	54.5	45.5	40.0
Bone	14.6	8.7	6.3	14.0
Adipose tissue	5.1	—	—	18.1
Total weight (kg)	308	16	39	70

Source: Adapted from reference 5.

Table 25-2. Half-Lives (in Hours) of Selected Drugs in Animals

Drug	Horse	Dog	Cat	Pig	Ruminant
Amphetamine	1.4	4.5	6.5	1.1	0.6
Ampicillin	1.6	0.8	—	—	1.2
Chloramphenicol	0.9	4.2	5.1	1.3	2.0
Kanamycin	1.5	1.0	—	—	1.9
Oxytetracycline	10.5	6.0	—	—	9.1
Penicillin G	0.9	0.5	—	—	0.7
Pentobarbital	1.5	4.5	4.9	—	0.8
Salicylate	1.0	8.6	37.6	5.9	0.8
Sulfadimethoxine	11.3	13.2	10.2	15.5	12.5
Sulfadoxine	14.0	—	—	8.2	11.7
Trimethoprim	3.2	3.0	—	2.3	0.8

Source: Adapted from reference 5.

Table 25-3. Drug Dosage Variations Among Different Species

Drug	Administration Route	Dose (mg/kg)			
		Ruminant	Horse	Dog	Cat
Xylazine	IM	0.2	2.0	2.0	2.0
Succinylcholine	IV	0.02	0.1	0.3	1.0

Key: IM = intramuscular; IV = intravenous.

Source: Reference 5.

The drug preparation to be used must be selected and administered at a dosage that is appropriate for a particular species of animal. Table 25-3 shows the dosage variations between animals for two different drugs administered by two different routes.

Table 25-4. Pharmacokinetic Parameters of Diazepam in the Human, Dog, and Rat

Pharmacokinetic Variable	Human	Dog	Rat
Half-life (in hours)	32.9	7.6	1.1
Body clearance (mL/kg-minute)	0.35	18.9	81.6
Plasma protein, binding (%)	96.81	6.0	86.3
Blood clearance (mL/kg-minute)	0.64	35.0	214.7
Hepatic extraction ratio	0.029	0.81	6.31
Fraction of free drug	0.032	0.04	0.14

Source: Adapted from reference 5.

The pharmacokinetic parameters of different drugs will vary among animals. Table 25-4 provides an example of the pharmacokinetic variations of diazepam in three animals, including humans.

Pharmaceutics

Variables that modify the rate and extent of absorption, thus changing the response to a drug, include the crystal habit of the drug, polymorphism, the specific salt used, the state of solvation or hydration, excipients and adjuvants, processing variations, and the formation of complexes. Choosing a flavoring for a drug can be a challenge because different animals prefer different flavors. Table 25-5 presents a variety of flavors that have been used in drugs for different animals.

Physiology

Physiologic considerations that affect drug response include drug sensitivity, age, sex, pregnancy, drug interactions in vivo, and disease states. The normal or distinctive habits of animals must be considered. For example, because cats are constantly grooming themselves, any drug placed on them topically is likely to be ingested.

Table 25-5. Suggested Flavors for Veterinary Medications

Animal	Comment	Flavor
Pets		
Avian	Birds prefer sweet and fruity flavors; use gels for birds that like to bite, or try adding fresh juice or flavored vehicle to bread balls or stuffing.	Tutti-frutti, piña colada, grape, orange, orange juice, tangerine, banana, molasses/millet, raspberry, honey/millet, nectar (and mixtures of these)
Parrots		Hot and spicy flavors (cayenne pepper)
Tropical birds		Tutti-frutti, piña colada, banana (and mixtures)
Canine	Dogs prefer meats, sweets, fixed oils, or a syringe of processed cheese spread as a vehicle. Use a mini ice cube tray for larger troches or make a milk bone for larger doses.	Bacon, beef, liver, chicken, turkey, cheese, chocolate (artificial), peanut butter, cod liver oil, honey, malt, molasses, caramel, anise, marshmallow, raspberry, strawberry
Feline	Cats usually do not like too much sweetness but hate bitter tastes. Flavored troches work, but make treats with square corners, not round. Flavored paste to the paw as an alternative is acceptable, but, if appropriate, consider transdermal administration.	Fish, fish/liver, tuna, cod liver oil, sardine, mackerel, salmon, beef, liver, chicken, cheese, cheese with fish, bacon, molasses, peanut butter, butter, butterscotch, marshmallow
Ferrets	In the wild, they prefer fish and meat, but if domesticated they can develop a sweet tooth.	Chocolate, peanut butter, molasses, honey, fish, beef, liver, bacon, raspberry, fruit punch, tutti-frutti, apple, strawberry, peas
Rabbits	Find their favorite vegetable or fruit and use it.	Lettuce, carrot, parsley, celery, banana cream, vanilla butternut, pineapple
Gerbils	As a rule, they like sweet and fruity flavors.	Orange, peach, tutti-frutti, tangerine, banana cream
Guinea pigs	Flavor a paste and spread it on their favorite vegetable.	Celery, pumpkin, lettuce, carrot
Reptiles	Smell can be more important than taste. (Snakes are the exception; administer drug by dropper.)	Lemon custard, banana cream, tutti-frutti, melon
Iguanas	Make the preparation smell good.	Cantaloupe, watermelon, other melons, kiwi, orange, banana, tangerine

Table 25-5. Suggested Flavors for Veterinary Medications (cont.)

Animal	Comment	Flavor
Rodents	Use a flavored paste or jelly.	Lemon custard, banana cream, cheese, peanut butter, vanilla butternut
Farm Animals		
Equine	Horses need large amounts in reasonable volumes. Use thick suspensions or pastes.	Apple, apple/caramel, caramel, cherry, butterscotch, molasses, honey, alfalfa, clover, maple, bluegrass, forage
Cattle		Eggnog, anise, anise/licorice, alfalfa, maple, molasses, honey, clover, bluegrass, meal, forage
Poultry		Vanilla butternut, watermelon, cantaloupe, milk, corn, meal
Emu	These birds are attracted to bright colors, especially yellow.	Cantaloupe, watermelon, kiwi, honeydew, strawberry, tutti-frutti
Swine	Try mixing the drug with peanut butter and rolling it in corn flakes.	Anisette, cherry, anise, meal, sarsaparilla, licorice, corn, peanut butter, honey, milk
Goat	It is not true that they will eat anything.	Molasses, honey, apple, caramel, cherry
Exotics and Zoo Animals		
Elephant	They differ in what they like, so check with the handler. Flavor and inject suspension into a favorite food. To neutralize the bitterness, use lots of stevia if needed. They need to avoid shots, which can easily cause abscesses. Check what handlers are able to do. Can they shoot the liquid in the mouth? If not, an option is to put nonbitter liquid on bread and cover with vegetables.	Apple, apple/peanut butter, cantaloupe, watermelon, raspberry, pumpkin, orange, chewing tobacco
Primates	Hide the bitterness; numerous flavors will work.	Banana, raspberry, apricot, orange, peach, chocolate
Colobus monkey		Carrot, sweet potato, leafy vegetables (spinach, lettuce), banana, apple
Baby monkey		Banana, apple, carrot
Ostrich	These birds are attracted to bright colors, especially green.	Strawberry, raspberry, tutti-frutti

(continued)

Table 25-5. Suggested Flavors for Veterinary Medications (cont.)

Animal	Comment	Flavor
Chinchilla		Banana, tutti-frutti
Armadillo		Canned dog food, bacon
Orangutan		Apricot nectar
Zebra		Apple, apple/caramel
Bear		Honey, licorice
Tiger, lion		Chicken, liver, beef, turkey, bacon, other meats (preferably freshly killed or live)
Coyote		Watermelon, meat flavors
Rhinoceros		Apple
Sea lion	Captive (inland) sea lions need sodium chloride supplementation. Place drug into a fish.	Whole fish

Compounded Veterinary Formulations

Bases

℞ Oral Paste Formulations (100 g)

	Formula 1	Formula 2	Formula 3	Formula 4
Polyethylene glycol 300	65 g	25 g		
Polyethylene glycol 3350	35 g	25 g	25 g	
Propylene glycol		50 g	25 g	
Peanut butter				65 g
Hydrogenated vegetable oil				35 g
Molasses			50 g	

1. Calculate the quantity of each ingredient required for the prescription.
2. Accurately weigh or measure each ingredient.
3. Generally, the polyethylene glycol formulas are prepared by heating the ingredients to a temperature of about 70°C, followed by cooling and stirring.
4. In formula 2, the propylene glycol is added while the preparation is hot, followed by cooling and stirring.
5. In formula 3, the molasses is added as the preparation is cooling.
6. Formula 4 can be prepared by simply mixing the ingredients.
7. Package and label.

Rx Nonaqueous Nonoleaginous Paste Base

Active drug	qs
Carbomer 934	1.0–1.5 g
Triethanolamine	0.23–0.35 g
Flavor	qs
Propylene glycol	qs 100 g

(Note: The consistency of this paste can be modified by altering the quantities of carbomer 934 and/or triethanolamine or by replacing up to half the propylene glycol with glycerin.)

For drugs soluble in propylene glycol:

1. Calculate the quantity of each ingredient required for the prescription.
2. Accurately weigh or measure each ingredient.
3. Place the propylene glycol in a suitable mixer and dissolve the drug and flavor.
4. Add the carbomer 934 and mix until dissolved.
5. Slowly add the triethanolamine and mix well; blend until smooth and homogeneous.
6. Package and label.

For drugs insoluble in propylene glycol:

1. Calculate the quantity of each ingredient required for the prescription.
2. Accurately weigh or measure each ingredient.
3. Dissolve the flavor in the propylene glycol; then add the carbomer 934 and mix until dissolved.
4. Slowly add the triethanolamine and mix well; blend until smooth and homogenous.
5. Slowly add the drug, as a fine powder, and mix until uniform.
6. Package and label.

Ophthalmics

Rx Veterinary Dexamethasone 0.1% Ophthalmic Ointment

Dexamethasone sodium phosphate	39.6 mg (equivalent to about 30 mg of dexamethasone)
Bacteriostatic water for injection	0.4 mL
Polysorbate 80	0.3 mL
Lacrilube	qs 30 g

(Note: This preparation should be prepared in a laminar airflow hood by validated, aseptic compounding pharmacists, using aseptic techniques.)

℞ **Veterinary Dexamethasone 0.1% Ophthalmic Ointment (cont.)**

1. Sterilize all equipment to be used before proceeding to the laminar airflow hood.
2. Accurately weigh or measure the ingredients.
3. Mix the dexamethasone sodium phosphate with the bacteriostatic water for injection.
4. Add the polysorbate 80 and mix well.
5. Aspirate the liquid into a syringe, attach a sterilizing filter, and filter into a sterile syringe.
6. Remove the barrel from a second sterile syringe and add the Lacrilube.
7. Connect the two syringes by using a sterile connector.
8. Thoroughly mix the product by alternately forcing the contents of one syringe into the other syringe.
9. Package and label.

Ointments/Creams/Gels

℞ **Dimethyl Sulfoxide 50% Cream, Veterinary (100 g)**

Dimethyl sulfoxide		50 g
Cetyl alcohol		6 g
Stearyl alcohol		6 g
Polysorbate 80		6 mL
Imidurea		100 mg
Preserved water (parabens)	qs	100 g

1. Calculate the quantity of each ingredient required for the prescription.
2. Accurately weigh or measure each ingredient.
3. Mix the dimethyl sulfoxide, polysorbate 80, and about 32 mL of preserved water.
4. Add the imidurea and heat to about 60°C while stirring.
5. In a separate container, heat the cetyl alcohol and stearyl alcohol until a clear melt is obtained.
6. Add the aqueous solution (step 4) to the oil solution (step 5) with stirring.
7. Remove from heat and mix until cooled.
8. If necessary, add sufficient preserved water to make 100 g, and mix well.
9. Package in glass containers and label.

R℞ **Antifungal Preparation for Animals**

Coal tar solution		5 mL
Resorcinol		2.5 g
Lanolin		6.5 g
Liquefied phenol		1.5 mL
Hydrophilic petrolatum		15 g
White petrolatum	qs	100 g

1. Calculate the quantity of each ingredient required for the prescription.
2. Accurately weigh or measure each ingredient.
3. Place the resorcinol powder on a pill tile.
4. Add 1 to 2 mL of coal tar solution at a time until the resorcinol powder is dissolved.
5. Add this mixture to about half of the hydrophilic petrolatum (Aquaphor or Aquabase can also be used). Using a spatula, incorporate the petrolatum until the mixture is smooth.
6. Add the lanolin and the remaining hydrophilic petrolatum until all of these ingredients are incorporated.
7. Add the liquefied phenol and mix until uniform.
8. Incorporate the white petrolatum and mix until homogenous.
9. Package and label.

R℞ **Hair Moisturizer/Conditioner for Horses and Other Animals**

Mineral oil, light	20 g
Hydrophilic petrolatum	80 g

1. Accurately weigh or measure the calculated quantity of each ingredient.
2. Using low heat, heat the light mineral oil.
3. Add the hydrophilic petrolatum (Aquaphor or Aquabase) and thoroughly mix.
4. Remove from heat and cool, with intermittent stirring.
5. Package and label.

℞ Sulfur and Peruvian Balsam Ointment for Mange/Ringworm in Animals

Peruvian balsam	12 g
Castor oil	12 g
Sulfur ointment	76 g

1. Calculate the quantity of each ingredient required for the prescription.
2. Accurately weigh or measure each ingredient.
3. Mix the Peruvian balsam with the castor oil.
4. Incorporate the sulfur ointment.
5. Mix until uniform.
6. Package and label.

℞ Sulfur Ointment

Precipitated sulfur	10 g
Liquid petrolatum	10 g
White ointment	80 g

1. Calculate the quantity of each ingredient required for the prescription.
2. Accurately weigh or measure each ingredient.
3. Levigate the precipitated sulfur with the liquid petrolatum until a smooth paste is formed.
4. Incorporate the white ointment and mix until uniform.
5. Package and label.

℞ Fleabite Gel (100 mL)

Dexamethasone sodium phosphate	50 mg
Quinine sulfate dihydrate	100 mg
Diphenhydramine HCl	1 g
Methylcellulose (1500 cP)	3 g
Purified water	qs 100 mL

1. Calculate the quantity of each ingredient required for the prescription.
2. Accurately weigh or measure each ingredient.
3. Dissolve the diphenhydramine HCl and dexamethasone sodium phosphate in about 40 mL of purified water.
4. Heat about 50 mL of purified water until steaming.
5. With rapid stirring, slowly sprinkle the methylcellulose onto the water until thoroughly dispersed.
6. Remove from heat and pour in the drug solution.
7. Add sufficient purified water to volume, followed by the quinine sulfate dihydrate, and mix well.
8. Store in the refrigerator for about 2 hours until gelling is complete.
9. Package and label.

R℞ Methimazole 5 mg/0.1 mL in Pluronic Lecithin Organogel (3 mL)

Methimazole	150 mg
Lecithin:isopropyl palmitate solution	0.66 mL
Pluronic F-127 gel 20%	qs 3 mL

(Note: The lecithin:isopropyl palmitate solution can be prepared by mixing 0.2 g of sorbic acid, 50 g of soy lecithin, and 50 g of isopropyl palmitate. The Pluronic F-127 gel can be prepared by mixing 0.2 g of sorbic acid, 20 g of Pluronic F-127, and sufficient purified water to make 100 mL.)

1. Calculate the quantity of each ingredient required for the prescription.
2. Accurately weigh or measure each ingredient.
3. Remove the plunger from a 3-mL Luer-Lok syringe (or appropriate size depending on quantity to be prepared) and attach a tip cap.
4. Pour the methimazole powder carefully into the syringe barrel.
5. Add the lecithin:isopropyl palmitate solution and replace the plunger.
6. In a second syringe, measure 2 mL of the Pluronic F-127 gel.
7. Attach a Luer-Lok/Luer-Lok Adapter to fit the two syringes together, and mix the contents back and forth between the two syringes.
8. Carefully (so as not to entrap air), force all the preparation into one syringe and measure the volume.
9. Remove the other syringe and obtain sufficient Pluronic F-127 gel to volume.
10. Reattach the syringes together, and mix the preparation back and forth until it is thoroughly mixed.
11. Package and label.

R℞ Veterinary Antiseptic Emollient (100 g)

Hydroxyquinoline	300 mg
Liquified phenol	2 mL
Methyl salicylate	1 mL
Lanolin	32 g
Petrolatum (white or yellow)	65 g

1. Calculate the quantity of each ingredient required for the prescription.
2. Accurately weigh or measure each ingredient.
3. Levigate the hydroxyquinoline into a small quantity of petrolatum and mix until smooth.
4. Gradually incorporate the remainder of the petrolatum into the mixture.
5. Incorporate the liquified phenol and methyl salicylate into the mixture.
6. Incorporate the lanolin and mix well.
7. Package and label.

Otics

℞ **Silver Sulfadiazine 1% Otic Lotion**

Silver sulfadiazine 1% cream	18 g
Silver sulfadiazine powder	315 mg
Propylene glycol	qs
Bacteriostatic water for injection	24 mL

1. Calculate the quantity of each ingredient required for the prescription.
2. Accurately weigh or measure each ingredient.
3. Wet the silver sulfadiazine powder with a few drops of propylene glycol to make a paste.
4. Add the silver sulfadiazine cream and mix well.
5. Add the bacteriostatic water for injection and mix well to make a lotion.
6. Package and label.

℞ **Gentamicin, Polymyxin, Neomycin, and Hydrocortisone Otic Drops (100 mL)**

Gentamicin sulfate activity	150 mg
Polymyxin B sulfate	150 mg
Neomycin sulfate	500 mg
Hydrocortisone	1 g
Propylene glycol	50 mL
Polysorbate 80	0.25 mL
Sodium bisulfite	100 mg
Purified water	30 mL
Glycerin	qs 100 mL

1. Calculate the required quantity of each ingredient for the total amount to be prepared. The quantity of gentamicin sulfate will be calculated from the activity labeled on the bulk container.
2. Accurately weigh or measure each ingredient.
3. Combine the hydrocortisone with the polysorbate 80 in a beaker and mix well. Slowly, with stirring, add the propylene glycol. A small quantity of heat may be required to dissolve the hydrocortisone.
4. In a separate container, dissolve the gentamicin sulfate, polymyxin B sulfate, neomycin sulfate, and sodium bisulfite in the purified water. Add about 10 mL of glycerin and mix well.
5. Add the solution from step 4 to the cooled solution from step 3 and mix well.
6. Add sufficient glycerin to volume and mix well.
7. Package and label.

℞ EDTA-TRIS Otic Solution

Edetate disodium		20 mg
TRIS (hydroxymethyl) aminomethane		605 mg
Sodium lauryl sulfate		190 mg
Sodium hydroxide 20% solution (fresh)		to adjust pH
Sterile water for irrigation	qs	100 mL

1. Calculate the quantity of each ingredient required for the prescription.
2. Accurately weigh or measure each ingredient.
3. Dissolve the TRIS in 90 mL of the sterile water for irrigation.
4. Dissolve the edetate disodium and sodium lauryl sulfate into the solution by using low heat and minimal stirring to avoid foaming.
5. Add sterile water for irrigation to a volume of about 98 mL.
6. Add sufficient sodium hydroxide 20% solution to obtain a pH of 8. (Note: Prepare the sodium hydroxide 20% solution by dissolving 2 g of sodium hydroxide in sufficient purified water to make 10 mL. Use within 5 days.)
7. Add sufficient sterile water for irrigation to volume and mix well.
8. Sterilize by autoclaving or sterile filtration (0.22-μm filter).
9. Package and label.

℞ Veterinary Antibiotic/Antifungal/Anti-inflammatory/Anesthetic Otic Drop

Gentamicin sulfate	300 mg (as gentamicin)
Betamethasone valerate	100 mg
Miconazole nitrate	1 g
Tetracaine hydrochloride	1 g
Propylene glycol	qs 100 mL

1. Calculate the required quantity of each ingredient for the total amount to be prepared. For the gentamicin sulfate, it will be necessary to calculate the quantity based on the labeled potency of the drug.
2. Accurately weigh or measure each ingredient.
3. Reduce the particle sizes of the powders, if necessary, and blend in a mortar with a pestle.
4. Add a small portion of the propylene glycol and form a smooth paste.
5. Geometrically, add the propylene glycol and mix until uniform.
6. Package and label.

Injections

R_X Iodine 2% in Oil Injection

Iodine, resublimed	2 g
Almond oil, sweet	qs 100 mL

(Note: This preparation should be prepared in a laminar airflow hood in a clean room by a validated, aseptic compounding pharmacist, using strict aseptic technique.)

1. Calculate the quantity of each ingredient required for the prescription.
2. Accurately weigh or measure each ingredient.
3. Place the iodine and sufficient almond oil to make 100 mL in a beaker.
4. Stir by using a magnetic stirrer and gentle heat until the iodine is dissolved, which can take several hours.
5. Filter the solution through a 0.22-μm sterile filter into sterile vials.
6. Package and label.

R_X Canine Methylpyrazole Intravenous Solution for Ethylene Glycol Poisoning

4-Methyl-pyrazole	1 g
Polyethylene glycol 300	9 mL
Bacteriostatic water for injection	qs 20 mL

1. Calculate the quantity of each ingredient required for the prescription.
2. Accurately weigh or measure each ingredient.
3. Place the 4-methyl-pyrazole and the polyethylene glycol 300 in a clean container and mix well.
4. Add sufficient bacteriostatic water for injection to make 20 mL and mix well.
5. Filter through a sterile 0.22-μm filter into a sterile container.
6. Package and label.

R_X Veterinary Electrolyte Injection

Sodium acetate trihydrate	4.333 g
Potassium chloride	467 mg
Calcium chloride dihydrate	200 mg
Magnesium chloride	133 mg
Benzyl alcohol	0.1 mL
5% Dextrose in water	50 mL
Sterile water for injection	qs 100 mL

(Note: This product should be prepared in a laminar airflow hood in a clean room by a validated, aseptic compounding pharmacist, using strict aseptic technique.)

℞ Veterinary Electrolyte Injection (cont.)

1. Calculate the quantity of each ingredient required for the prescription.
2. Accurately weigh or measure each ingredient.
3. Dissolve the electrolytes and the benzyl alcohol in the 5% dextrose in water.
4. Add sufficient sterile water for injection to volume.
5. Filter through a sterile 0.2-μm filter into a sterile container (or) package in clean vials and autoclave at 121°C, 15 psi, for 20 minutes.
6. Package and label.

℞ Sterile Vehicle for a Mastitis Preparation for Animals

Aluminum monosterate	2 g
Methylparaben	200 mg
Propylparaben	40 mg
Sesame oil	100 mL

1. Calculate the quantity of each ingredient required for the prescription.
2. Accurately weigh or measure each ingredient.
3. Using moderate agitation, dissolve the parabens in about 100 mL of the sesame oil. Make sure the ingredients are at room temperature.
4. Place mixture in a container that, when closed, allows almost no headspace.
5. Add the aluminum monostearate and stir rapidly until dispersion is complete.
6. Replace the container cap with a piece of aluminum foil and, using dry heat, sterilize the mixture at 140°C for 2 hours.
7. Remove heat source; allow mixture to cool to 100°C without agitation.
8. When the temperature of the mixture reaches 100°C, resume slow agitation; continue this action until the product reaches room temperature.
9. Using a clean air environment, add the active ingredient, which has been previously sterilized.
10. Package in a sterile container and label.

Topical Sprays

℞ Sucrose Octaacetate and Capsicum Spray for Pets (100 mL)

Sucrose octaacetate	1 g
Capsicum oleoresin	1 g
Polysorbate 60	2 mL
Propylene glycol	10 mL
Isopropyl alcohol 70%	31.4 mL
Preserved water	qs 100 mL

Sucrose Octaacetate and Capsicum Spray for Pets (100 mL) (cont.)

1. Calculate the quantity of each ingredient required for the prescription.
2. Accurately weigh or measure each ingredient.
3. Dissolve the sucrose octaacetate, polysorbate 60, and propylene glycol in the isopropyl alcohol.
4. Disperse the capsicum oleoresin in the solution.
5. Add sufficient preserved water to volume and stir until a homogenous mixture is obtained.
6. Package and label.

Oral Liquids/Gels

 Amitriptyline Hydrochloride 1 mg/mL Oral Liquid and Gel

	Liquid	Gel
Amitriptyline hydrochloride	100 mg	100 mg
Glycerin	2 mL	10 mL
Flavor	qs	qs
Simple syrup	qs	100 mL
Methylcellulose 4000 cP	4 g	
Sodium benzoate	200 mg	
Citric acid	200 mg	
Purified water	qs	100 mL

Oral Liquid

1. Calculate the quantity of each ingredient required for the prescription.
2. Accurately weigh or measure each ingredient.
3. Mix the amitriptyline hydrochloride and the flavor with the glycerin.
4. Add sufficient simple syrup to volume and mix well.
5. Package and label.

Oral Gel

1. Calculate the quantity of each ingredient required for the prescription.
2. Accurately weigh or measure each ingredient.
3. Mix the amitriptyline hydrochloride, flavor, sodium benzoate, citric acid, and methylcellulose with the glycerin.
4. Add sufficient purified water to volume and mix well.
5. Package and label.

℞ Veterinary Phenobarbital 22 mg/mL Oral Liquid

Phenobarbital	2.2 g
Propylene glycol	3.2 mL
Xanthan gum	200 mg
Aspartame	500 mg
Sodium saccharin	100 mg
Stevia powder	100 mg
Raspberry concentrate	3.33 mL
Peppermint spirit	13 drops
Simple syrup	qs 100 mL

1. Calculate the quantity of each ingredient required for the prescription.
2. Accurately weigh or measure each ingredient.
3. In a mortar, combine the phenobarbital, xanthan gum, aspartame, sodium saccharin, and stevia powder.
4. Add the propylene glycol and mix until a smooth paste is formed.
5. Add the flavors and mix well.
6. Add sufficient simple syrup to volume and mix well.
7. Package and label.

℞ Potassium Bromide 500 mg/mL Oral Solution

Potassium bromide	50 g
Purified water	qs 100 mL

1. Accurately weigh the potassium bromide.
2. Add sufficient purified water to volume and mix until dissolved.
3. Package and label.

℞ Sulfadiazine Sodium 333 mg/mL and Pyrimethamine 16.7 mg/mL Oral Liquid

Sulfadiazine sodium	33.3 g
Pyrimethamine	1.67 g
Diethanolamine	1.033 mL
Polysorbate 80	0.1 mL
Xanthan gum	100 mg
Hydroxyethylcellulose 5000 cP	0.925 g
Sodium saccharin	100 mg
Appleade flavor (or other)	1.5 mL
Potassium sorbate	200 mg
Sodium metabisulfite	99 mg
Propylene glycol	1.5 g
Purified water	qs 100 mL

℞ **Sulfadiazine Sodium 333 mg/mL and Pyrimethamine 16.7 mg/mL Oral Liquid (cont.)**

1. Calculate the quantity of each ingredient required for the prescription.
2. Accurately weigh or measure each ingredient.
3. On a magnetic stirrer, add the sodium metabisulfite to about 40 mL of purified water in a beaker.
4. Slowly add sodium sulfadiazine until dissolved. (Note: This task can take 30 minutes; a small amount of sodium hydroxide can be used if needed.)
5. Add diethanolamine, polysorbate 80, and flavor with continued stirring.
6. Dissolve the sodium saccharin and potassium sorbate in a small quantity of purified water and add to the mixture.
7. Mix propylene glycol with xanthan gum; add this to mixture and mix well.
8. Add the pyrimethamine and mix well.
9. Increase the speed of the stirrer and slowly add the hydroxyethylcellulose (sprinkle through a sieve) and stir until uniform.
10. Package and label.

Capsules

℞ **Canine Diarrhea Capsules (for 100 capsules)**

Neomycin sulfate	1.44 g
Sulfaguanidine	14.8 g
Sulfadiazine	920 mg
Sulfamerazine	920 mg
Sulfathiazole	920 mg
Kaolin	30 g
Pectin	1 g

1. Calculate the quantity of each ingredient required for the prescription.
2. Accurately weigh each ingredient.
3. Mix the sulfadiazine, sulfamerazine, and sulfathiazole together.
4. Add the pectin, followed by the neomycin sulfate, with mixing.
5. Geometrically, add the sulfaguanidine and then the kaolin.
6. Mix thoroughly.
7. Fill 100 capsules, size 0, with a tight pack.
8. Check for uniform capsule weights.
9. Package and label.

℞ Gelatin Base

Gelatin	43.4 g
Glycerin	155 mL
Purified water	21.6 mL

1. Accurately weigh or measure the calculated quantity of each ingredient.
2. Heat the glycerin using a boiling water bath.
3. Add the purified water and continue heating for 5 minutes, while stirring.
4. Slowly add the gelatin over a 3-minute period, stirring until mixed thoroughly and free of lumps.
5. Continue to heat for 45 minutes only.
6. Remove from heat and cool.

Chewable Treats/Troches

℞ Chewable Treat Base

Powdered animal food		65 g
Gelatin base, melted	qs	100 g
Active drug		qs

1. Accurately weigh or measure the calculated quantity of each ingredient.
2. Pulverize a nugget-type animal food of choice.
3. Melt the gelatin base (see previous formula "Gelatin Base").
4. Incorporate the powdered animal food and mix well.
5. Add drug and mix well.
6. Pour into molds and allow to set.
7. Package and label.

℞ Animal Treats for Drug Ingestion

Powdered animal food	13.2 g
Glycerin	2 mL
Flavor (chicken, beef, and the like)	1 mL
Gelatin base	6.6 g
Active drug	qs

R℞ **Animal Treats for Drug Ingestion (cont.)**

1. Accurately weigh or measure the calculated quantity of each ingredient.
2. Cut the gelatin base (see formula "Gelatin Base") into small pieces and put into a beaker in a water bath.
3. Mix the powdered animal food with the active drug powder.
4. Mix the flavor with the glycerin and add to the melted gelatin.
5. Incorporate the powdered animal food:active drug.
6. Fill the desired molds and allow to set until hardened. (Note: Blister molds, suppository molds, and the like will work.)

R℞ **Phenylpropanolamine Hydrochloride 10 mg Chewable Troches for Dogs**

Phenylpropanolamine HCl	240 mg
Silica gel	240 mg
Acacia powder	480 mg
Peanut butter	14.4 g
Hydrogenated vegetable oil	9.6 g

1. Accurately weigh or measure the calculated quantity of each ingredient.
2. Mix the phenylpropanolamine HCl, silica gel, and acacia powders together.
3. Using low heat, mix the peanut butter and hydrogenated vegetable oil.
4. Incorporate the powders and mix well. Pour into troche molds and allow to cool.

Implantable Pellets

 Implantable Pellet

2-Hydroxyethyl methacrylate	4200 parts
Ethylene glycol dimethacrylate	43 parts
Diisopropyl dicarbonate	750 parts
Active drug	750 parts (approximately)

1. Accurately weigh or measure the calculated quantity of each ingredient.
2. Mix the above ingredients thoroughly and place into molds, preferably cylindrical in shape.
3. Place mold in water bath maintained at 75°C for approximately 25 minutes to effect polymerization. The amount of cross-linking will determine the release rate: the more cross-linking, the longer the release rate. Cross-linking can be increased or decreased by altering the amount of diisopropyl dicarbonate present and the length of time the mold remains in the water bath.

References

1. Drug Compounding Task Force. Guidelines for pharmaceutical compounding. *J Am Vet Med Assoc* 1992;200(2):172–3.
2. American Veterinary Medical Association. *AVMA Guidelines for Supervising Use and Distribution of Veterinary Prescription Drugs.* Schaumburg, Ill: American Veterinary Medical Association; 1991.
3. Food and Drug Administration. *1993 Pasteurized Milk Ordinance.* Available at: http://vm.cfsan.fda.gov/~ear/pmo-1993.html. Accessed May 11, 1998.
4. Food and Drug Administration. Veterinary medicine; §615.100 Extra-label use of new animal drugs in food-producing animals. In: *FDA Compliance Policy Guides.* Rockville, Md: United States Department of Health, Education, and Welfare; Food and Drug Administration; August 1996.
5. Blodinger J. *Formulation of Veterinary Dosage Forms.* New York: Marcel Dekker; 1983.

Additional References

Bennett K, ed. *Compendium of Veterinary Products.* Port Huron, Mich: North American Compendiums; 1995–1996.

Birchard SJ, Sherding RG, eds. *Small Animal Practice.* Philadelphia: WB Saunders; 1994.

Ettinger SJ. *Textbook of Veterinary Internal Medicine.* Vols I and II. Philadelphia: WB Saunders; 1995.

Kirk, RW. *Current Veterinary Therapy XII: Small Animal Practice.* Philadelphia: WB Saunders; 1995.

Plumb, DC. *Veterinary Drug Handbook.* 2nd ed. White Bear Lake, Minn: PharmaVet Publishing; 1995.

Robinson NE, ed. *Current Therapy in Equine Medicine.* Philadelphia: WB Saunders; 1992.

Talbot RB, ed. *Veterinary Pharmaceuticals and Biologicals.* 12th ed. Lenexa, Kans: Veterinary Medicine Publishing; 1996.

Appendix 1

Agents Withdrawn by FDA Because of Safety/Efficacy Concerns

As a result of the Federal Food and Drug Administration Modernization Act of 1997 (FDAMA), Section 503A(a), the Food and Drug Administration (FDA) must develop numerous lists relating to compounding, including (1) a list of bulk-drug substances for compounding that are not already approved for compounding, (2) a list of products not to be compounded because of withdrawal from the market due to safety or efficacy concerns, and (3) a list of difficult-to-compound products.

The FDA is proposing that the drug products listed below be included on the list of drug products withdrawn or removed from the market because they have been found to be unsafe or ineffective. Therefore, compounding a drug product that appears on this list will not be covered by the exemption provided in Section 503A(a) of FDAMA and will be subject to enforcement action.

The proposed list and some discussion appeared in the October 8, 1998, *Federal Register* (63[195]:54083–54087). This listing is alphabetically arranged by established name of the active ingredient. Unless otherwise noted, all drug products containing a specific ingredient have been removed. (Compounding may still be permitted for other dosage forms of the product or for other indications.) Reasons for withdrawal and withdrawal dates are also provided.

FDA-Withdrawn Agents

Drug	Reason for Withdrawal	Withdrawal Date	Comments
Adenosine phosphate	Neither safe nor effective for intended uses as a vasodilator and anti-inflammatory	1973 (FDA)	Formerly marketed as a component of Adeno for injection, Adco for injection, and other drug products
Adrenal cortex	Low level of corticosteroids in the injection and extract presented a substantial risk of undertreatment of serious conditions such as adrenal cortical insufficiency, burns and hypoglycemia and thus a significant potential hazard	January 1978 (FDA)	
Azaribine	Associated with very serious thromboembolic events	Approval of NDA withdrawn June 10, 1977	Formerly marketed as Triazure tablets
Benoxaprofen	Associated with fatal cholestatic jaundice and other serious adverse reactions	Voluntarily withdrawn by mfr. August 5, 1982	Formerly marketed as Oraflex tablets
Bithionol	Shown to be a potent photosensitizer with potential to cause serious skin disorders	Approval of NDA withdrawn October 24, 1967	
Bromfenac sodium	Associated with fatal hepatic failure	Voluntarily withdrawn by mfr. June 22, 1998	Formerly marketed as Duract capsules
Butamben (all parenteral drug products)	Associated with severe adverse reactions such as severe tissue slough and transverse myelitis	Approval of NDA withdrawn August 7, 1964	Formerly marketed as Efocaine
Camphorated oil	Associated with poisoning in infants and young children due to accidental ingestion	1982 (FDA)	

FDA-Withdrawn Agents (cont.)

Drug	Reason for Withdrawal	Withdrawal Date	Comments
Carbetapentane citrate (all oral-gel drug products)	Not safe because of inexact methods of measuring the gel by consumers, which were potentially dangerous	Approval of NDA withdrawn November 19, 1972	Formerly marketed as Candette Cough Jel
Casein (iodinated)	Associated with thyrotoxic side effects	Approval of NDA withdrawn October 22, 1964	Formerly marketed as component of Neo-Barine
Chlorhexidine gluconate (all tinctures formulated for use as patient preoperative skin preparation)	Associated with chemical and thermal burns when used as patient preoperative skin preparation	Voluntarily withdrawn early 1984; removed for safety reasons	Chlorhexidine gluconate topical tincture 0.5% formerly marketed as Hibitane
Chlormadione acetate	Associated with development of mammary tumors in dogs	Mfr. ceased marketing in 1970; approvals of NDAs withdrawn March 16, 1972	Formerly marketed as component of combination drug products Estalor-21 and C-Quens tablets
Chloroform	National Cancer Institute studies demonstrated carcinogenicity in animals	1976 (FDA)	
Cobalt (cobalt salts [except radioactive forms of cobalt and its salts and cobalamin and its derivatives])	Not safe or effective for treatment of iron-deficiency anemia; toxic effects include liver damage, claudication and myocardial damage	1967 (FDA)	
Dexfenfluramine hydrochloride	Associated with valvular heart disease	Voluntarily withdrawn by mfr. September 1997	Formerly marketed as Redux capsules
Diamthazole dihydrochloride	Associated with neurotoxicity	Approvals of NDAs withdrawn on July 19, 1977	Formerly marketed as Asterol ointment, powder and tincture

(continued)

FDA-Withdrawn Agents (cont.)

Drug	Reason for Withdrawal	Withdrawal Date	Comments
Dibromsalan	Found to be potent photosensitizer capable of causing disabling skin disorders	Removed from market 1975 (FDA)	Formerly marketed in a number of products, mainly antibacterial soaps; as an anti-microbial or preservative, or for other purposes
Diethylstilbestrol (all oral and parenteral drug products containing 25 mg or more per unit dose)	Associated with adenocarcinoma of the vagina in offspring of patients when used in early pregnancy	Approvals of NDAs withdrawn February 18, 1975 (FDA)	
Dihydrostreptomycin sulfate	Associated with ototoxicity	Approvals of NDAs withdrawn September 3, 1970 (FDA)	
Dipyrone	Associated with potentially fatal agranulocytosis	Approvals of NDAs withdrawn June 17, 1977 (FDA)	Formerly marketed as Dimethone tablets and injection, Protemp oral liquid and others
Encainide hydrochloride	Associated with increased death rates in patients with asymptomatic heart rhythm abnormalities following a recent heart attack	Voluntarily withdrawn by mfr. December 16, 1991	Formerly marketed as Enkaid capsules
Fenfluramine hydrochloride	Associated with valvular heart disease	Voluntarily withdrawn by mfr. September 1997	Formerly marketed as Pondimin tablets
Flosequinan	Study indicated drug was associated with adverse effects on survival and that beneficial effects on symptoms of heart failure did not last beyond first three months of therapy, after which time patients had higher rate of hospitalization than patients on placebo	Voluntarily withdrawn by mfr. July 1993	Formerly marketed as Manoplax tablets

FDA-Withdrawn Agents (cont.)

Drug	Reason for Withdrawal	Withdrawal Date	Comments
Gelatin (all IV products)	Found not suitable as plasma expander because drug caused increased blood viscosity, reduced blood clotting and prolonged bleeding time	Approval of NDA withdrawn April 19, 1978 (FDA)	Formerly marketed as Knox Special Gelatin Solution Intravenous 6%
Glycerol (iodinated)	Found to have carcinogenic potential April 1993 (FDA)		Formerly marketed as Iodur Elixir and others
Gonadotropin chorionic (of animal origin)	Shown to produce allergic reactions	Approval of NDA withdrawn July 6, 1972	Formerly marketed as Synapoidin Steri-Vial
Mepazine	Associated with granulocytopenia, granulocytosis, paralytic ileus, urinary retention, seizures, hypotension and jaundice	Approval of NDA withdrawn May 28, 1970	Mepazine HCI formerly marketed as Pacatal tablets; mepazine acetate formerly marketed as Pacatal for injection
Metabromsalan	Found to be potent photosensitizer capable of causing disabling skin disorders	Removed from market 1975 (FDA)	Formerly marketed in number of products, mainly antibacterial soaps; as an antimicrobial or preservative, or for other purposes
Methamphetamine hydrochloride (parenteral products)	Found to have history of serious abuse and severe risk of dependence	Approvals of NDAs withdrawn March 30, 1973	Formerly marketed as Methedrine injection and Drinalfa injection and used as adjunct treatment for weight reduction
Methapyrilene	Shown to be potent carcinogen	Voluntarily withdrawn by mfr. May, June 1979	Formerly marketed in many drug products
Methopholine	Associated with ophthalmic changes and corneal opacities in dogs	Approval of NDA withdrawn March 22, 1965	Formerly marketed as Versidyne tablets

(continued)

FDA-Withdrawn Agents (cont.)

Drug	Reason for Withdrawal	Withdrawal Date	Comments
Mibefradil dihydrochloride	Associated with potentially harmful interactions with other drugs; and reduced activity of certain liver enzymes important in helping the body eliminate many other drugs, which can cause some of these drugs to accumulate to dangerous levels in the body	Voluntarily removed by mfr. June 8, 1998	Formerly marketed as Posicor tablets
Neomycin sulfate (parenteral products)	Found to present toxicity problems when used to irrigate wounds and found not to be acceptable for treatment of urinary tract infections due to availability of newer, safer antibiotics that were as effective or more effective	Approvals of marketing applications withdrawn January 5, 1989 (FDA)	
Nitrofurazone (except topical products formulated for dermatologic applications)	Associated with mammary neoplasia in rats	Approvals of NDAs withdrawn December 4, 1974, and June 10, 1975	Formerly marketed in nasal drops, otic drops and vaginal suppositories
Nomifensine maleate	Associated with increased incidence of hemolytic anemia	Voluntarily removed by approved application holder January 23, 1986; approval of NDA withdrawn March 20, 1992 (FDA)	Formerly marketed as Merital capsules
Oxyphenisatin	Associated with hepatitis and jaundice	Approvals of NDAs withdrawn March 9, 1973	Formerly marketed in Lavema Compound Solution and Lavema Enema Powder
Oxyphenisatin acetate	Associated with hepatitis and jaundice	Approvals of NDAs withdrawn February 1, 1972	Formerly marketed in Dialose Plus capsules, Noloc capsules and others

FDA-Withdrawn Agents (cont.)

Drug	Reason for Withdrawal	Withdrawal Date	Comments
Phenacetin	Associated with high potential for harm to kidneys and possibility of hemolytic anemia and methemoglobinemia resulting from abuse	Approvals of NDAs withdrawn on November 4, 1983	Formerly marketed in A.P.C. with Butalbital tablets and capsules and other drug products
Phenformin hydrochloride	Associated with lactic acidosis	Approvals of NDAs withdrawn November 15, 1978 (FDA)	Formerly marketed as D.B.I. tablets, Meltrol-50 capsules and others
Pipamazine	Associated with hepatic lesions	Approval of NDA withdrawn July 17, 1969	Formerly marketed as Mornidine tablets and injection
Potassium arsenite	Toxic and highly carcinogenic	FDA determined Fowler's Solution a new drug in April 1980; voluntarily removed by mfr. from market	Formerly marketed as Fowler's Solution (oral)
Potassium chloride (all solid oral dosage form products that supply 100 mg or more per dosage unit, except for controlled-release dosage forms and products formulated for preparation of solution prior to ingestion)	Concentrated forms of the salt associated with small-bowel lesions	Approvals of NDAs withdrawn July 29, 1977 and April 29, 1992	
Povidone (all IV products)	Found unsafe for use as plasma expander in emergency treatment of shock because povidone accumulates in the body and may cause storage disease with formation of granulomas; also interferes with blood coagulation, hemostasis and blood typing and cross matching	Approval of NDA withdrawn April 19, 1978	Formerly marketed as Polyvinylpyrrolidone in Normal Saline

(continued)

FDA-Withdrawn Agents (cont.)

Drug	Reason for Withdrawal	Withdrawal Date	Comments
Reserpine (all oral dosage forms containing more than 1 mg)	Associated with greater frequency and severity of adverse effects in strengths greater than 1 mg	Approvals of NDAs or portions of NDA for solid oral dosage-form products with more than 1 mg withdrawn May 9, 1977	Formerly marketed as Reserpoid tablets, Rau-Sed tablets and others
Sparteine sulfate	Found to have unpredictable effects and to be associated with tetanic uterine contractions and obstetrical complications	Approvals of NDAs withdrawn August 17, 1979	Formerly marketed as Spartocin injection and Tocosamine sterile solution
Sulfadimethoxine	Associated with Stevens-Johnson syndrome and fatalities	Approval of NDA withdrawn March 11, 1966	Formerly marketed in Madricidin capsules
Sulfathiazole (all products except those for vaginal use)	Associated with renal complications, rash, fever, blood dyscrasias and liver damage	Approvals of NDAs withdrawn September 28, 1970	Formerly marketed in Tresamide tablets and others
Suprofen	Associated with flank pain syndrome	Voluntarily removed by mfr. May 1987	Formerly marketed as Suprol capsules
Sweet spirits of nitre	Associated with methemoglobinemia in infants	1980 (FDA)	Also known as spirit of nitre, spirit of nitrous ether and ethyl nitrite spirit
Temafloxacin hydrochloride	Associated with hypoglycemia in elderly patients, as well as a constellation of multisystem organ involvements characterized by hemolytic anemia, frequently associated with renal failure, markedly abnormal liver tests and coagulopathy	Voluntarily removed by approved application holder spring 1992; approval of NDA withdrawn September 25, 1997	Formerly marketed as Omniflox tablets

FDA-Withdrawn Agents (cont.)

Drug	Reason for Withdrawal	Withdrawal Date	Comments
Terfenadine	Associated with serious heart problems when used concurrently with certain drugs, including certain antibiotics and antifungals	Voluntarily removed by mfr. February 1998	Formerly marketed in Seldane and Seldane-D tablets
3.3.4.5-tetrachloro-salicylanilide	Found to be potent photosensitizer capable of causing disabling skin disorders	1975 (FDA)	Formerly marketed in a number of drug products, such as antibacterial soaps, as antimicrobial, preservative or for other purposes
Tetracyline (all liquid oral products formulated for pediatric use containing a concentration greater than 25 mg/mL)	Associated with temporary inhibition of bone growth, permanent staining of teeth and enamel hypoplasia in children		FDA amended antibiotic drug regulations so that drug products containing tetracycline formulated for pediatric use in concentrations greater than 25 mg/mL would not be certified
Ticrynafen	Associated with liver toxicity	Voluntarily withdrawn by mfr. January 16, 1980	Formerly marketed as Selacryn tablets
Tibromsalan	Found to be potent photosensitizer capable of causing disabling skin disorders	Removed from market 1975 (FDA)	Formerly marketed in a number of drug products, largely antibacterial soaps, as antimicrobial or preservative, or for other purposes
Trichloroethane (all aerosol products intended for inhalation)	Potentially toxic to the cardiovascular system and associated with deaths from misuse or abuse	1977 (FDA)	
Urethane	Determined to be carcinogenic	Approval of NDA withdrawn March 18, 1977	Also known as urethan and ethyl carbamate; formerly marketed as inactive ingredient in Profinel injection
Vinyl chloride (all aerosol products)	Inhalation associated with acute toxicity manifested by dizziness, headache, disorientation and unconsciousness	1974 (FDA)	

(continued)

FDA-Withdrawn Agents (cont.)

Drug	Reason for Withdrawal	Withdrawal Date	Comments
Zirconium (all aerosol products)	Associated with human skin granulomas and toxic effects in the lungs and other internal organs of test animals	Withdrawn 1977 (FDA)	Formerly used in several aerosol drug products as antiperspirant
Zomepirac sodium	Associated with fatal and near-fatal anaphylactoid reactions	Voluntarily withdrawn by mfr. March 1983	Formerly marketed as Zomax tablets

Key: mfr. = manufacturer.

Specific Gravity Values

Specific Gravity Values of Selected Liquids

Liquid	Specific Gravity
Acetic acid, glacial	1.05
Acetic acid, NF	1.04
Acetone	0.79
Alcohol, ethyl	0.82
Alkyl (C12–C15) benzoate	0.92
Almond oil	0.91
Ammonium solution, strong	0.90
Amylene hydrate	0.81
Benzoin tincture	0.85
Benzyl benzoate	1.12
Castor oil	0.96
Chloroform	1.48
Coal tar solution (LCD)	0.87
Compound benzoin tincture	0.91
Corn oil	0.92
Cottonseed oil	0.92
Diethanolamine	1.09
Diethylene glycol monoethyl ether	0.99
Dimethicone 20	0.95
Dimethicone 100	0.966
Dimethicone 200	0.968
Dimethicone 350	0.969
Dimethicone 500	0.971
Dimethicone 1000	0.971
Dimethicone 30,000	0.973
Ethyl acetate	0.90
Ethyl oleate	0.87
Glycerin	1.25
Hexylene glycol	0.92
Hydrochloric acid	1.18

Specific Gravity Values of Selected Liquids (cont.)

Liquid	Specific Gravity
Hydrochloric acid, diluted	1.05
Isopropyl alcohol	0.78
Isopropyl myristate	0.85
Isopropyl palmitate	0.85
Lactic acid	1.20
Liquefied phenol	1.06
Methylene chloride	1.32
Methylsalicylate	1.18
Mineral oil, heavy	0.88
Mineral oil, light	0.85
Monoethanolamine	1.01
Nitric acid	1.41
Olive oil	0.91
Peanut oil	0.92
Peppermint oil	0.91
Phosphoric acid	1.71
Phosphoric acid, diluted	1.06
Polyethylene glycol 300	1.12
Polyethylene glycol 400	1.12
Polyethylene glycol 600	1.12
Propylene glycol	1.04
Resorcinol monoacetate	1.20
Rose soluble	1.16
Sesame oil	0.92
Simethicone	0.967
Soybean oil	0.92
Squalane	0.80
Trolamine	1.12
Water	1.00
Witch hazel	0.98

Sodium Chloride Equivalent Values of Selected Agents

Substance	NaCl E1%
A	
Acetrizoate methylglucamine	0.08
Acetrizoate sodium	0.10
Acetylcysteine	0.20
Acriflavine	0.10
Adenosine phosphate	0.41
Alcohol, 95%	0.65
Alcohol, 100%	0.70
Alphaprodine hydrochloride	0.19
Alum (potassium)	0.18
Amantadine hydrochloride	0.31
Aminacrine hydrochloride	0.17
Aminoacetic acid	0.41
Aminocaproic acid	0.26
Aminohippuric acid	0.13
Aminophylline	0.17
p-Aminosalicylate sodium	0.29
Ammonium carbonate	0.70
Ammonium chloride	1.08
Ammonium lactate	0.33
Ammonium nitrate	0.69
Ammonium phosphate, dibasic	0.55
Ammonium sulfate	0.55
Amobarbital sodium	0.25
Amphetamine Phosphate	0.34
Amphetamine sulfate	0.22
Amylcaine hydrochloride	0.22

Anileridine hydrochloride	0.19
Antimony potassium tartrate	0.18
Antipyrine	0.17
Antistine hydrochloride	0.18
Apomorphine hydrochloride	0.14
Arecoline hydrobromide	0.27
Arginine glutamate	0.17
L-Arginine hydrochloride	0.30
Arsenic trioxide	0.30
Ascorbic acid	0.18
Atropine methylbromide	0.14
Atropine sulfate	0.13
Aurothioglucose	0.03

B

Bacitracin	0.05
Baclofen	0.27
Barbital sodium	0.29
Benoxinate hydrochloride	0.18
Benzalkonium chloride	0.16
Benzethonium chloride	0.05
Benztropine mesylate	0.21
Benzyl alcohol	0.17
Bethanechol chloride	0.39
Bismuth potassium tartrate	0.09
Bismuth sodium tartrate	0.13
Boric acid	0.50
Brompheniramine maleate	0.09
Bupivacaine hydrochloride	0.17
Butabarbital sodium	0.27
Butacaine sulfate	0.20

C

Caffeine	0.08
Caffeine and sodium benzoate	0.25
Caffeine and sodium salicylate	0.12
Calcium aminosalicylate	0.27
Calcium chloride	0.51
Calcium chloride (6 H_2O)	0.35
Calcium chloride, anhydrous	0.68
Calcium chloride, dihydrate	0.51
Calcium disodium edetate	0.21
Calcium gluconate	0.16
Calcium lactate	0.23
Calcium lactate pentahydrate	0.23
Calcium lactobionate	0.08
Calcium levulinate	0.27
Camphor	0.20

Capreomycin sulfate	0.04
Carbenicillin sodium	0.20
Carboxymethylcellulose sodium	0.03
Cephaloridine	0.07
Chloramine-T	0.23
Chloramphenicol	0.10
Chloramphenicol sodium succinate	0.14
Chlorobutanol	0.24
Chlordiazepoxide hydrochloride	0.22
Chlorobutanol (hydrated)	0.24
Chloroprocaine hydrochloride	0.20
Chloroquine phosphate	0.14
Chloroquine sulfate	0.09
Chlorpheniramine maleate	0.15
Chlortetracycline hydrochloride	0.11
Chlortetracycline sulfate	0.13
Citric acid	0.18
Clindamycin phosphate	0.08
Clonidine hydrochloride	0.22
Cocaine hydrochloride	0.16
Codeine phosphate	0.14
Colistimethate sodium	0.15
Congo red	0.05
Cromolyn sodium	0.14
Cupric sulfate	0.18
Cupric sulfate, anhydrous	0.27
Cupric sulfate, pentahydrate	0.18
Cyclophosphamide	0.10
Cytarabine	0.11

D

Deferoxamine mesylate	0.09
Demecarium bromide	0.12
Dexamethasone sodium phosphate	0.17
Dextroamphetamine hydrochloride	0.34
Dextroamphetamine phosphate	0.25
Dextroamphetamine sulfate	0.23
Dextrose	0.16
Dextrose (anhydrous)	0.18
Dextrose, monohydrate	0.16
Diatrizoate sodium	0.09
Dibucaine hydrochloride	0.13
Dicloxacillin sodium (1 H_2O)	0.10
Diethanolamine	0.31
Dihydrostreptomycin sulfate	0.06
Dimethpyrindene maleate	0.12
Dimethyl sulfoxide	0.42
Diperodon hydrochloride	0.14

Diphenhydramine hydrochloride	0.20
Diphenidol hydrochloride	0.16
Disodium edetate	0.23
Dopamine hydrochloride	0.30
Doxapram hydrochloride	0.12
Doxycycline hyclate	0.12
Dyphylline	0.10

E

Echothiophate iodide	0.16
Edetate disodium	0.23
Edetate trisodium monohydrate	0.29
Emetine hydrochloride	0.10
Ephedrine hydrochloride	0.30
Ephedrine sulfate	0.23
Epinephrine bitartrate	0.18
Epinephrine hydrochloride	0.29
Ergonovine maleate	0.16
Erythromycin lactobionate	0.07
Ethylenediamine	0.44
Ethylhydrocupreine hydrochloride	0.17
Ethylmorphine hydrochloride	0.16
Eucatropine hydrochloride	0.18
Evans blue	0.06

F

Fentanyl citrate	0.11
Ferric ammonium citrate, green	0.17
Ferrous gluconate	0.15
Ferrous lactate	0.21
Floxuridine	0.13
Fluorescein sodium	0.31
Fluorouracil	0.13
Fluphenazine 2-hydrochloride	0.14
D-Fructose	0.18
Furtrethonium iodide	0.24

G

Galactose, anhydrous	0.18
Gentamicin sulfate	0.05
D-Glucuronic acid	0.20
L-Glutamic acid	0.25
Glutathione	0.34
Glycerin	0.34
Glycine	0.41
Glycopyrrolate	0.15
Gold sodium thiomalate	0.10
Guanidine hydrochloride	0.65

H

Heparin sodium	0.07
Hetacillin potassium	0.17
Hexafluorenium bromide	0.11
Hexamethonium tartrate	0.16
Hexamethylene sodium acetaminosalicylate	0.18
Histamine phosphate	0.25
Histamine 2 hydrochloride	0.40
Histidine monohydrochloride	0.29
Holocaine hydrochloride	0.20
Homatropine hydrobromide	0.17
Homatropine methylbromide	0.19
Hyaluronidase	0.01
Hydromorphone hydrochloride	0.22
Hydroxyamphetamine hydrobromide	0.26
Hydroxystilbamidine isethionate	0.16

I

Imipramine hydrochloride	0.20
Indigotindisulfonate sodium	0.30
Iopamidol	0.03
Isopropyl Alcohol	0.53
Isometheptene mucate	0.18
Isoproterenol sulfate	0.14

K

Kanamycin sulfate	0.07

L

Lactic acid	0.41
Lactose	0.07
Lactose, anhydrous	0.07
Levallorphan tartrate	0.13
Levorphanol tartrate	0.12
Lircomycin hydrochloride	0.16
Lithium carbonate	—
Lithium chloride	—
Lyapolate sodium	0.09

M

Magnesium chloride	0.45
Magnesium sulfate	0.17
Magnesium sulfate, anhydrous	0.32
Magnesium sulfate, septahydrate	0.17
Mannitol	0.17
Maphenide hydrochloride	0.075
Menthol	0.20
Meperidine hydrochloride	0.22
Mepivacaine hydrochloride	0.21

Merbromin	0.14
Methacholine bromide	0.28
Methenamine	0.23
Methionine	0.28
Monoethanolamine	0.53
Morphine hydrochloride	0.15
Mercuric chloride	0.13
Mercuric cyanide	0.15
Mesoridazine besylate	0.07
Metaraminol bitartrate	0.20
Methacholine chloride	0.32
Methadone hydrochloride	0.17
Methamphetamine hydrochloride	0.37
Methdilazine hydrochloride	0.10
Methenamine	0.23
Methiodal sodium	0.24
Methitural sodium	0.25
Methocarbamol	0.10
Methotrimeprazine hydrochloride	0.10
Methoxyphenamine hydrochloride	0.26
p-Methylaminoethanolphenol tartrate	0.17
Methyldopate hydrochloride	0.21
Methylergonovine maleate	0.10
N-Methylglucamine	0.20
Methylphenidate hydrochloride	0.22
Methylprednisolone Na succinate	0.09
Metycaine hydrochloride	0.20
Mild silver protein	0.18
Minocycline hydrochloride	0.10
Monoethanolamine	0.53
Morphine hydrochloride	0.15
Morphine hydrochloride trihydrate	0.15
Morphine nitrate	0.19
Morphine sulfate	0.14

N

Nafcillin sodium	0.14
Nalbuphine hydrochloride	0.16
Nalorphine hydrochloride	0.21
Naloxone hydrochloride	0.14
Naphazoline hydrochloride	0.27
Neomycin sulfate	0.11
Neomycin sulfate pentahydrate	0.11
Neostigmine bromide	0.22
Neostigmine methylsulfate	0.20
Nicotinamide	0.26
Nicotinic acid	0.25
Novobiocin sodium	0.10

O

Oleandomycin phosphate	0.08
Orphenadrine citrate	0.13
Oxymetazoline hydrochloride	0.22
Oxyquinoline sulfate	0.21

P

d-Pantothenyl alcohol	0.18
Papaverine hydrochloride	0.10
Paraldehyde	0.25
Pargyline hydrochloride	0.29
Penicillin G, potassium	0.18
Penicillin G procaine	0.10
Penicillin G, sodium	0.18
Pentazocine lactate	0.15
Phenacaine hydrochloride	0.20
Phenobarbital sodium	0.24
Phenol	0.35
Phentolamine mesylate	0.17
Phenylephrine hydrochloride	0.32
Phenylethyl alcohol	0.25
Phenylpropanolamine hydrochloride	0.38
Physostigmine salicylate	0.16
Pilocarpine hydrochloride	0.24
Pilocarpine nitrate	0.23
Piperocaine hydrochloride	0.21
Polyethylene glycol 300	0.12
Polyethylene glycol 400	0.08
Polyethylene glycol 1500	0.06
Polyethylene glycol 1540	0.02
Polyethylene glycol 4000	0.02
Polymyxin B sulfate	0.09
Polysorbate 80	0.02
Polyvinyl alcohol (99% hydrol)	0.02
Polyvinylpyrrolidone	0.01
Potassium acetate	0.59
Potassium chlorate	0.49
Potassium chloride	0.76
Potassium iodide	0.34
Potassium nitrate	0.56
Potassium permanganate	0.39
Potassium sorbate	0.41
Potassium phosphate	0.46
Potassium phosphate, dibasic	0.46
Potassium phosphate, monobasic	0.44
Potassium sulfate	0.44
Povidone	0.01
Pralidoxime chloride	0.32

Prilocaine hydrochloride	0.22
Procainamide hydrochloride	0.22
Procaine hydrochloride	0.21
Prochlorperazine edisylate	0.06
Promazine hydrochloride	0.13
Proparacaine hydrochloride	0.15
Propiomazine hydrochloride	0.15
Propylene glycol	0.43
Pyrathiazine hydrochloride	0.17
Pyridostigmine bromide	0.22
Pyridoxine hydrochloride	0.36

Q

Quinine bisulfate	0.09
Quinine dihydrochloride	0.23
Quinine hydrochloride	0.14
Quinine and urea hydrochloride	0.23

R

Resorcinol	0.28
Riboflavin phosphate, sodium	0.08
Rolitetracycline	0.11
Rose Bengal	0.07
Rose Bengal B	0.08

S

Scopolamine hydrobromide	0.12
Scopolamine methylnitrate	0.16
Secobarbital sodium	0.24
Silver nitrate	0.33
Silver protein, mild	0.17
Sodium acetate	0.46
Sodium acetate, anhydrous	0.77
Sodium acetazolamide	0.23
Sodium ampicillin	0.16
Sodium antimonyl tartrate	0.13
Sodium ascorbate	0.32
Sodium benzoate	0.40
Sodium bicarbonate	0.65
Sodium biphosphate, anhydrous	0.46
Sodium biphosphate (H_2O)	0.40
Sodium biphosphate (2 H_2O)	0.36
Sodium bismuth thioglycollate	0.19
Sodium bisulfite	0.61
Sodium borate	0.42
Sodium borate, decahydrate	0.42
Sodium bromide	0.58
Sodium cacodylate	0.32
Sodium carbonate, anhydrous	0.70

Sodium carbonate, monohydrated	0.60
Sodium carboxymethyl cellulose	0.03
Sodium cephalothin	0.17
Sodium chloride	1.00
Sodium citrate	0.31
Sodium colistimethate	0.15
Sodium folate	0.12
Sodium iodide	0.39
Sodium lactate	0.55
Sodium lauryl sulfate	0.08
Sodium metabisulfite	0.67
Sodium methicillin	0.18
Sodium nafcillin	0.14
Sodium nitrate	0.68
Sodium nitrite	0.84
Sodium oxacillin	0.17
Sodium phenylbutazone	0.18
Sodium phosphate	0.29
Sodium phosphate, dibasic, anhydrous	0.53
Sodium phosphate, dibasic, dodecahydrate	0.22
Sodium phosphate, dibasic, septahydrate	0.29
Sodium phosphate, dibasic (2 H_2O)	0.42
Sodium phosphate, dibasic (12 H_2O)	0.22
Sodium phosphate, dihydrate	0.42
Sodium phosphate, monobasic	0.43
Sodium propionate	0.61
Sodium ricinoleate	0.10
Sodium salicylate	0.36
Sodium succinate	0.32
Sodium sulfate	0.26
Sodium sulfate, anhydrous	0.58
Sodium sulfite, exsiccated	0.65
Sodium sulfobromophthalein	0.06
Sodium tartrate	0.33
Sodium thiosulfate	0.31
Sodium warfarin	0.17
Sorbitol hemihydrate	0.16
Sparteine sulfate	0.10
Spectinomycin hydrochloride	0.16
Streptomycin sulfate	0.07
Strong silver protein	0.08
Sucrose	0.08
Sulfacetamide sodium	0.23
Sulfadiazine sodium	0.24
Sulfamerazine sodium	0.23
Sulfanilamide	0.22
Sulfapyridine sodium	0.23
Sulfathiazole sodium	0.22

T

Tannic acid	0.03
Tartaric acid	0.25
Tetracaine hydrochloride	0.18
Tetracycline hydrochloride	0.14
Thiamine hydrochloride	0.25
Thiethylperazine maleate	0.09
Thiopropazate dihydrochloride	0.16
Thioridazine hydrochloride	0.05
Thiotepa	0.16
Tridihexethyl chloride	0.16
Triethanolamine	0.21
Trifluoperazine 2hydrochloride	0.18
Triflupromazine hydrochloride	0.09
Trimeprazine tartrate	0.06
Trimethadione	0.23
Trimethobenzamide hydrochloride	0.10
Tripelennamine hydrochloride	0.30
Trisodium edetate, monohydrate	0.29
Tromethamine	0.26
Tropicamide	0.09
Trypan blue	0.26
Tubocurarine chloride	0.13

U

Urea	0.59
Uridine	0.12

V

Valethamate bromide	0.15
Vancomycin sulfate	0.05
Viomycin sulfate	0.08

W

Warfarin sodium	0.17

X

Xylometazoline hydrochloride	0.21

Z

Zinc chloride	0.62
Zinc phenolsulfonate	0.18
Zinc sulfate	0.15
Zinc sulfate (dried)	0.23
Zinc sulfate, septahydrate	0.15

Key: E%NaCl = sodium chloride equivalents based on a 1% solution

Buffers and Buffer Solutions

 Boric Acid Buffer (pH 5)

Boric acid		19 g
Purified water	qs	1000 mL

 Boric Acid–Sodium Borate Buffer

Boric acid		0.43 g
Sodium borate		4.2 g
Purified water	qs	1000 mL

 Sorensen's Modified Phosphate

Acid stock solution (1/15 M sodium biphosphate):

Sodium biphosphate, anhydrous		8.006 g
Purified water	qs	1000 mL

Alkaline stock solution (1/15 M sodium phosphate):

Sodium phosphate, anhydrous		9.473 g
Purified water	qs	1000 mL

Preparation of Sorensen's Modified Phosphate Buffer with Specific pH

	Required Volume of Stock Solutions		Grams of Sodium
pH	mL of Acid Stock Solution	mL of Alkaline Stock Solution	Chloride Required for Tonicity
5.9	90	10	0.52
6.2	80	20	0.51
6.5	70	30	0.50
6.6	60	40	0.49
6.8	50	50	0.48
7.0	40	60	0.46
7.2	30	70	0.45
7.4	20	80	0.44
7.7	10	90	0.43
8.0	5	95	0.42

Gilford Ophthalmic Buffer

Acid stock solution:

Boric acid		12.4 g
Potassium chloride		7.4 g
Purified water	qs	1000 mL

Alkaline stock solution:

Sodium carbonate, monohydrate		24.8 g
Purified water	qs	1000 mL

Preparation of Gilford Ophthalmic Buffer with Specific pH

	Required Volume of Stock Solutions	
pH	mL of Acid Stock Solution	mL of Alkaline Stock Solution
6.0	30	0.05
6.2	30	0.1
6.6	30	0.2
6.8	30	0.3
6.9	30	0.5
7.0	30	0.6
7.2	30	1.0
7.4	30	1.5
7.6	30	2.0
7.8	30	3.0
8.0	30	4.0
8.5	30	8.0

Palitzsch Buffer

Acid stock solution (0.2 M boric acid solution):

Boric acid		12.404 g
Purified water	qs	1000 mL

Alkaline stock solution (0.05 M sodium borate solution):

Sodium borate, decahydrate		19.108 g
Purified water	qs	1000 mL

Preparation of Palitzsch Buffer with Specific pH

	Required Volume of Stock Solutions	
pH	**mL of Acid Stock Solution**	**mL of Alkaline Stock Solution**
6.8	97	3
7.1	94	6
7.4	90	10
7.6	85	15
7.8	80	20
7.9	75	25
8.1	70	30
8.2	65	35
8.4	55	45
8.6	45	55
8.7	40	60
8.8	30	70
9.0	20	80
9.1	10	90

Sodium Acetate–Boric Acid Stock Solution

Acid stock solution (pH 7.6):

Sodium acetate, trihydrate		20 g
Purified water	qs	1000 mL

Alkaline stock solution (pH approx. 5):

Boric acid crystals		19 g
Purified water	qs	1000 mL

Preparation of Sodium Acetate–Boric Acid Stock Solution with Specific pH

	Required Volume of Stock Solutions	
pH	**mL of Acid Stock Solution (pH 7.6)**	**mL of Acid Stock Solution (pH 5)**
5.0	—	100
5.7	5	95
6.05	10	90
6.3	20	80
6.5	30	70
6.65	40	60
6.75	50	50
6.85	60	40
6.95	70	30
7.1	80	20
7.25	90	10
7.4	100	5
7.6	100	0

Atkins and Pantin Buffer Solution

Acid stock solution (0.2 M boric acid solution):

Boric acid		12.405 g
Sodium chloride		7.5 g
Purified water	qs	1000 ml

Alkaline stock solution (0.2 M sodium carbonate solution):

Sodium carbonate, anhydrous		21.2 g
Purified water	qs	1000 mL

Preparation of Atkins and Pantin Buffer Solution with Specific pH

	Required Volume of Stock Solutions	
pH	mL of Acid Stock Solution	mL of Alkaline Stock Solution
7.6	93.8	6.2
7.8	91.7	8.3
8.0	88.8	11.2
8.2	85.0	15.0
8.4	80.7	19.3
8.6	75.7	24.3
8.8	69.5	30.5
9.0	63.0	37.0
9.2	56.4	43.6
9.4	49.7	50.3
9.6	42.9	57.1
9.8	36.0	64.0
10.0	29.1	70.9
10.2	22.1	77.9
10.4	15.4	84.6
10.6	9.8	90.2
10.8	5.7	94.3
11.0	3.5	96.5

Feldman Buffer

Acid stock solution:

Boric acid		12.368 g
Sodium chloride		2.925 g
Purified water	qs	1000 ml

Alkaline stock solution:

Sodium borate, decahydreate		19.07 g
Purified water	qs	1000 mL

Preparation of Feldman Buffer with Specific pH

	Required Volume of Stock Solutions	
pH	mL of Acid Stock Solution	mL of Alkaline Stock Solution
5.0	100	0
6.0	100	0.4
7.0	95	5
7.1	94	6
7.2	93	7
7.3	91	9
7.4	89	11
7.5	87	13
7.6	85	15
7.7	82	18
7.8	80	20
7.9	76	24
8.0	73	27
8.1	69	31
8.2	65	35

Viscosity-Increasing Agents for Aqueous Systems

Properties of Commonly Used Suspending/Thickening Agents

Substance	Solubility[a]			Usual Suspension Concentration (%)	pH of Aqueous Solution (%)	Most Effective pH Range	Recommended Preservatives
	Water	Alcohol	Glycerin				
Acacia NF	2.7	PrIn	20	5.0–10.0	4.5–5 (5%)	—	Benzoic acid 0.1%, sodium benzoate 0.1%, methylparaben 0.17% with propylparaben 0.03%
Agar NF	Swells	IS	—	<1.0	—	—	—
Alginic acid NF	Swells	PrIn	—	—	1.5–3.5 (3%)	—	Benzoic acid 0.1%–0.2%, sodium benzoate 0.1%–0.2%, sorbic acid 0.1%–0.2%, parabens
Attapulgite, colloidal/activated	PrIn	PrIn	—	—	7.5–9 (5%)	6–8.5	—
Bentonite NF	PrIn	PrIn	PrIn	0.5–5.0	9.5–10.5 (2%)	>6	—
Carbomer 910, 934, 934P, 940, 941, 1342 NF	Sol	Sol (after neutralization)	—	0.5–1.0	2.5–3 (1%)	6–11	Chlorocresol 0.1%, methylparaben 0.1%, thimerosal 0.1%
Carboxymethylcellulose calcium NF	IS	PrIn	—	0.25–5.0	4.5–6 (1%)	2–10	—
Carboxymethylcellulose sodium USP	Sol	PrIn	—	0.25–5.0	6.5–8.5 (1%)	2–10	—
Carrageenan NF	1:100[b]	—	—	—	—	—	—
Cellulose, microcrystalline NF	PrIn	—	—	0.5–5.0	5–7	—	—

Material							
Microcrystalline cellulose and carboxymethylcellulose sodium NF	PartSol	—	—	—	6–8 (1.2%)	—	—
Dextrin NF	Sol	PrIn	—	—	—	—	—
Gelatin NF	Sol	PrIn	Sol	—	3.8–6 (type A), 5–7.4 (type B)	—	—
Guar gum NF	FS	—	—	2.5	5–7 (1%)	4–10.5	Methylparaben 0.15% with propylparaben 0.02%
Hydroxyethyl cellulose NF	Sol	PrIn	—	1.0–5.0	5.5–8.5 (1%)	2–12	—
Hydroxypropyl cellulose NF	2	2.5	PrIn	—	5–8 (1%)	6–8	—
Hydroxypropyl methylcellulose USP	Sol	PrIn	—	0.5–5.0	5.5–8 (1%)	3–11	—
Magnesium aluminum silicate NF	PrIn	PrIn	—	0.5–10.0	9–10 (5%)	—	—
Methylcellulose USP	Sol	PrIn	—	—	5.5–8 (1%)	3–11	—
Pectin USP	20	PrIn	—	—	5% acidic	—	—
Poloxamer NF	Varies	Varies	—	10.0–40.0	6–7.4 (2.5%)	—	—
Polyethylene oxide NF	—	—	—	1.0	—	—	—

Properties of Commonly Used Suspending/Thickening Agents

Substance	Solubility[a]			Usual Suspension Concentration (%)	pH of Aqueous Solution (%)	Most Effective pH Range	Recommended Preservatives
	Water	Alcohol	Glycerin				
Polyvinyl alcohol USP	FS	—	—	0.5–3.0	5–8 (4%)	—	—
Povidone USP	FS	FS	—	2.0–10.0	3–7 (5%)	—	—
Propylene glycol alginate NF	Sol	—	—	1.0–5.0	—	3–6	—
Silicon dioxide NF, colloidal	PrIn	IS	—	2.0–10.0	3.5–4.4 (4%)	1–7.5	—
Sodium alginate NF	Sol (slowly)	PrIn	—	1.0–5.0	7.2 (1%)	4–10	Chlorocresol 0.1%, chloroxylenol 0.1%, parabens, benzoic acid (if acidic)
Tragacanth NF	PrIn	PrIn	—	—	5–6 (1%)	4–8	Benzoic acid 0.1%, sodium benzoate 0.1%, methylparaben 0.17% with propylparaben 0.03%
Xanthan gum NF	Sol	PrIn	—	1.0–2.0	6–8 (1%)	3–12	—

[a]Amount (mL) required to dissolve 1 g of material.

[b]Hot water.

Index

Page numbers preceded by a capital A indicate material located in an appendix. Page numbers followed by a lowercase, italic *b, f,* or *t* indicate material located in a box, figure, or table, respectively.

Q

R